# Public Health 101

**THIRD EDITION**

*Improving Community Health*

**Richard Riegelman, MD, MPH, PhD**
Professor and Founding Dean
Milken Institute School of Public Health
The George Washington University
Washington, DC

**Brenda Kirkwood, MPH, DrPH**
Clinical Associate Professor
School of Public Health
University at Albany, State University of New York
Albany, NY

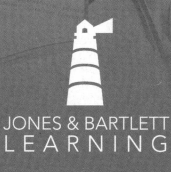

JONES & BARTLETT
LEARNING

*World Headquarters*
Jones & Bartlett Learning
5 Wall Street
Burlington, MA 01803
978-443-5000
info@jblearning.com
www.jblearning.com

Jones & Bartlett Learning books and products are available through most bookstores and online booksellers. To contact Jones & Bartlett Learning directly, call 800-832-0034, fax 978-443-8000, or visit our website, www.jblearning.com.

13474-2

**Production Credits**
VP, Product Management David D. Cella
Director of Product Management: Michael Brown
Product Specialist: Danielle Bessette
Production Manager: Carolyn Rogers Pershouse
Vendor Manager: Molly Hogue
Director of Vendor Management: Amy Rose
Senior Marketing Manager: Sophie Fleck Teague
Manufacturing and Inventory Control Supervisor: Amy Bacus
Composition: codeMantra U.S. LLC
Project Management: codeMantra U.S. LLC
Cover Design: Kristin E. Parker
Director of Rights & Media: Joanna Gallant
Rights & Media Specialist: Wes DeShano
Media Development Editor: Troy Liston
Cover Image: ©Jack Berman/Moment/Getty
Printing and Binding: LSC Communications
Cover Printing: LSC Communications

**Library of Congress Cataloging-in-Publication Data**
Names: Riegelman, Richard K., author. | Kirkwood, Brenda, author.
Title: Public health 101: improving community health / Richard Riegelman, Brenda Kirkwood.
Other titles: Public health one hundred one
Description: Third edition. | Burlington, MA: Jones & Bartlett Learning, [2019] | Includes bibliographical references and index.
Identifiers: LCCN 2017044501 | ISBN 9781284118445 (pbk.: alk. paper)
Subjects: | MESH: Public Health
Classification: LCC RA425 | NLM WA 100 | DDC 362.1—dc23
LC record available at https://lccn.loc.gov/2017044501

6048

Printed in the United States of America
22 21 20 19 18    10 9 8 7 6 5 4 3 2

*To Nancy Alfred Persily, whose enthusiasm for teaching public health to undergraduates inspired* Public Health 101: Improving Community Health

# Contents

Image credits: ©Jack Berman/Moment/Getty; © Mc Satori/Shutterstock; © KidStock/Blend Images/Getty;
© Christian Delbert/Shutterstock; © Jovanmandic/iStock/Getty Images Plus/Getty

## SECTION IV  Cases and Discussion Questions    237

## SECTION V  Public Health Institutions and Systems    245

### Chapter 12  Public Health Institutions
and Systems. . . . . . . . . . . . . . . . 247

## SECTION V  Cases and Discussion Questions    309

# Acknowledgments

*Public Health 101: Improving Community Health, Third Edition* is the culmination of two decades of effort aimed at introducing public health to undergraduates. The effort originated with the teaching of an introductory course in public health in 1998 at the then newly created George Washington University School of Public Health and Health Services. The new course, organized by associate dean Nancy Alfred Persily, inspired efforts to teach and to learn from a new generation. The approach was designed as part of a liberal arts education, stimulating the movement that came to be called the Educated Citizen and Public Health.

Efforts to think through the content of an introductory course in public health have involved a large number of people throughout the United States. Public health, arts and sciences, and clinical educators all participated in the 2006 Consensus Conference on Public Health Education, which put forward the framework for Public Health 101 upon which this book is based. Among those who led and continue to lead this effort is Susan Albertine, whose insights into the relationship between public health and liberal education have formed the basis for much of the Educated Citizen and Public Health movement.

I have taught Public Health 101 since 2002, which has provided me with an opportunity to teach and to learn from well over 500 undergraduate students at The George Washington University. Their feedback and input has been central to writing and rewriting this book. I would also like to thank Alan Greenberg and Heather Young, the chair and vice chair of the Department of Epidemiology and Biostatistics at The George Washington University Milken Institute School of Public Health, for their support of my efforts to expand the audience for undergraduate public health.

I am pleased that Brenda Kirkwood has joined me as a co-author. I first had the opportunity to work with Brenda while she was a DrPH student at The George Washington University. Dr. Kirkwood has made extraordinary contributions to Public Health 101. Her insights and careful reviews and dedication to getting the details right have been key to the quality of this edition. Brenda is truly exceptional and a pleasure to work with, as will be confirmed by all who work with her.

Mike Brown, Director of Product Management of the Public Health and Health Administration line of products for Jones & Bartlett Learning, has made special contributions to this book and the *Essential Public Health* series as a whole. His vision has helped craft the series, and his publishing expertise made it happen. The production, marketing, and editorial staff of Jones & Bartlett Learning deserve special recognition. Their commitment to this book and the entire *Essential Public Health* series has gone well beyond the expectations of their jobs.

Last, but by no means least, is my wife, Linda Riegelman, who encouraged this book and the *Essential Public Health* series from the beginning. She saw the need to reach out to students and make real the roles that public health plays in their everyday lives.

Confronting the challenge of putting together *Public Health 101* has been one of the great joys of my professional life. I hope it will bring both joy and challenge to you as you enter into the important and engaging world of public health.

*Richard Riegelman, MD, MPH, PhD*

# Preface: What Is *Public Health 101: Improving Community Health* All About?

Public health is more than a profession; it is a way of thinking. *Public Health 101: Improving Community Health* introduces you to the profession and also the way of thinking that we will call population health. Population health is an important way of looking at the world, whether you are going into public health as a profession, a clinically oriented health profession, business, law, international affairs, or a range of other professions.

Population health is also a key way of thinking, which prepares you for the challenges of citizenship in a democracy. Many of the issues that come before us as a society stem from or benefit from a population health perspective. Whether we are dealing with AIDS, the impact of aging, climate change, or the costs of health care, the population perspective can help us frame the issues and analyze the options to intervene. Population health requires an evidence-based approach to collecting and using the facts to develop and implement approaches to improve community health.

In addition, the population perspective leads us to look broadly at the way issues intertwine and interact with each other. We call this systems thinking. In population health, systems thinking is taking center stage as we increasingly struggle with complex problems that require us to look beyond the traditional boundaries of health and disease and the traditional lines between the roles of the health professions.

Until recently, public health was considered a discipline taught only at the graduate level. Today, undergraduate public health is booming at 4-year colleges and is beginning to take hold at community colleges as well. Its roots in general and liberal education go back to the 1980s, when David Fraser, the president of Swarthmore and an epidemiologist who led the investigation of Legionnaires' disease, wrote a now classic article called "Epidemiology as a Liberal Art."[1]

In 2003, the National Academy of Medicine, formerly called the Institute of Medicine, recommended that "all undergraduates should have access to education in public health."[2] That recommendation encouraged the development of the Educated Citizen and Public Health initiative, a collaboration of undergraduate educators and public health educators to define and stimulate public health curricula for all undergraduates. *Public Health 101* was written to implement the recommendations that came out of this initiative and continues to form the basis for undergraduate education in public health.

The third edition of *Public Health 101* has a new subtitle, *Improving Community Health. Improving Community Health* is designed to highlight the importance of community-wide collaboration to promote and protect health as well as to prevent disease and disability. The third edition more fully addresses the work of a wide range of health professionals whose roles are an indispensable part of improving community health.

This third edition of *Public Health 101* has been thoroughly updated and expanded. Each chapter includes new material designed to expand your understanding of public health. From e-cigarettes to the opioid epidemic, from aging as a public health issue to the One Health movement, *Public Health 101* aims to make public health relevant to today's students and today's world. Each of the five sections includes new case studies challenging you to apply what you have learned.

*Public Health 101: Improving Community Health* will not try to overload your mind with facts. It is about providing you with frameworks for thinking, and applying these frameworks to real situations and thought-provoking scenarios. Each chapter begins and ends with vignettes designed to show you the types of situations you will confront in public health. After each section, there are case studies that relate to one or more chapters in the section. They provide realistic, engaging exercises and open-ended questions to help you think through the application of the key concepts presented in each section.

Hopefully, you will come away from reading *Public Health 101* with an appreciation of how the health of the public is influenced by and can be improved by efforts directed at the population level, as well as at the individual level. Let us begin in Chapter 1 by exploring the ways that public health affects everyone's daily life.

## ▶ References

1.  Fraser DW. Epidemiology as a liberal art. *N Engl J Med.* 1987; 316:309–314.
2.  Gebbie K, Rosenstock L, Hernandez LM. *Who Will Keep the Public Healthy? Educating Public Health Professionals for the 21st Century.* Washington, DC: National Academy Press; 2003.

# About the Authors

**Richard Riegelman, MD, MPH, PhD**, is professor of epidemiology–biostatistics, medicine, and health policy, and founding dean of The George Washington University Milken Institute School of Public Health. His education includes an MD from the University of Wisconsin, plus an MPH and PhD in epidemiology from The Johns Hopkins University. Dr. Riegelman practiced primary care internal medicine for over 20 years.

Dr. Riegelman has over 75 publications, including 6 books for students and practitioners of medicine and public health. He is editor of the Jones & Bartlett Learning *Essential Public Health* series. The series provides books and ancillary materials for the full spectrum of curricula for undergraduate public health education.

Dr. Riegelman has spearheaded efforts to fulfill the National Academy of Medicine's recommendation that "all undergraduates should have access to education in public health." He continues to work with public health and undergraduate education associations to integrate public health into the mainstream of undergraduate education at 2-year as well as 4-year colleges and universities. Richard Riegelman teaches undergraduate and graduate public health courses, which include Public Health 101 and Epidemiology 101.

**Brenda Kirkwood, MPH, DrPH**, works in academic administration and is clinical associate professor at the School of Public Health, University at Albany, State University of New York. Dr. Kirkwood has experience in higher education spanning public and private institutions on the associate, baccalaureate, and graduate levels, including development and teaching of undergraduate and graduate public health courses, development and management of public health academic programs, student advisement and mentorship, and contributing to public health education research. Prior to her career in higher education, Dr. Kirkwood held positions within the New York State Department of Health. She received a BS from Ithaca College, MPH from the University at Albany, State University of New York, and DrPH from The George Washington University.

Dr. Kirkwood has been actively involved in national efforts to expand public health education and strengthen the public health workforce. Her numerous publications and presentations have focused on the roles of, and opportunities for, public health education in 2-year and 4-year colleges and universities as well as at the graduate level.

Image credits: ©Jack Berman/Moment/Getty; © Mc Satori/Shutterstock; © KidStock/Blend Images/Getty; © Christian Delbert/Shutterstock; © Jovanmandic/iStock/Getty Images Plus/Getty

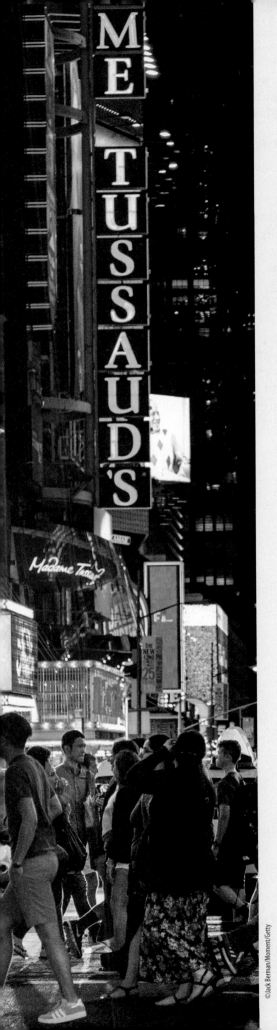

# SECTION I
# Principles of Population Health

Section I of *Public Health 101: Improving Community Health* introduces you to the ways that public health affects your every waking moment, from the food you eat, to the water you drink, to the car you drive. Even sleep matters. In public health, we use bed nets to prevent malaria, we use beds that prevent back pain, and put infants to sleep on their backs to prevent sudden infant death syndrome (SIDS).

In Section I, we will examine a range of approaches to public health that have been used over the centuries. Then we will focus on a 21st century approach known as **population health**. Population health considers the full range of options for intervention to address health problems, from community control of communicable disease and environmental health, to healthcare delivery systems, to public policies such as taxation and laws designed to reduce cigarette smoking. Population health takes a life cycle approach, considering how risks to health affect the population throughout the life span. We will also look at how populations are changing and aging by examining three important transitions that affect population health today and will continue to do so for years to come.

In this section, we will also examine an evidence-based approach to population health that focuses on defining the problem, establishing the etiology, making evidence-based recommendations, implementing these recommendations in practice, and evaluating the impacts of interventions. The population health and evidence-based approaches introduced in Section I provide an underpinning for all that follows.

At the end of Section I (and at the end of every section), there are cases with discussion questions that draw on chapters from the section. Each case is designed as a realistic description of the types of problems we face as we seek to improve community health.

So with no further ado, let us take a look at how public health can and does affect all of our daily lives.

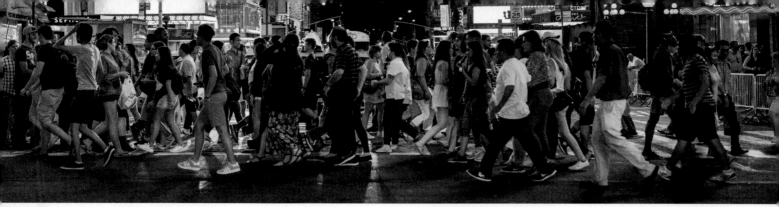

# CHAPTER 1

# Public Health: The Population Health Approach

## LEARNING OBJECTIVES

By the end of this chapter, the student will be able to:

- identify multiple ways that public health affects daily life.
- define eras of public health from ancient times to the present.
- define the meaning of "population health."
- illustrate the uses of health care, traditional public health, and social interventions in population health.
- identify a range of determinants of disease.
- identify ways that populations change over time and how this affects health.

I woke up this morning, got out of bed, and went to the bathroom. There I used the toilet, washed my hands, brushed and flossed my teeth, drank a glass of water, and took my blood pressure medicine, cholesterol medication, and an aspirin. Then I did my exercises and took a shower.

On the way to the kitchen, I didn't even notice the smoke detector I passed or the old ashtrays in the closet. I took a low-fat yogurt out of the refrigerator and prepared hot cereal in the microwave oven for my breakfast.

Then I walked out my door into the crisp, clean air and got in my car. I put on my seat belt, saw the light go on for the airbag, and safely drove to work. I got to my office, where I paid little attention to the new defibrillator at the entrance, the "no smoking" signs, or the absence of asbestos. I arrived safely in my well-ventilated office and got ready to teach Public Health 101.

It wasn't a very eventful morning, but then it's all in a morning's work when it comes to public health.

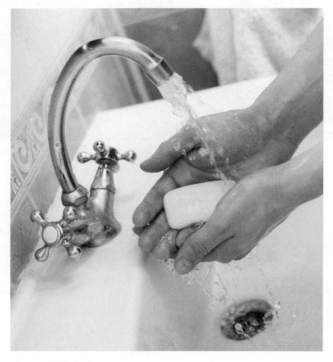

© Champion studio/Shutterstock

This rather mundane morning is made possible by a long list of achievements that reflect the often-ignored history of public health.[1] We take for granted the fact that water chlorination, hand washing, and indoor plumbing largely eliminated the transmission of common bacterial diseases, which for centuries killed the young and not so young. Do not overlook the impact of prevention on our teeth and gums. Teeth brushing, flossing, and fluoridation of water have made a dramatic impact on the dental health of children and adults.

The more recent advances in the prevention of heart disease have been a major public health achievement. Preventive successes include the reduction of blood pressure and cholesterol, cigarette smoking prevention and cessation efforts, the use of low-dose aspirin, an understanding of the role of exercise, and the widespread availability of defibrillators. These can be credited with at least half of the dramatic reductions in heart disease that have reduced the death rate from coronary artery disease by approximately 50% in the United States and most other developed countries in the last half century.

The refrigerator was one of the most important advances in food safety, which illustrates the impact of social change and innovation not necessarily intended to improve health. Food and product safety are public health achievements that require continued attention. It was public pressure for food safety that in large part brought about the creation of the U.S. Food and Drug Administration. The work of this public health agency continues to affect all of our lives from the safety of the foods we eat to the drugs and cosmetics we use.

Radiation safety, like radiation itself, usually goes unnoticed, from the regulation of microwave ovens to the reduction of radon in buildings. We rarely notice when disease does not occur.

Highway safety illustrates the wide scope of activities required to protect the public's health. From seat belts, child restraints, and airbags to safer cars, highways, designated driver programs, and enforcement of drunk driving laws, public health efforts require collaboration with professionals not usually thought of as having a health focus. New technologies produce new challenges as our constant communications lead to inattention to the road. However, technology also offers new opportunities which help compensate for some of our "blind spots."

The physical environment also has been made safer by the efforts of public health. Improvement in the quality of the air we breathe both outdoors and indoors has been an ongoing accomplishment of what we will call "population health." Our lives are safer today because of interventions ranging from installation of smoke detectors to removal of asbestos from buildings.

However, the challenges continue. Globalization increases the potential for the spread of existing and emerging diseases and raises concerns about the safety of the products we use. Climate change and ongoing environmental deterioration continue to produce new territory for "old" diseases, such as malaria, dengue fever, and, more recently, Zika. Overuse of technologies, such as antibiotics, has encouraged the emergence of resistant bacteria. Overprescription of opioids has led to an epidemic of fatal overdoses among the young and not so young.

The 1900s saw an increase in life expectancy of almost 30 years in most developed countries, much of it due to the successes of public health initiatives.[2] We cannot assume that these trends will continue indefinitely. The epidemic of obesity already threatens to slow down or reverse the progress we have been making. The challenges of 21st century public health include the protection of health and continued improvement in quality of life, not just the quantity of years individuals are living.

To understand the role of public health in these achievements and other, ongoing challenges, let us start at the beginning and ask: What do we mean by "public health"?

# ▶ What Do We Mean by "Public Health"?

Ask your parents what "public health" means, and they might say, "Health care for the poor." They are right that public health has always been about providing services for **vulnerable populations** or those at higher than average risk of disease and/or bad outcomes of disease, either directly or through the healthcare system. Public health approaches to vulnerable populations range from reducing exposure to lead paint in deteriorating buildings, to food supplementation, to preventing birth defects and goiters. Addressing the needs of vulnerable populations has always been a cornerstone of public health. As we will see, however, the definition of "vulnerable populations" continues to change, as do the challenges of addressing their needs.

Ask your grandparents what "public health" means, and they might say, "Washing your hands." Well, they are right too—public health has always been about determining risks to health and providing successful interventions that are applicable to everyone. But hand washing is only the tip of the iceberg. The types of interventions that apply to everyone and benefit everyone span an enormous range: from food and drug safety to controlling air pollution, from measures to prevent the spread of tuberculosis to vaccinating against childhood diseases, from prevention and response to disasters to detection of contaminants in our water.

The concerns of society as a whole are always in the forefront of public health though traditionally the focus of public health has been on prevention among mothers and children and the working aged population. These concerns keep changing and the methods for addressing them keep expanding. New technologies and global, local, and national interventions are becoming a necessary part of public health. To understand what public health has been and what it is becoming, let us look at some definitions of "public health." The following are two definitions of "public health"—one from the early 1900s and one from more recent years.

> Public health is "the science and art of preventing disease, prolonging life and promoting health through organized community effort."[3]

> The substance of public health is the "organized community efforts aimed at the prevention of disease and the promotion of health."[4]

These definitions show how little the concept of public health changed throughout the 1900s; however, the concept of public health in the 21st century is beginning to undergo important changes in a number of ways, including:

- The goal of prolonging life is being complemented by an emphasis on the quality of life. Protection of health when it already exists is becoming a focus along with promoting health when it is at risk.
- Use of new technologies, such as the Internet, is redefining "community," as well as offering us new ways to communicate.
- The enormous expansion in the options for intervention, as well as the increasing awareness of potential harms and costs of intervention programs, requires a new science of "evidence-based" public health.
- Public health and clinical care, as well as public and private partnerships, are coming together in new ways to produce collaborative efforts rarely seen in the 1900s.
- Complex public health problems need to be viewed as part of larger health and social systems, which require efforts to simultaneously examine multiple problems and multiple solutions rather than one problem or one solution at a time.
- Public health increasingly needs to pay attention to the full range of health issues, not just prevention among mothers and children and the working aged population but prevention of disability among our growing elderly populations. A full life cycle approach is now needed to improve community health.

A new 21st century definition of public health is needed. One such definition might read as follows:

> The totality of all evidence-based public and private efforts throughout the life cycle that preserve and promote health and prevent disease, disability, and death.

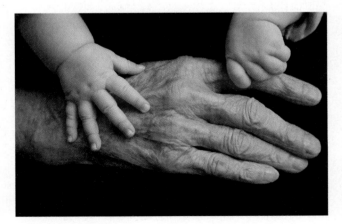

© AnnettVauteck/E+/Getty Images

This broad definition recognizes public health as the umbrella for a range of approaches that need to be viewed as a part of a big picture or population perspective. Specifically, this definition enlarges the traditional scope of public health to include an examination of the full range of environmental, social, and economic determinants of health—not just those traditionally addressed by public health and clinical health care. An examination of the full range of interventions to address health issues, including the structure and function of healthcare delivery systems, plus the role of public policies that affect health even when health is not their intended effect. This is being called a "health in all policies" approach.

If your children ask you what public health is, you might respond: "It is about the big picture issues that affect our own health and the health of our community every day of our lives. It is about protecting health in the face of disasters, preventing disease from addictions such as cigarettes and opioids, controlling infections such as the human immunodeficiency virus (HIV) and Zika, and developing systems to ensure the safety of the food we eat and the water we drink."

A variety of terms have been used to describe this big picture perspective that takes into account the full range of factors that affect health and considers their interactions.[5] We will use the term population health. Before exploring what we mean by the **population health approach**, let us examine how the approaches to public health have changed over time.[a]

## ▶ How Has the Approach of Public Health Changed Over Time?

### Health Protection (Antiquity—1830s)

Organized community efforts to promote health and prevent disease go back to ancient times.[6,7] The earliest human civilizations integrated concepts of prevention into their culture, their religion, and their laws. Prohibitions against specific foods—including pork, beef, and seafood—plus customs for food preparation, including officially designated

methods of killing cattle and methods of cooking, were part of the earliest practices of ancient societies. Prohibitions against alcohol or its limited use for religious ceremony have long been part of societies' efforts to control behavior, as well as prevent disease. Prohibition of cannibalism, the most universal of food taboos, has strong grounding in the protection of health.[b]

The earliest civilizations have viewed sexual practices as having health consequences. Male circumcision, premarital abstinence, and marital fidelity have all been shown to have impacts on health.

Quarantine or isolation of individuals with disease or those exposed to disease has likewise been practiced for thousands of years. The intuitive notion that isolating individuals with disease could protect individuals and societies led to some of the earliest organized efforts to prevent the spread of disease. At times they were successful but without a solid scientific basis. Efforts to separate individuals and communities from epidemics sometimes led to misguided efforts, such as the unsuccessful attempts to control the black plague by barring outsiders from walled towns while not recognizing that it was the rats and fleas that transmitted the disease.

During the 1700s and the first half of the 1800s, individuals occasionally produced important insights into the prevention of disease. In the 1740s, British naval commander James Lind demonstrated that lemons and other citrus fruit could prevent and treat scurvy, a then-common disease among sailors, whose daily nourishment was devoid of citrus fruit, the best source of vitamin C.

In the last years of the 1700s, English physician Edward Jenner recognized that cowpox, a common mild ailment among those who milked cows, protected those who developed it against life-threatening smallpox. He developed what came to be called a vaccine—derived from the Latin *vacca*, meaning "cow." He placed fluid from cowpox sores under the skin of recipients, including his son, and exposed them to smallpox. Despite the success of these smallpox prevention efforts, widespread use of vaccinations was slow to develop, partially because at that time there was not an adequate scientific basis to explain the reason for its success.

---

a Turnock[2] has described several meanings of "public health." These include the system and social enterprise, the profession, the methods, the government services, and the health of the public. The population health approach used in this text may be thought of as subsuming all of these different perspectives on public health.

b In recent years, this prohibition has been indirectly violated by feeding beef products containing bones and brain matter to other cattle. The development of "mad cow" disease and its transmission to humans has been traced to this practice, which can be viewed as analogous to human cannibalism.

## Hygiene Movement (1840–1870s)

All of these approaches to disease prevention were known before organized public health existed. Public health awareness began to emerge in Europe and the United States in the mid-1800s. The U.S. public health movement has its origins in Europe, where concepts of disease as the consequence of social conditions took root in the 1830s and 1840s. This movement, which put forth the idea that disease emerges from social conditions of inequality, produced the concept of **social justice**. Many attribute public health's focus on vulnerable populations to this tradition.

While early organized public health efforts paid special attention to vulnerable members of society, they also focused on the hazards that affected everyone, such as contamination of the environment. This focus on sanitation and public health was often called the hygiene movement, which began even before the development of the germ theory of disease. Despite the absence of an adequate scientific foundation, the hygiene movement made major strides in controlling communicable diseases, such as tuberculosis, cholera, and waterborne diseases, largely through alteration of the physical environment.

The fundamental concepts of epidemiology also developed during this era. In the 1850s, John Snow, often called the father of epidemiology, helped establish the importance of careful data collection and documentation of rates of disease before and after an intervention in order to evaluate effectiveness. He is known for his efforts to close down the Broad Street pump, which supplied water contaminated by cholera to a district of London. His actions quickly helped terminate that epidemic of cholera. John Snow's approach has become a symbol of the earliest formal epidemiological thinking.

Ignaz Semmelweis, an Austrian physician, used much the same approach in the mid-1800s to control puerperal fever—or fever of childbirth—then a major cause of maternal mortality. Noting that physicians frequently went from the autopsy room to the delivery room without washing their hands, he instituted a handwashing procedure and was able to document a dramatic reduction in the frequency of puerperal fever. Unfortunately, he was unable to convince many of his contemporaries to accept this intervention without a clear mechanism of action. Until the acceptance of the germ theory of disease, puerperal fever continued to be the major cause of maternal deaths in Europe and North America.

The mid-1800s in England also saw the development of birth and death records, or vital statistics, which formed the basis of population-wide assessment of health status. From the beginning of this type of data collection, there was controversy over how to define the cause of death. Two key figures in the early history of organized public health took opposing positions that reflect this continuing controversy. Edwin Chadwick argued that specific pathological conditions or diseases should be the basis for the cause of death. William Farr argued that underlying factors, including what we would today call social determinants of health, should be seen as the actual causes of death.

## Contagion Control (1880–1940s)

The methods of public health were already being established before the development of the germ theory of disease by Louis Pasteur and his European colleagues in the second half of the 1800s. The revolutions in biology that they ignited ushered in a new era in public health. U.S. physicians and public health leaders often went to Europe to study new techniques and approaches and brought them back to the United States to use at home.

After the Civil War, U.S. public health began to produce its own advances and organizations. In 1872, the American Public Health Association (APHA) was formed. According to its own historical account, the APHA's "founders recognized that two of the association's most important functions were advocacy for adoption by the government of the most current scientific advances relevant to public health, and public education on how to improve community health."[8]

The biological revolution of the late 1800s and early 1900s that resulted from the germ theory of disease laid the groundwork for the modern era of public health. An understanding of the contributions of bacteria and other organisms to disease produced novel diagnostic testing capabilities. For example, scientists could now identify tuberculosis cases through skin testing, bacterial culture, and the newly discovered chest X-ray. Concepts of vaccination advanced with the development of new vaccines against toxins produced by tetanus- and diphtheria-causing bacteria. Without antibiotics or other effective cures, much of public health in this era relied on prevention, isolation of those with disease, and case-finding methods to prevent further exposure.

In the early years of the 1900s, epidemiology methods continued to contribute to the understanding of disease. The investigations of pellagra by Goldberger and the United States Public Health Service overthrew the assumption of the day that pellagra was an infectious disease and established that it was a nutritional deficiency that could be prevented or easily cured with vitamin B-6 (niacin) or a balanced diet. Understanding the role of nutrition was central to public health's emerging focus on prenatal care and childhood growth and development. Incorporating key scientific advances, these efforts matured in the 1920s and 1930s and introduced a growing alphabet of vitamins and nutrients to the U.S. vocabulary.

## Filling Holes in the Medical Care System (1950s–mid-1980s)

A new era of effective medical intervention against active disease began in force after World War II. The discovery of penicillin and its often miraculous early successes convinced scientists, public health practitioners, and the general public that a new era in medicine and public health had arrived.

During this era, public health's focus was on filling the holes in the healthcare system. In this period, the role of public health was often seen as assisting clinicians to effectively deliver clinical services to those without the benefits of private medical care and helping to integrate preventive efforts into the practice of medicine. Thus, the great public health success of organized campaigns for the eradication of polio was mistakenly seen solely as a victory for medicine. Likewise, the successful passage of Medicaid and Medicare, outgrowths of public health's commitment to social justice, was simply viewed as efforts to expand the private practice of medicine.

This period, however, did lay the foundations for the emergence of a new era in public health. Epidemiological methods designed for the study of noncommunicable diseases demonstrated the major role that cigarette smoking plays in lung cancer and a variety of other diseases. The emergence of the randomized controlled trial and the regulation of drugs, vaccines, and other interventions by the Food and Drug Administration developed the foundations for what we now call evidence-based public health and evidence-based medicine.

## Health Promotion/Disease Prevention (Mid-1980s–2000)

The 1980s and much of the 1990s were characterized by a focus on individual responsibility for health and interventions at the individual level. Often referred to as health promotion and disease prevention, these interventions targeted individuals to effect behavioral change and combat the risk factors for diseases. As an example, to help prevent coronary artery disease, efforts were made to help individuals address high blood pressure and cholesterol, cigarette smoking, and obesity.

Behavioral change strategies were also used to help prevent the spread of the newly emerging HIV/AIDS epidemic. Efforts aimed at individual prevention and early detection as part of medical practice began to bear some fruit with the widespread introduction of mammography for detection of breast cancer and the worldwide use of Pap smears for the detection of cervical cancer. Newborn screening for genetic disease became a widespread and often legally mandated program, combining individual and community components.

Major public health advances during this era resulted from the environmental movement, which brought public awareness of the health dangers of lead in gasoline and paint. The environmental movement also focused on reducing cancer by controlling radiation exposure from a range of sources, including sunlight and radon, both naturally occurring radiation sources. In a triumph of global cooperation, governments worked together to address the newly discovered hole in the ozone layer. In the United States, reductions in air pollution levels and smoking rates during this era had an impact on the frequency of chronic lung disease, asthma, and most likely coronary artery disease.

## Population Health (2000s)

The heavy reliance on individual interventions that characterized much of the last half of the 1900s changed rapidly in the beginning of the 21st century. The current era in public health that is often called "population health" has begun to transform professional and public thought about health and the relationship between traditional public health and the healthcare system. From the potential for bioterrorism, to the high costs of health care, to the control of pandemic influenza, AIDS, and Ebola, the need for community-wide or population-wide public health efforts has become increasingly evident. This new era is characterized by a global perspective and the need to address international health issues. The concept of One Health, which focuses on the connections between human health, animal health, and ecosystem health, is providing a framework for understanding the global health impacts that affect all of us. One Health includes a focus on the potential impacts of climate change, emerging and reemerging infectious diseases, and the consequences of trade in potentially contaminated or dangerous products, ranging from food to toys.

**TABLE 1.1** outlines these eras of public health, identifies their key defining elements, and highlights important events that symbolize each era.[9]

**TABLE 1.1** Eras of Public Health

| Eras of public health | Focus of attention/ paradigm | Action framework | Notable events and movements in public health and epidemiology |
|---|---|---|---|
| Health protection (Antiquity–1830s) | Authority-based control of individual and community behaviors | Religious and cultural practices and prohibited behaviors | Quarantine for epidemics; sexual prohibitions to reduce disease transmission; dietary restrictions to reduce food-borne disease |
| Hygiene movement (1840–1870s) | Sanitary conditions as basis for improved health | Environmental action on a community-wide basis distinct from health care | Snow on cholera; Semmelweis and puerperal fever; collection of vital statistics as empirical foundation for public health and epidemiology |
| Contagion control (1880–1940s) | Germ theory: demonstration of infectious origins of disease | Communicable disease control through environmental control, vaccination, sanatoriums, and outbreak investigation in general population | Linkage of epidemiology, bacteriology, and immunology to form tuberculosis (TB) sanatoriums; outbreak investigation, e.g., Goldberger and pellagra |
| Filling holes in the medical care system (1950s–mid-1980s) | Integration of control of communicable diseases, modification of risk factors, and care of high-risk populations as part of medical care | Public system for control of specific communicable diseases and care for vulnerable populations distinct from general healthcare system, beginning of integrated healthcare systems with integration of preventive services into general healthcare system | Antibiotics; randomized controlled trials; concept of risk factors; surgeon general reports on cigarette smoking; Framingham study on cardiovascular risks; health maintenance organizations and community health centers with integration of preventive services into general healthcare system |
| Health promotion/ Disease prevention (Mid-1980s–2000) | Focus on individual behavior and disease detection in vulnerable and general populations | Clinical and population-oriented prevention with focus on individual control of decision-making and multiple interventions | AIDS epidemic and need for multiple interventions to reduce risk; reductions in coronary heart disease through multiple interventions |
| Population health (2000s) | Coordination of public health and healthcare delivery based upon shared evidence-based systems thinking | Evidence-based recommendations and information management, focus on harms and costs as well as benefits of interventions, globalization | Evidence-based medicine and public health; information technology; antibiotic resistance; global collaboration, e.g., one health; tobacco control; climate change, and a full life cycle approach to improving community health |

Data from Awofeso N. What's New About the "New Public Health"? *American Journal of Public Health.* 2004;94(5):705–709.

Today we have entered an era in which a focus on the individual is increasingly coupled with a focus on what needs to be done at the community and population level. This era of public health can be viewed as "the era of population health."

## What Is Meant by "Population Health"?

The concept of population health has emerged in recent years as a broader concept that stresses collaboration between traditional public health professions, healthcare delivery professionals, and a range of other professions that affect health. Population health provides an intellectual umbrella for thinking about the wide spectrum of factors that can and do affect the health of individuals and the population as a whole. **FIGURE 1.1** provides an overview of what falls under the umbrella of population health.

Population health also provides strategies for considering the broad range of potential **interventions** to address these issues. By "intervention" we mean the full range of strategies designed to protect health and prevent disease, disability, and death. Interventions include preventive efforts, such as nutrition and vaccination; curative efforts, such as antibiotics and cancer surgery; and efforts to prevent complications and restore function, from chemotherapy to physical therapy. Thus, population health is about improving community health.

The concept of population health can be seen as a comprehensive way of thinking about the modern scope of public health. It utilizes an evidence-based approach to analyze the determinants of health and disease and the options for intervention to preserve and improve health throughout the life cycle. Population health requires us to define what we mean by "health issues" and what we mean by "population(s)." It also requires us to define what we mean by "society's shared health concerns," as well as "society's vulnerable groups." To understand population health, we therefore need to define what we mean by each of these four components:

- Health issues
- Population(s)
- Society's shared health concerns
- Society's vulnerable groups

## What Are the Implications of Each of the Four Components of Public Health?

All four of the key components of public health have changed in recent years. Let us take a look at the historical, current, and emerging scopes of each component and consider their implications.

For most of the history of public health, the term "health" focused solely on physical health. Mental health has now been recognized as an important part of the definition; conditions such as depression and substance abuse make enormous contributions to disability in populations throughout the world. The boundaries of what we mean by "health" continue to expand, and the limits of health are not clear. Many novel medical interventions—including modification of genes and treatments to increase height, improve cosmetic appearance, and improve sexual performance—confront us with the question: Are these health issues?

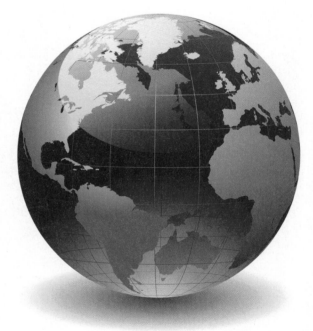

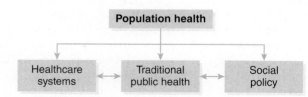

**FIGURE 1.1** The Full Spectrum of Population Health

© rtguest/Shutterstock

The definition of "population," likewise, is undergoing fundamental change. For most of recorded history, a population was defined geographically. Geographic communities, such as cities, states, and countries, defined the structure and functions of public health. The current definition of "population" has expanded to include the idea of a global community, recognizing the increasingly interconnected issues of global health. The definition of "population" is also focusing more on nongeographic communities. Universities now speak of an online-learning community, health care is delivered to members of a health plan community, and the Internet is constantly creating new social media communities. All of these new definitions of "population" are affecting the thinking and approaches needed to address public health issues.

What about the meaning of society-wide concerns—have they changed as well? Historically, public health and communicable disease were nearly synonymous, as symbolized by the field of epidemiology, which actually derives its name from the study of communicable disease epidemics. In recent decades, the focus of society-wide concerns has greatly expanded to include toxic exposures from the physical environment, transportation safety, and the costs of health care. However, communicable disease never went away as a focus of public health, and there is a recent resurgence in concern over emerging infectious diseases, including HIV/AIDS, pandemic flu, Ebola, and Zika as well as newly drug-resistant diseases, such as staph infections and tuberculosis. Additional concerns, ranging from the impact of climate change to the harms and benefits of new technologies, are altering the meaning of society-wide concerns.

Finally, the meaning of "vulnerable populations" continues to transform. For most of the 1900s, public health focused on maternal and child health and high-risk occupations as the operational definition of "vulnerable populations." While these groups remain important to public health, additional groups now receive more attention, including the disabled, the frail elderly, and those without health insurance. Attention is also beginning to focus on the immunosuppressed among those living with HIV/AIDS, who are at higher risk of infection and illness, and those whose genetic code documents their special vulnerability to disease and reactions to medications.

Public health has always been about our shared health concerns as a society and our concerns about vulnerable populations. These concerns have changed over time, and new concerns continue to emerge. **TABLE 1.2** outlines historical, current, and emerging components of the population health approach to public health. As illustrated by communicable diseases, past concerns cannot be relegated to history.

**TABLE 1.2** Components of Population Health

|  | Health | Population | Examples of society-wide concerns | Examples of vulnerable groups |
|---|---|---|---|---|
| Historical | Physical | Geographically limited | Communicable disease | High-risk maternal and child, high-risk occupations |
| Current | Physical and mental | Local, state, national, global, governmentally defined | Toxic substances, product and transportation safety, communicable diseases, costs of health care | Disabled, frail elderly, individuals with pain, uninsured |
| Emerging | Cosmetic, genetic, social functioning | Defined by local, national, and global communications | Disasters, climate change, technology hazards, emerging infectious diseases | Immunosuppressed, genetic vulnerability |

## Should We Focus on Everyone or on Vulnerable Groups?

Public health is often confronted with the potential conflict of focusing on everyone and addressing society-wide concerns versus focusing on the needs of vulnerable populations.[10] This conflict is reflected in the two different approaches to addressing public health problems. We will call them the **high-risk approach** and the **improving-the-average approach**.

The high-risk approach focuses on those with the highest probability of developing disease and aims to bring their risk close to the levels experienced by the rest of the population. **FIGURE 1.2A** illustrates the high-risk approach.

The success of the high-risk approach, as shown in **FIGURE 1.2B**, assumes that those with a high probability of developing disease are heavily concentrated among those with exposure to what we call **risk factors**. Risk factors include a wide range of exposures, from cigarette smoke and other toxic substances to high-risk sexual behaviors.

The improving-the-average approach focuses on the entire population and aims to reduce the risk for everyone. **FIGURE 1.3** illustrates this approach.

The improving-the-average approach assumes that everyone is at some degree of risk and the risk

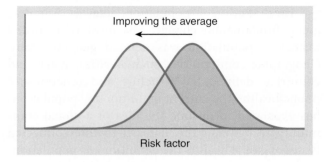

**FIGURE 1.3** Improving the Average

increases with the extent of exposure. In this situation, most of the disease occurs among the large number of people who have only modestly increased exposure. The successful reduction in average cholesterol levels through changes in the U.S. diet and the anticipated reduction in diabetes via a focus on weight reduction among children illustrate this approach.

One approach may work better than the other in specific circumstances, but in general, both approaches are needed if we are going to successfully address today's and tomorrow's health issues. These two approaches parallel public health's long-standing focus on both the health of vulnerable populations and society-wide health concerns.[c]

Now that we understand what we mean by "population health,"[d] let us take a look at the range of approaches that may be used to promote and protect health.

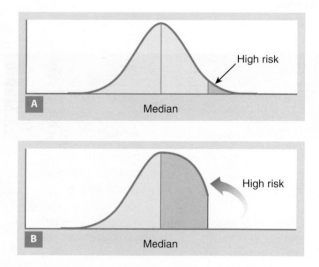

**FIGURE 1.2** (A) High Risk and (B) Reducing High Risk

## What Do We Mean by Population Health's Focus on the Life Cycle?

To improve community health, population health approaches need to consider the impacts on health throughout the life cycle. Issues of health risks actually extend from prenatal to postmortem. The prenatal in utero environment has long been known to affect health after birth, while the Ebola epidemic reminded us that direct contact with the recently deceased can be a major source of spread of disease.

---

c  An additional approach includes reducing disparities by narrowing the curve so that the gap is reduced between the lowest of the low-risk and the highest of the high-risk. For instance, this might be accomplished by transferring financial resources and/or health services from the low-risk to the high-risk category through taxation or other methods. Depending on the distribution of the factors affecting health, this approach may or may not reduce the overall frequency of disease more than the other approaches. The distribution of risk in Figures 1.2 and 1.3 assumes a bell-shaped or normal distribution. The actual distribution of factors affecting health may not follow this distribution.

d  The term population health is increasingly begin used by a wide range of health professionals and now carries a range of meanings. It may be used to refer to the health of a clinical population served by a hospital, a group practice, or a health plan. It may also be used to refer to a high-risk group or those who already have a specific disease. All these uses of the term population health share a focus on a defined population. Whenever the term population health is used it is important to ask "which population"?

Age is the single most important factor influencing the causes of death and disability. To allow us to focus on age, public health has long divided age into groups. These age groups may be defined by biological impact such as the different impacts which occur among the very young and the very old. They may also be defined by changing social issues, the most common of which is the age for entering and leaving the workforce.

The way we divide populations by age has changed over time and continues to change. The category we call adolescents and youth is evolving as the transition to the workforce is occurring at an older age. As the healthy life span increases, a new age category, sometimes called the young elderly, is emerging between the traditional end of full-time work and the onset of the stage we will call the old elderly.

**TABLE 1.3** presents one way of dividing the age groups in the United States and describing leading causes of death and disability.

**TABLE 1.3** Leading Causes of Death and Disability by Age Groups in the United States[11–13]

| Age Group (Age) | Age Group Name | Unique features of the age group and death rates per 1,000 in the United States | Major causes of death and disability in the United States |
| --- | --- | --- | --- |
| Birth to 28 days | Neonatal | Highest death rate of any age group until over 50. Approximately 4/1,000. Nearly two-thirds of deaths during first year of life occur in this period | Most deaths due to conditions present at birth including premature birth, low birthweight, and birth defects. |
| Birth to 1 year | Infancy | Infant mortality rates approximately 6/1,000 live births with approximately 2/1,000 after 1 month | Sudden infant death syndrome and infectious diseases are important causes of death after 1 month. |
| 1–5 years | Early childhood | Death rates fall dramatically in the United States and developed countries where infectious disease and malnutrition deaths are low. Rates approximately 0.2–0.4/1,000 per year | Unintentional injuries are the leading cause of death and disability. |
| 5–14 years | Childhood | Lowest death rates of any period with most years approximately 0.1/10,000 | Unintentional injury remains the leading cause of death and disability, with cancer being the second leading cause of death. Suicide is the third leading cause of death among those 10–14. |
| 15–24 years | Adolescents and Youth | Increasing death rates with nearly 1/1,000 deaths per year by age 24 | Dramatic increase in unintentional injuries and intentional injuries with homicide and suicide as the second and third leading causes of death. Behavior and mental disorders are the single largest cause of disability, and remain so until after age 65. |
| 25–65 years | Working age | Rates gradually increase from approximately 1/1,000 at age 30 to 1.5/1,000 at age 40 to 3/1,000 at age 50 to 8/1,000 at age 60 to 12/10,000 at age 65 | Causes of death change with increases in cancer and heart disease as the first and second leading causes of death by age 45 and remaining so through age 65. Chronic obstructive pulmonary disease is the third leading cause of death by age 55 and remains so until age 85.<br><br>Muscular-skeletal diseases are the greatest cause of disability during this period. |

*(continues)*

**TABLE 1.3** Leading Causes of Death and Disability by Age Groups in the United States[11–13]    *(continued)*

| Age Group (Age) | Age Group Name | Unique features of the age group and death rates per 1,000 in the United States | Major causes of death and disability in the United States |
|---|---|---|---|
| 66–85 years | Young elderly/ Senior citizens | Rates gradually increase from approximately 20/10,000 at age 70 to 30/1,000 at age 75 to 50/1,000 at age 80 | Cancer remains the leading cause of death until age 80 when it is exceeded by heart disease. Strokes and Alzheimer's increase as cause of death and disability after age 75. |
| 85+years | Old elderly/ Frail elderly | Rates rapidly increase from approximately 80/1,000 at age 85 to 140/1,000 at age 90 to 225/1,000 at age 95 to 300 per 1,000 at age 100 | Heart disease and cancer remain the first and second leading causes of death followed by Alzheimer's and strokes until age 95 when Alzheimer's becomes the second leading cause of death. Alzheimer's becomes the leading cause of disability in this age group. |

Data from Centers for Disease Control and Prevention. National Center for Health Statistics. Deaths, percent of total deaths, and death rates for the 15 leading causes of death in 5-year age groups, by race and sex: United States, 2014. Available at https://www.cdc.gov/nchs/nvss/mortality/lcwk2.htm. Accessed July 23, 2017; Centers for Disease Control and Prevention. National Center for Injury Prevention and Control. 10 Leading Causes of Death by Age Group, United States—2010. Available at https://www.cdc.gov/injury/wisqars/pdf/10lcid_all_deaths_by_age_group_2010 -a.pdf. Accessed July 23, 2017; National Institute of Mental Health. Cumulative U.S. DALYs for the Leading Disease/Disorder Categories by Age (2010). Available at https://www.nimh.nih.gov/health /statistics/disability/us-leading-disease-disorder-categories-by-age.shtml. Accessed July 23, 2017.

## ▶ What Are the Approaches Available to Protect and Promote Health?

The wide range of strategies that have been, are being, and will be used to address health issues can be divided into three general categories: health care, traditional public health, and social interventions.

Health care includes the delivery of services to individuals on a one-on-one basis. It includes services for those who are sick or disabled with illness or diseases, as well as for those who are asymptomatic. Services delivered as part of clinical prevention have been categorized as vaccinations, behavioral counseling, screening for disease, and preventive medications.[14]

Traditional public health efforts have a population-based preventive perspective utilizing interventions targeting communities or populations, as well as defined high-risk or vulnerable groups. Communicable disease control, reduction of environmental hazards, food and drug safety, and nutritional and behavioral risk factors have been key areas of focus of traditional public health approaches.

Both health care and traditional public health approaches share a goal to directly affect the health of those they reach. In contrast, social interventions are primarily aimed at achieving other nonhealth goals, such as increasing convenience, pleasure, economic growth, and social justice. Social interventions range from improving housing, to improving education and services for the poor, to increasing global trade. These interventions may have dramatic and sometimes unanticipated positive or negative health consequences. Social interventions, like increased availability of high-quality food, may improve health, while the availability of convenient high-fat or high-calorie foods may pose a risk to health.

**TABLE 1.4** describes the characteristics of health care, traditional public health, and social approaches to population health and provides examples of each approach.

None of these approaches is new. However, they have traditionally been separated or put into silos in our thinking process, with the connections between them often ignored. Thinking in systems and connecting the pieces is an important part of the 21st century challenge of defining public health.

Now that we have explained what we mean by "public health" and seen the scope and methods that we call "population health," let us continue our big picture approach by taking a look at what we mean by the "determinants of health and disease."

**TABLE 1.4** Approaches to Population Health

| | Characteristics | Examples |
|---|---|---|
| Health care | Systems for delivering one-on-one individual health services, including those aimed at prevention, cure, palliation, and rehabilitation | Clinical preventive services, including vaccinations, behavioral counseling, screening for disease, and preventive medications |
| Traditional public health | Group- and community-based interventions directed at health promotion and disease prevention | Communicable disease control, control of environmental hazards, food and drug safety, reduction in risk factors for disease |
| Social interventions | Interventions with another non-health-related purpose, which have secondary impacts on health | Interventions that improve the built environment, increase education, alter nutrition, or address socioeconomic disparities through changes in tax laws; globalization and mobility of goods and populations |

## ▶ What Factors Determine the Occurrence of Disease, Disability, and Death?

To complete our look at the big picture issues in public health, we need to gain an understanding of the forces that determine disease and the outcome of disease, including what in public health has been called morbidity (disability) and mortality (death).[e]

We need to establish what are called contributory causes based on evidence. **Contributory causes** can be thought of as immediate causes of disease. For instance, the HIV virus and cigarette smoking are two well-established contributory causes of disease, disability, and death. They directly produce disease, as well as disability and death. However, knowing these contributory causes of disease is often not enough. We need to ask: What determines whether people will smoke or come in contact with the HIV virus? What determines their course once exposed to cigarettes or HIV? In public health, we use the term **determinants** to identify these underlying factors, or "causes of causes" that ultimately bring about disease.

Determinants look beyond the known contributory causes of disease to factors that are at work often years before a disease develops.[15,16] These underlying factors may be thought of as "upstream" forces. Like great storms, we know the water will flow downstream, often producing flooding and destruction along the way. We just do not know exactly when and where the destruction will occur.

There is no official list or agreed-upon definition of what is included in determinants of disease.[f] Nonetheless, there is wide agreement that the following factors are among those that can be described as determinants in that they increase or at times decrease the chances of developing conditions that threaten the quantity and/or quality of life. Some but not all of

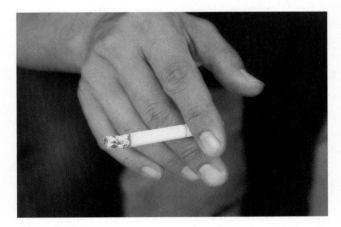

© Cherngchay Donkhuntod/Shutterstock

---

e   We will use the term "disease" as shorthand for the broad range of outcomes that includes injuries and exposures that result in death and disability.

f   Health Canada15 has identified 12 determinants of health, which are: (1) income and social status, (2) employment, (3) education, (4) social environments, (5) physical environments, (6) healthy child development, (7) personal health practices and coping skills, (8) health services, (9) social support networks, (10) biology and genetic endowment, (11) gender, and (12) culture. Many of these are subsumed under socioeconomic-cultural determinants in the BIG GEMS framework. The World Health Organization's Commission on Social Determinants of Health has also produced a list of determinants that is consistent with the BIG GEMS framework.16

these factors are related to socioeconomic status and are categorized as social determinants of health.

Behavior

Infection

Genetics

Geography

Environment

Medical care

Socioeconomic-cultural

**BIG GEMS** provides a convenient device for remembering these determinants of disease. Let us see what we mean by each of the determinants.

Behavior—Behavior implies actions that increase exposure to the factors that produce disease or protect individuals from disease. Actions such as smoking cigarettes, exercising, eating a particular diet, consuming alcohol, having unprotected intercourse, and using seat belts are all examples of the ways that behaviors help determine the development of disease.

Infection—Infections are often the direct cause of disease. In addition, we are increasingly recognizing that early or long-standing exposures to infections may contribute to the development of disease or even protection against disease. Diseases as diverse as gastric and duodenal ulcers, gallstones, and hepatoma or cancer originating in the liver are increasingly thought to have infection as an important determinant. Early exposure to infections may actually reduce diseases ranging from polio to asthma through their impact on the microbial environment in our gastrointestinal track, increasingly referred to as our microbiome.

Genetics—The revolution in genetics has focused our attention on roles that genetic factors play in the development and outcome of disease. Even when contributory causes, such as cigarettes, have been clearly established as producing lung cancer, genetic factors also play a role in the development and progression of the disease. While genetic factors play a role in many diseases, they are only occasionally the most important determinant of disease.

Geography—Geographic location influences the frequency and even the presence of disease. Infectious diseases such as malaria, Chagas disease, schistosomiasis, and Lyme disease occur only in defined geographic areas. Geography may also imply local geological conditions, such as those that produce high levels of radon—a naturally occurring radiation that contributes to the development of lung cancer. Geography implies that special locations are required to produce disease, such as altitude sickness, frostbite in cold climates, or certain types of snake bites in the tropics.

Environment—Environmental factors determine disease and the course of disease in a number of ways. The unaltered or "natural" physical world around us may produce disability and death from sudden natural disasters, such as earthquakes and volcanic eruptions, to iodine deficiencies due to low iodine content in the food-producing soil. The altered physical environment produced by human intervention includes exposures to toxic substances in occupational or nonoccupational settings. The physical environment built for use by humans—the **built environment**—produces determinants ranging from indoor air pollution, to "infant-proofed" homes, to hazards on the highway.

Medical care—Access to and the quality of medical care can be a determinant of disease. When a high percentage of individuals are protected by vaccination, nonvaccinated individuals in the population may be protected as well. Cigarette smoking cessation efforts may help smokers to quit, and treatment of infectious disease may reduce the spread to others. Medical care, however, often has its major impact on the course of disease by attempting to prevent or minimize disability and death once disease develops.

Socioeconomic-cultural—In the United States, socioeconomic factors have been defined as education, income, and occupational status. These measures have all been shown to be determinants of diseases as varied as breast cancer, tuberculosis, and occupational injuries. Cultural and religious factors are increasingly being recognized as determinants of diseases because beliefs sometimes influence decisions

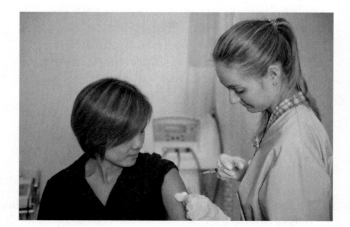

© MAGNIFIER/Shutterstock

about treatments, in turn affecting the outcome of the disease. While most diseases are more frequent in lower socioeconomic groups, others, such as breast cancer, may be more common in higher socioeconomic groups.

Determinants of disease come up again and again as we explore the work of population health. Historically, understanding determinants has often allowed us to prevent diseases and their consequences even when we did not fully understand the mechanism by which the determinants produced their impact. For instance:

- Scurvy was controlled by citrus fruits well before vitamin C was identified.
- Malaria was partially controlled by clearing swamps before the relationship to mosquito transmission was appreciated.

- Hepatitis B and HIV infections were partially controlled even before the organisms were identified through the reduction in use of contaminated needles and the establishment of standards for blood transfusions.
- Tuberculosis death rates were greatly reduced through less crowded housing, the use of TB sanitariums, and better nutrition.

Using asthma as an example, **BOX 1.1** illustrates the many ways that determinants can affect the development and course of a disease.

Determinants of health may change over time, and the composition of populations may change in ways that affect health. Let us take a look at some of the ways that populations have changed and are changing that affect population health.

---

**BOX 1.1** Asthma and the Determinants of Disease

*Jennifer, a teenager living in a rundown urban apartment in a city with high levels of air pollution, develops severe asthma. Her mother also has severe asthma, yet both of them smoke cigarettes. Her clinician prescribed medications to prevent asthma attacks, but she takes them only when she experiences severe symptoms. Jennifer is hospitalized twice with pneumonia due to common bacterial infections. She then develops an antibiotic-resistant infection. During this hospitalization, she requires intensive care on a respirator. After several weeks of intensive care and every known treatment to save her life, she dies suddenly.*

Asthma is an inflammatory disease of the lung coupled with an increased reactivity of the airways, which together produce a narrowing of the airways of the lungs. When the airways become swollen and inflamed, they become narrower, allowing less air through to the lung tissue and causing symptoms such as wheezing, coughing, chest tightness, breathing difficulty, and predisposition to infection. Once considered a minor ailment, asthma is now the most common chronic disorder of childhood. It affects over 6 million children under the age of 18 in the United States alone.

Jennifer's tragic history illustrates how a wide range of determinants of disease may affect the occurrence, severity, and development of complications of a disease. Let us walk through the BIG GEMS framework and see how each determinant had impacts on Jennifer.

Behavior—Behavioral factors play an important role in the development of asthma attacks and in their complications. Cigarette smoking makes asthma attacks more frequent and more severe. It also predisposes individuals to developing infections such as pneumonia. Treatment for severe asthma requires regular treatments along with more intensive treatment when an attack occurs. It is difficult for many people, especially

teenagers, to take medication regularly, yet failure to adhere to treatment greatly complicates the disease.

Infection—Infection is a frequent precipitant of asthma, and asthma increases the frequency and severity of infections. Infectious diseases, especially pneumonia, can be life-threatening in asthmatics, requiring prompt and high-quality medical care. The increasing development of antibiotic-resistant infections poses special risks to those with asthma.

Genetics—Genetic factors predispose people to childhood asthma. However, many children and adults without a family history develop asthma.

Geography—Asthma is more common in geographic areas with high levels of naturally occurring allergens due to flowering plants. However, today even populations in desert climates in the United States are often affected by asthma, as irrigation results in the planting of allergen-producing trees and other plants.

Environment—The physical environment, including that built for use by humans, has increasingly been recognized as a major factor affecting the development of asthma and asthma attacks. Indoor air pollution due to wood burning is the most common form of air pollution in many developing countries. Along with cigarette smoke, air pollution inflames the lungs acutely and chronically. Cockroaches often found in rundown buildings have been found to be highly allergenic and predisposing to asthma. Other factors in the built environment, including mold and exposure to pet dander, can also trigger wheezing in susceptible individuals.

Medical care—The course of asthma can be greatly affected by medical care. Management of the acute and chronic effects of asthma can be positively affected by efforts to understand an individual's exposures, reducing the chronic inflammation with medications, managing the acute symptoms, and avoiding life-threatening complications.

   Socioeconomic-cultural—Disease and disease progression are often influenced by an individual's socioeconomic status. Air pollution is often greater in lower socioeconomic neighborhoods of urban areas. Mold and cockroach infestations may be greater in poor neighborhoods. Access to and the quality of medical

care may be affected by social, economic, and cultural factors.

   Asthma is a condition that demonstrates the contributions made by the full range of determinants included in the BIG GEMS framework. No one determinant alone explains the bulk of the disease. The large number of determinants and their interactions provide opportunities for a range of health care, traditional public health, and social interventions.

## ▶ What Changes in Populations Over Time Can Affect Health?

A number of important trends or transitions in the composition of populations that affect the pattern of disease have been described in recent years. These transitions have implications for what we can expect to happen throughout the 21st century. We will call these the demographic, epidemiological, and nutritional transitions.

The **demographic transition** describes the impact of falling childhood death rates and extended life spans on the size and the age distribution of populations.[17] During the first half of the 20th century, death rates among the young fell dramatically in today's developed countries. Death rates continued their dramatic decline in most parts of the developing world during the second half of the 20th century.

Birth rates tend to remain high for years or decades after the decline in deaths. High birth rates paired with lower death rates lead to rapid growth in population size, as we have seen in much of the developing world. This trend continues today and is expected to go on in many parts of the world well into the 21st century. **Population pyramids** are often useful for displaying the changes in the age distribution that occur over time. Population pyramids display the number of males and females that are present or expected to be present for each age group in a particular year. The population pyramids in **FIGURE 1.4** illustrate how the population of Nigeria is expected to grow through 2050 due to a high birth rate and a lowered death rate.

Despite the delay, a decline in birth rates reliably occurs following the decline in childhood deaths. This decline in births gradually leads to aging of the population and can eventually lead to declining population numbers in the absence of large-scale immigration. We are now seeing societies in much of Europe and Japan as well as the United States with rapidly growing

elderly populations. Over 25% of the population of Japan is currently over 65 compared to approximately 15% in the United States.

Take a look at the population pyramids in **FIGURE 1.5**, which show what is expected to occur in the coming years in much of Europe and Japan. Japan is used as an example of the emergence of an inverted population pyramid, with a smaller young population and a larger older population. Populations with a large number of the elderly relative to the number of younger individuals have a heavier burden of disease and create the conditions for aging to become a public health issue.

The large number of immigrants to the United States and their generally higher birth rates have slowed this process in the United States, but the basic trend of a growing elderly population continues. The population pyramids for the United States are displayed in **FIGURE 1.6**.

**BOX 1.2** looks at the impacts that an increasing elderly population can be expected to have in the United States in the coming years and the challenges faced by public health.

A second transition has been called the **epidemiological transition**,[20] or public health transition. The epidemiological transition implies that as social and economic development occurs, different types of diseases become prominent. Deaths in less developed societies are often dominated by epidemic communicable diseases and diseases associated with malnutrition and childhood infections. As a country develops, communicable diseases often come under control, and noncommunicable and chronic diseases, such as heart disease, often predominate.

A related transition known as the **nutritional transition**[21] implies that countries frequently move from poorly balanced diets often deficient in nutrients, proteins, and calories to a diet of highly processed food, including fats, sugars, and salt. The consequences of both under- and overnutrition affect and will continue to affect the public's health well into the 21st century.

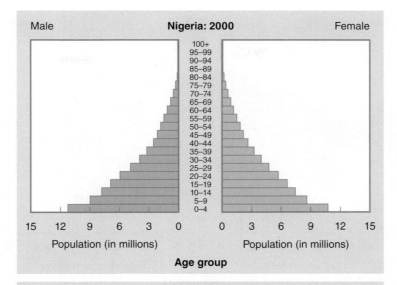

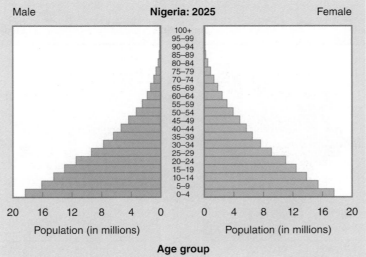

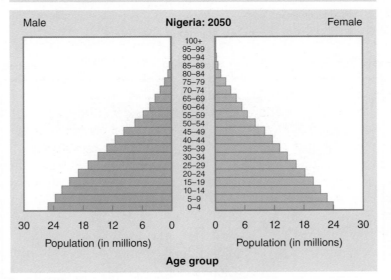

**FIGURE 1.4** Population Pyramid Expected for Nigeria

Reproduced from U.S. Census Bureau. International Database. Available at http://www.census.gov/population/international/data/idb/informationGateway.php. Accessed July 14, 2017

As we have seen, population health focuses on the big picture issues and the determinants of disease. Increasingly, public health also emphasizes a focus on research evidence as a basis for understanding the cause or etiology of disease and the interventions that can improve the outcome. Let us now explore what we mean by "evidence-based public health."

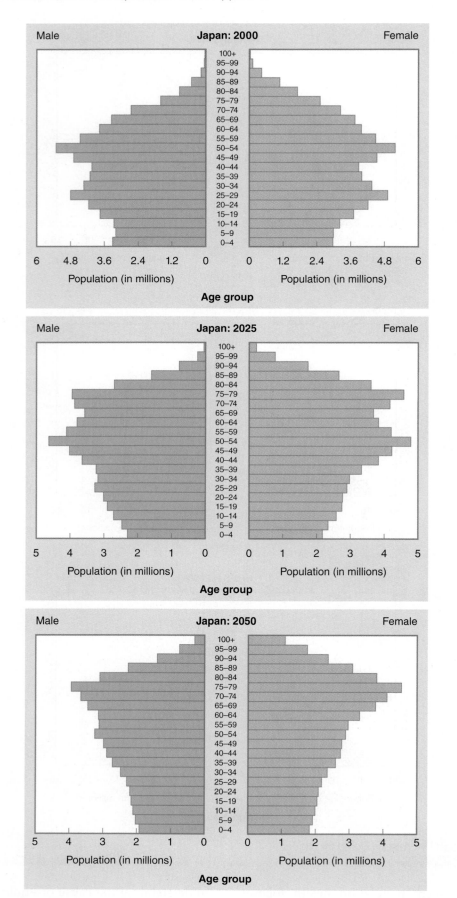

**FIGURE 1.5** Population Pyramid Expected for Japan

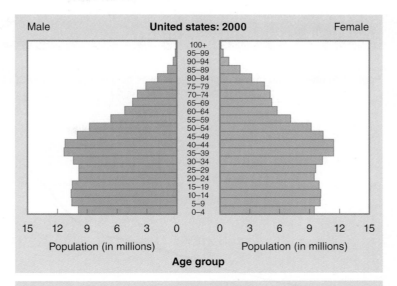

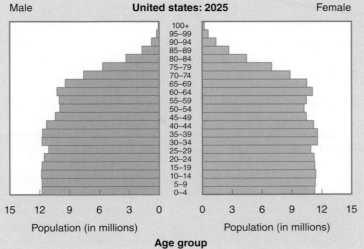

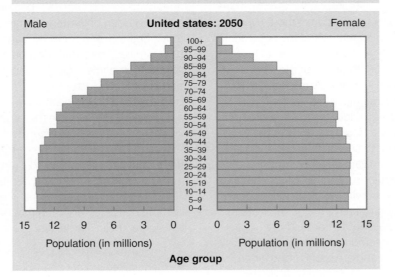

**FIGURE 1.6** Population Pyramid Expected for the United States

Reproduced from U.S. Census Bureau. International Database. Available at http://www.census.gov/population/international/data/idb/informationGateway.php. Accessed July 14, 2017

**BOX 1.2**  Aging as a Public Health Issue

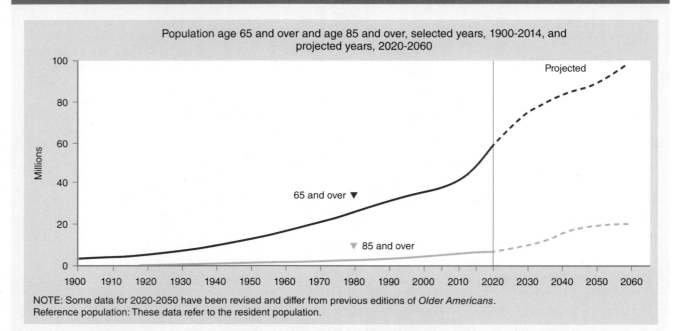

Population age 65 and over and age 85 and over, selected years, 1900-2014, and projected years, 2020-2060

NOTE: Some data for 2020-2050 have been revised and differ from previous editions of *Older Americans*.
Reference population: These data refer to the resident population.

**FIGURE 1.7**  Population Aged 65 and Over and Age 85 and Over, Selected Years 1900–2014 and Projected Years 2020–2060

Reproduced from Federal Interagency Forum on Aging-Related Statistics. *Older Americans 2016: Key Indicators of Well-Being*. Federal Interagency Forum on Aging-Related Statistics. Washington, DC: U.S. Government Printing office. August 2016 page 2. Available at: https://agingstats.gov/docs/LatestReport/Older-Americans-2016-Key-Indicators-of-WellBeing.pdf. Accessed July 14, 2017.

The proportion of the elderly in the United States is increasing rapidly in the second decade of the 21st century as the "baby boomers" born between 1946 and 1964 enter the 65- to 74-year-old age group. **FIGURE 1.7** illustrates the rapid increase that is occurring and is expected to continue in the coming decades among those 65 and over and 85 and over. By 2030 the proportion of those over 65 is expected to reach approximately 25% of the population compared to the current level of approximately 15%.

The impact of aging is felt throughout the life span as working aged adults are increasingly responsible for taking care of their aging parents as well as their own children, and all taxpayers shoulder the costs of programs for the elderly. Government programs for the elderly are already under financial strain. The finances of Social Security, Medicare, and Medicaid-financed nursing home care have become key issues in national political debates.

The ability of a slowly growing workforce to support a rapidly aging population will have major implications in the United States for decades to come. These impacts, though great, are not expected to have the same consequences as in Japan and areas of Europe where overall population numbers are declining, while the elderly, especially those over 85, continue to increase.

The social and economic consequences of an aging population will be felt personally by most of today's college students. They will face a future with elderly parents and a society which is challenged to help address their needs.

The most dramatic impacts of an aging population will occur as a higher percentage of the elderly

population reach age 85 and over. Dementia, including Alzheimer's disease and other conditions that chronically impair memory, rapidly increases among those 85 and older. Less than 4% of those 65 to 69 are diagnosed with dementia, but the percentage rises to almost 25% from ages 85 to 90 and over 35% beginning at age 90.[18]

The burden of dementia is rapidly becoming a major financial and social burden to the elderly and their families. The social isolation and depression that often accompanies aging in general and dementia in particular is one factor that can and should be addressed by public health and healthcare interventions.

Those 85 and over are the largest contributor to a vulnerable population known as the frail elderly. Over 25% of those over 85 can be classified as frail elderly. The frail elderly are susceptible to a range of health issues including falls, infection, and depression.

Gerontologists suggest that if someone has three or more of five factors, then that person should be considered frail.[19] These factors are:

- Unintentional weight loss (10 pounds or more in a year)
- General feeling of exhaustion
- Weakness (as measured by grip strength)
- Slow walking speed
- Low levels of physical activity

Fortunately there are a number of public health, healthcare, and social interventions that can prevent frailty or minimize its consequences; they are often described as follows:

**F**ood- maintain intake
**R**esistance exercises
**A**therosclerosis prevention (e.g., blood pressure, low-density lipoprotein cholesterol reduction, smoking cessation, etc.)
**I**solation prevention
**L**imit pain
**T**ai Chi or other balance exercises
**Y**early check for testosterone deficiency

Impaired vision, impaired hearing, and dental problems are perhaps the most common modifiable

incapacitating impairments of the elderly. Yet Medicare does not generally provide coverage for these treatable conditions. Efforts to support the frail elderly and prevent falls, social isolation, and other preventable conditions are increasingly seen as part of the population health's commitment to improving the health of the elderly.

Focusing on the health of the elderly is an increasingly important part of population health. It is becoming an important way to improve the health of the community both for the elderly and for those who hope to live a long life.

## Key Words

BIG GEMS
Built environment
Contributory causes
Demographic transition
Determinants

Epidemiological transition
High-risk approach
Interventions
Improving-the-average approach
Nutritional transition

Population health approach
Population pyramid
Risk factor
Social justice
Vulnerable populations

## Discussion Question

Think about a typical day in your life and identify ways that public health affects it.

## References

1. Pfizer Global Pharmaceuticals. *Milestones in Public Health: Accomplishments in Public Health over the Last 100 Years*. New York, NY: Pfizer Global Pharmaceuticals; 2006.
2. Turnock BJ. *Public Health: What It Is and How It Works*. 4th ed. Sudbury, MA: Jones and Bartlett Publishers; 2009.
3. Winslow CEA. The untilled field of public health. *Modernizing Medicine*. 1920;920(2):183–191.
4. Institute of Medicine. *The Future of Public Health*. Washington, DC: National Academy Press; 1988:41.
5. Young TK. *Population Health: Concepts and Methods*. New York, NY: Oxford University Press; 1998.
6. Rosen G. *A History of Public Health*. Baltimore, MD: Johns Hopkins University Press; 1993.
7. Porter D. *Health, Civilization, and the State: A History of Public Health from Ancient to Modern Times*. Oxford: Rutledge; 1999.
8. American Public Health Association. APHA history and timeline. https://www.apha.org/news-and-media/newsroom/online-press-kit/apha-history-and-timeline. Accessed July 14, 2017.
9. Awofeso N. What's new about the "New Public Health"? *American Journal Public Health*. 2004;94(5):705–709.
10. Rose G, Khaw KT, Marmot M. *Rose's Strategy of Preventive Medicine*. New York, NY: Oxford University Press; 2008.
11. Centers for Disease Control and Prevention. National Center for Health Statistics. Deaths, percent of total deaths, and death rates for the 15 leading causes of death in 5-year age groups, by race and sex: United States, 2014. Available at https://www.cdc.gov/nchs/nvss/mortality/lcwk2.htm. Accessed July 23, 2017.
12. Centers for Disease Control and Prevention. National Center for Injury Prevention and Control. 10 Leading Causes of Death by Age Group, United States—2010. Available at https://www.cdc.gov/injury/wisqars/pdf/10lcid_all_deaths_by_age_group_2010-a.pdf. Accessed July 23, 2017.
13. National Institute of Mental Health. Cumulative U.S. DALYs for the leading disease/disorder categories by age, 2010. Available at https://www.nimh.nih.gov/health/statistics/disability/us-leading-disease-disorder-categories-by-age.shtml. Accessed July 23, 2017.
14. U.S. Preventive Services Task Force. Recommendations for primarycarepractice.https://www.uspreventiveservicestaskforce.org/Page/Name/recommendations. Accessed July 14, 2017.
15. Public Health Agency of Canada. Population health approach—what determines health? http://www.phac-aspc.gc.ca/ph-sp. Accessed July 14, 2017.
16. Commission on Social Determinants of Health. Closing the gap in a generation: health equity through action on the social determinants of health. *Final Report of the Commission on Social Determinants of Health*. Geneva: World Health Organization; 2008.
17. U.S. Census Bureau. International database. http://www.census.gov/ipc/www/idb/pyramids.html. Accessed July 14, 2017.
18. Reproduced from Federal Interagency Forum on Aging-Related Statistics. *Older Americans 2016: Key Indicators of Well-Being*. Federal Interagency Forum on Aging-Related Statistics. Washington, DC: U.S. Government Printing office. August 2016, page 2. Available at https://agingstats.gov/docs/LatestReport/Older-Americans-2016-Key-Indicators-of-WellBeing.pdf. Accessed July 14, 2017.
19. Xue Q-L. The frailty syndrome: Definition and natural history. *Clinics in Geriatric Medicine*. 2011;27(1):1–15. doi:10.1016/j.cger.2010.08.009.
20. Omran AR. The epidemiologic transition: a theory of the epidemiology of population change. *The Milbank Memorial Fund Quarterly*. 1971;49(4):509–538.
21. Skolnik R. *Global Health 101*. 3rd ed. Burlington, MA: Jones & Bartlett Learning; 2016.

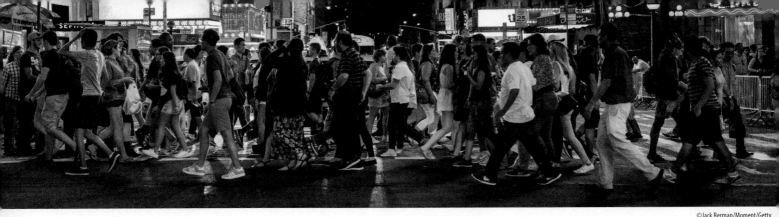

# CHAPTER 2
# Evidence-Based Public Health

## LEARNING OBJECTIVES

By the end of this chapter, the student will be able to:

- explain the steps in the evidence-based public health process.
- describe a public health problem in terms of morbidity and mortality.
- describe the course of a disease in terms of incidence, prevalence, and case-fatality.
- describe how the distribution of disease may be used to generate hypotheses about the cause of a disease.
- describe an approach used in public health to identify a contributory cause of a disease or other condition and establish the efficacy of an intervention.
- describe the uses of qualitative data that complement quantitative data.
- describe the process of grading evidence-based recommendations.
- use an approach to identify options for intervention based on "when, who, and how."
- explain the role that evaluation plays in establishing effectiveness as part of evidence-based public health.

Tobacco was introduced to Europe as a new world crop in the early 1600s. Despite the availability of pipe tobacco and, later, cigars, the mass production and consumption of tobacco through cigarette smoking did not begin until the development of the cigarette rolling machine by James Duke in the 1880s. This invention allowed mass production and distribution of cigarettes for the first time. Men were the first mass consumers of cigarettes. During World War I, cigarettes were widely distributed free of charge to U.S. soldiers.

Cigarette smoking first became popular among women in the 1920s—an era noted for changes in the role and attitudes of women—and at this time, advertising of cigarettes began to focus on women. The mass consumption of cigarettes by women, however, trailed that of men by at least

two decades. By the 1950s, over 50% of adult males and approximately 25% of adult females were regular cigarette smokers.

The health problems of cigarette smoking were not fully recognized until decades after the habit became widespread. As late as the 1940s, R.J. Reynolds advertised that "more doctors smoke Camels than any other cigarette."

Epidemiologists observed that lung cancer deaths were increasing in frequency in the 1930s and 1940s. The increase in cases did not appear to be due to changes in efforts to recognize the disease, the ability to recognize the disease, or the definition of the disease. Even after the increasing average life span and aging of the population was taken into account, it was evident that the rate of death from lung cancer was increasing—and more rapidly for men than women. In addition, it was noted that residents of states with higher rates of smoking had higher rates of lung cancer. In the 1950s, the number of lung cancer deaths in females also began to increase, and by the 1960s, the disease had become the most common cause of cancer-related deaths in males and was still rising among women.[1,2]

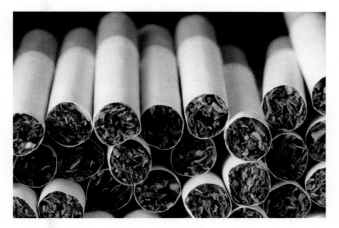
© underworld/Shutterstock

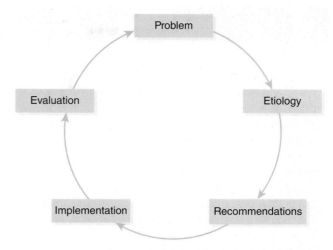

**FIGURE 2.1** Evidence-Based Public Health: The P.E.R.I.E. Approach

This type of information was the basis for describing the problems of cigarette smoking and lung cancer and developing ideas or hypotheses about its etiology, or cause. Let us take a look at how the evidence-based public health approach has been used to address the problem of cigarette smoking. There are five basic questions that we need to ask that together make up what we will call the evidence-based public health approach.[3]

1. **P**roblem: What is the health problem?
2. **E**tiology: What is/are the contributory cause(s)?
3. **R**ecommendations: What works to reduce the health impacts?
4. **I**mplementation: How can we get the job done?
5. **E**valuation: How well does/do the intervention(s) work in practice?

These five questions provide a framework for defining, analyzing, and addressing a wide range of public health issues and can be applied to cigarette smoking for the purposes of this chapter.[4] We will call this framework the **P.E.R.I.E. process**. This process is actually circular, as illustrated in **FIGURE 2.1**. If the evaluation suggests that more needs to be done, the cycle

can and should be repeated. Thus, it is an ongoing process.

Using cigarette smoking as an example, we will illustrate the steps needed to apply the evidence-based public health approach.

## ▶ How Can We Describe a Health Problem?

In describing a health problem, we need to address the burden, course, and distribution of disease. The first step in addressing a health problem is to describe its **burden of disease**, which is the occurrence of disability and death due to a disease. In public heath, disability is often called **morbidity** and death is called **mortality**. We will want to know the current burden of disease and whether there has been a recent change in the burden of the disease.

In addition to describing the burden of disease, it is important to describe what we call the **course of a disease**. The course of the disease asks how often the disease occurs, how likely it is to be present currently, and what happens once it occurs. Describing the course of a disease as well as the burden of disease requires us to use measurements known as rates. **BOX 2.1** discusses what we mean by "rates" and how we can use them to describe the burden and course of disease.

In addition to describing the burden and the course of a disease or other health problem, we need to ask: What is the **distribution of disease**? Distribution of disease asks such questions as: Who gets the disease? Where are they located? When does the disease occur? Let us see how understanding the

## BOX 2.1 Rates and the Description of a Health Problem

The term "**rate**" is often used to describe any type of measurement that has a numerator and a denominator where the numerator is a subset of the denominator—that is, the numerator includes only individuals who are also included in the denominator. In a rate, the numerator measures the number of times an event, such as the diagnosis of lung cancer, occurs. The denominator measures the number of times the event could occur. We often use the entire population in the denominator, but at times, we may only use the **at-risk population**. For instance, when measuring the rate of cervical cancer, we would only use the population of women in the denominator, and when measuring rates of prostate cancer, we would only use the population of men in the denominator.[a]

There are two basic types of rates that are key to describing a disease.[5,6] These are called **incidence** rates and **prevalence**. Incidence rates measure the chances of developing a disease over a period of time—usually one year. That is, incidence rates are the number of new cases of a disease that develop during a year divided by the number of people in the at-risk population at the beginning of the year, as in the following equation:

$$\text{Incidence rate} = \frac{\#\ of\ new\ cases\ of\ a\ disease\ in\ a\ year}{\#\ of\ people\ in\ the\ at\text{-}risk\ population}$$

We often express incidence rates as the number of events per 100,000 people in the denominator. For instance, the incidence rate of lung cancer might be 100 per 100,000 per year. In evidence-based public health, comparing incidence rates is often a useful starting point when trying to establish the **etiology**, or cause, of a problem.

Mortality rates are a special type of incidence rate that measure the incidence of death due to a disease during a particular year. Mortality rates are often used to measure the burden of disease. When most people who develop a disease die from the disease, as is the situation with lung cancer, the mortality rate and the incidence rates are very similar. Thus, if the incidence rate of lung cancer is 100 per 100,000 per year, the mortality rate might be 95 per 100,000 per year. When mortality rates and incidence rates are similar and mortality rates are more easily or reliably obtained, epidemiologists may substitute mortality rates for incidence rates.[b]

The relationship between the incidence rate and the mortality rate is important because it estimates the chances of dying from the disease once it is diagnosed. We call this the **case-fatality**. In our example, the chances of dying from lung cancer—the morality rate divided by the incidence rate—is 95%, which indicates that lung cancer results in a very poor prognosis once it is diagnosed.

Prevalence is the number of individuals who have a disease at a particular time divided by the number of individuals who could potentially have the disease. It can be represented by the following equation:

$$\text{Prevalence} = \frac{\#\ of\ living\ with\ a\ particular\ disease}{\#\ of\ people\ in\ the\ at\text{-}risk\ population}$$

Thus, prevalence tells us the **proportion** or percentage of individuals who have the disease at a point in time.[5,6]

Despite the fact that lung cancer has become the most common cancer, the prevalence will be low—perhaps one-tenth of 1% or less—because those who develop lung cancer do not generally live for a long period of time. Therefore, you will rarely see people with lung cancer. The prevalence of chronic diseases of prolonged duration, such as asthma or chronic obstructive pulmonary disease (COPD), is often relatively high; hence you will often see people with these diseases.[c]

Prevalence is often useful when trying to assess the total impact or burden of a health problem in a population and can help identify the need for services. For example, knowledge that there is a high prevalence of lung cancer in a certain region may indicate that there is a need for special types of healthcare services in that

---

a  When talking about the term "rate," many epidemiologists also include a unit of time, such as a day or a year, over which the number of events in the numerator is measured. This may also be called a **true rate**. The term "rate" as used in this text includes true rates, as well as proportions. A proportion is a fraction in which the numerator is a subset of the denominator. A time period is not required for a proportion; however, it often reflects the situation at one point in time.

b  This is an example of the pragmatic approach that is often taken by epidemiologists when they are limited by the available data. The question facing epidemiologists is frequently: Is the data good enough to address the question? Thus, epidemiology can be thought of as an approximation science.

c  The relationship between incidence and prevalence rates is approximately the incidence rate × average duration of the disease = the prevalence rate. Both the incidence rate and the average duration affect the prevalence of the disease. Together, the incidence, prevalence, and case-fatality rates provide a population-based summary of the course of a disease. Incidence reflects the chance of developing the disease, prevalence indicates the chances of having the disease, and case-fatality indicates the prognosis or chance of dying from the disease.

area. Prevalence is also very useful in clinical medicine as the starting point for screening and diagnosis.

When using rates to describe a problem, we often use the rates of mortality and morbidity to describe the burden of disease. We use the incidence, prevalence, and case-fatality as the three key rates or measures that together provide a description of the course of disease. Together,

these three measures address the key issues that we need to know in describing the course of a health problem: How likely it is to occur? How likely it is to be present currently? What happens once it occurs? Thus, understanding the burden of disease and the course of disease require us to understand and use rates. As we will see, rates are also key to understanding the distribution of disease.

distribution of disease may help generate ideas or hypotheses about the disease's etiology (cause).

## ▶ How Can Understanding the Distribution of Disease Help Us Generate Ideas or Hypotheses About the Cause Of Disease?

Public health professionals called **epidemiologists** investigate factors known as "person" and "place" to see if they can find patterns or **associations** in the frequency of a disease. We call these **group associations** or ecological associations. Group associations may suggest ideas or hypotheses about the cause, or etiology, of a disease.

"Person" includes demographic characteristics that describe people, such as age, gender, race, and socioeconomic factors. It also includes behaviors or exposures, such as cigarette smoking, exercise, radiation exposure, and use of medications. "Place" traditionally implies geographic location, such as a city or state. Place matters in the occurrence of disease. The term "healthography" has recently been introduced to reflect the importance of geographic location to health. Place also includes nonphysical connections between people, such as a university community or a shared Internet site. When these types of factors occur more frequently among groups with the disease than among groups without the disease, we call them **risk indicators** or risk markers.[a]

**BOX 2.2** illustrates how person and place can be used to generate hypotheses about the cause of a disease.

In looking at the distribution of lung cancer and the potential risk factors, epidemiologists found some important relationships. In terms of person,

the increases in lung cancer mortality observed in the 1930s–1950s were far more dramatic among men than among women, though by the 1950s, the mortality rate among women had begun to increase as well. It was noted that cigarette use had increased first in men and later among women. There appeared to be a delay of several decades between the increase in cigarette smoking and the increase in lung cancer mortality among both men and women. This illustrates that "time" along with "person" and "place" is important in generating hypotheses.

In terms of place, it was found that the relationship between cigarette smoking and lung cancer mortality was present throughout the United States, but was strongest in those states where cigarette smoking was most common. Therefore, changes over time and the distribution of disease using person and place led epidemiologists to the conclusion that there was an association between groups of people who smoked more frequently and the same group's mortality rates due to lung cancer. These relationships generated the idea that cigarettes might be a cause of lung cancer.

It is important to realize that these mortality rates are group rates. These data did not include any information about whether those who died from lung cancer were smokers. It merely indicated that groups who smoked more, such as males, also had higher mortality rates from lung cancer. The most that we can hope to achieve from these data is to generate hypotheses based on associations between groups, or group associations. When we try to establish causation or etiology, we will need to go beyond group association and focus on associations at the individual level.

Finally, epidemiologists take a scientific approach to addressing public health problems. They are often skeptical of initial answers to a question and ask: Could there be another explanation for the differences or changes in the distribution of disease?

---

a  The term "risk indicator" or "risk marker" needs to be distinguished from the term "risk factor." A risk factor is a candidate for being a contributory cause and implies that at least an association at the individual level has been established.

**BOX 2.2**   Generating Hypotheses from Distributions of Person and Place

An increased frequency of disease based upon occupation has often provided the initial evidence of a group association based upon a combination of "person" and "place." The first recognized occupational disease was found among chimney sweeps often exposed for long periods of time to large quantities of coal dust and who were found to have a high incidence of testicular cancer.

The Mad Hatter described in *Alice's Adventures in Wonderland* by Lewis Carroll made infamous the 19th-century recognition that exposure to mercury fumes was associated with mental changes. Mercury fumes were created when making the felt used for hats, hence the term "mad as a hatter."

The high frequency of asbestosis among those who worked in shipyards suggested a relationship decades before the dangers of asbestos were fully recognized and addressed. A lung disease known as silicosis among those who worked in the mining industry likewise suggested a relationship that led to an in-depth investigation and greater control of the risks.

More recently, a rare tumor called angiosarcoma was found to occur among those exposed over long periods to polyvinyl chloride (PVC), a plastic widely used in construction. The initial report of four cases of this unusual cancer among workers in one PVC plant

was enough to strongly suggest a cause-and-effect relationship based upon place alone.

An important example of the impact that place can have on generating ideas or hypotheses about causation is the history of fluoride and cavities. In the early years of the 1900s, children in the town of Colorado Springs, CO, were found to have a very high incidence of brown discoloration of the teeth. It was soon recognized that this condition was limited to those who obtained their water from a common source. Ironically, those with brown teeth were also protected from cavities. This clear relationship to place was followed by over two decades of research that led to the understanding that fluoride in the water reduces the risk of cavities, while very high levels of the compound also lead to brown teeth. Examination of the levels of fluoride in other water systems eventually led to the establishment of levels of fluoride that could protect against cavities without producing brown teeth.

Such strong and clear-cut relationships are important, but relatively unusual. Often, examinations of the characteristics of person and place in populations suggests hypotheses that can be followed up among individuals to establish cause-and-effect relationships.[4,5]

# How Do Epidemiologists Investigate Whether There Is Another Explanation for the Difference or Changes in the Distribution of Disease?

Epidemiologists ask: Are the differences or changes real or are they **artifactual**? There are three basic reasons that changes in rates may be artifactual rather than real:

- Differences or changes in the interest in identifying the disease
- Differences or changes in the ability to identify the disease
- Differences or changes in the definition of the disease

For some conditions, such as HIV/AIDS, these changes have all occurred. New and effective treatments have increased the interest in detecting the infection. Improved technology has increased the

ability to detect HIV infections at an earlier point in time. In addition, there have been a number of modifications of the definition of AIDS based on new opportunistic infections and newly recognized complications. Therefore, with HIV/AIDS, we need to be especially attentive to the possibility that artifactual changes have occurred.

In describing the distribution of a problem, epidemiologists ask: Are the differences or changes used to suggest group associations and generate hypotheses artifactual or real?

Let us see how this applies to our lung cancer example. As we have seen, lung cancer is a disease with a very poor prognosis; therefore, the burden of disease is high as measured by its high mortality rate. This was the situation in the past and to a large extent continues to be the situation.

Mortality rates have been obtained from death certificates for many years. The cause of death on death certificates is classified using a standardized coding system known as the International Classification of Diseases (ICD). No equally complete or accurate system has been available for collecting data on the incidence rates of lung cancer. However, as we

---

**BOX 2.3** Age Adjustment

Despite the existence of a real change in the rates of lung cancer between 1930 and 1960, it was still possible that the increased mortality rates from lung cancer were due to the increasing life span that was occurring between 1930 and 1960, leading to the aging of the population and an older population on average. Perhaps older people are more likely to develop lung cancer and the aging of the population itself explains the real increase in the rates. To address this issue, epidemiologists use what is called **age adjustment**. To conduct age adjustment, epidemiologists look at the rates of the disease in each age group and also the **age distribution**, or the number of people in each age group in the population. Then they combine the rates for each age group, taking into account or adjusting for the age distribution of a population.[a]

Taking into account the older average age of the population in 1960 compared to 1930 slightly reduced the apparent increase in lung cancer but large differences between 1930 and 1960 remained. As a result, epidemiologists concluded that lung cancer mortality rates changed over this period, especially among men; the changes in rates were real; and the changes could not be explained simply by the aging of the population. Thus, epidemiologists had established the existence of a group association between groups that smoked more cigarettes and groups that developed lung cancer.

---

a  Adjustment for age is often performed by combining the rates in each age group using the age distribution of what is called a **standard population**. The age distribution of the U.S. population in 2000 is currently used as the standard population. Adjustment is not limited to age and may at times be conducted using other characteristics that may differ among the groups, such as gender or race, which may affect the probability of developing a disease.

---

learned in our discussion of rates, the incidence rates and mortality rates for lung cancer are very similar. Therefore, we can use mortality data as a substitute for incidence data when evaluating the overall burden of lung cancer in a population. By the 1930s, epidemiologists had concluded from the study of death certificates that lung cancer deaths were rapidly increasing. This increase continued through the 1950s—with the increase in lung cancer occurring two decades or more after the increase in consumption of cigarettes. Therefore, it was not immediately obvious that the two were related. In order to hypothesize that cigarettes are a cause of lung cancer, one needed to conclude that there was a long delay and/or a need for long-term exposure to cigarettes before lung cancer developed. There was a need for more **evidence** linking cigarettes and lung cancer.

From the 1930s through the 1950s, a large number of studies established that lung cancer deaths were increasing among men, but not among women. That is, there was a change over time and a difference between groups. Epidemiologists, therefore, considered whether the changes or differences in rates were real, or whether they could be artificial or artifactual.

With lung cancer, the diagnosis at the time of death has been of great interest for many years. The ability to diagnose the disease has not changed substantially over the years. In addition, the use of ICD codes on death certificates has helped standardize the definition of the disease. Epidemiologists concluded that it was unlikely that changes in interest, ability, or definition explained the changes in the rates of lung cancer observed in males, thus they concluded that the changes were not artifactual, but real.[b]

**BOX 2.3** discusses age adjustment, which is one additional step that epidemiologists frequently make when looking at rates.

## ▶ What Is the Implication of a Group Association?

Group associations are established by investigations that use information on groups or a population without having information on the specific individuals within the group. These studies have been called **population comparisons** or ecological studies. Having established the existence of a group association, we still do not know if the individuals who smoke cigarettes are the same ones who develop lung cancer. We can think of a group association as a hypothesis that requires investigation at the individual

---

b  There are actually several types of lung cancer defined by the ICD codes. Most, but not all, types of lung cancer are strongly associated with cigarette smoking.

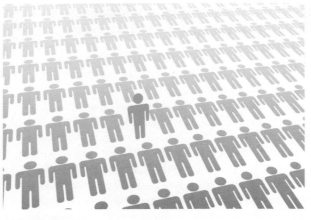

level. The group association between cigarettes and lung cancer was the beginning of a long road to establish that cigarettes are a cause of lung cancer.

Not all group associations are also individual associations. Imagine the following situation: the mortality rates from drowning are higher in southern states than in northern states in the United States. The per capita consumption of ice cream is also higher in southern states than in northern states. Thus, a group association was established between ice cream consumption and drowning. In thinking about this relationship, you will soon realize that there is another difference between southern and northern states. The average temperature is higher in southern states, and higher temperatures are most likely associated with more swimming and also more ice cream consumption. Ice cream consumption is therefore related both to swimming and to drowning. We call this type of factor a possible **confounding variable**. In this situation, there is no evidence that those who drown actually consumed ice cream. That is, there is no evidence of an association at the individual level. Thus, group associations can be misleading if they suggest relationships that do not exist at the individual level.

Epidemiology research studies that look at associations at the individual level are key to establishing etiology, or cause. Etiology is the second component of the P.E.R.I.E. approach. Let us turn our attention to how to establish etiology.

## ▶ Etiology: How Do We Establish Contributory Cause?

Understanding the reasons for disease is fundamental to the prevention of disability and death.

We call these reasons etiology or causation. In evidence-based public health, we use a very specific definition of causation—**contributory cause**. The evidence-based public health approach relies on epidemiological research studies to establish a contributory cause. This requires that we go beyond group association and establish three definitive requirements:[6]

1.  The "cause" is associated with the "effect" at the individual level. That is, the potential "cause" and the potential "effect" occur more frequently in the same individual than would be expected by chance. Therefore, we need to establish that individuals with lung cancer are more frequently smokers than individuals without lung cancer.
2.  The "cause" precedes the "effect" in time. That is, the potential "cause" is present at an earlier time than the potential "effect." Therefore, we need to establish that cigarette smoking comes before the development of lung cancer.
3.  Altering the "cause" alters the "effect." That is, when the potential "cause" is reduced or eliminated, the potential "effect" is also reduced or eliminated. Therefore, we need to establish that reducing cigarette smoking reduces lung cancer rates.

**BOX 2.4** illustrates the logic behind using these three criteria to establish a cause-and-effect relationship, as well as the implications of a contributory cause.

These three definitive requirements may be established using three different types of studies, all of which relate potential "causes" to potential "effects" at the individual level. That is, they investigate whether individuals who smoke cigarettes are the same individuals who develop lung cancer.[5] The three basic types of investigations are called **case-control studies, cohort studies**, and **randomized controlled trials**.

Case-control studies are most useful for establishing requirement number one; that is, the "cause" is associated with the "effect" at the individual level. Case-control studies can demonstrate that cigarettes and lung cancer occur together more frequently than would be expected by chance alone. To accomplish this, cases with the disease (lung cancer) are compared to controls without the disease to determine whether the cases and the controls previously were exposed to the potential "cause" (cigarette smoking).

**BOX 2.4** Lightning, Thunder, and Contributory Cause

The requirements for establishing the type of cause-and-effect relationship known as contributory cause used in evidence-based public health can be illustrated by the cause-and-effect relationship between lightning and thunder that human beings have recognized from the earliest times of civilization.

First, lightning is generally associated with thunder; that is, the two occur together far more often than one would expect if there were no relationship. Second, with careful observation, it can be concluded that the lightning is seen a short time before the thunder is heard. That is, the potential "cause" (the lightning) precedes in time the "effect" (the thunder). Finally, when the lightning stops, so does the thunder—thus, altering the "cause" alters the "effect."

Notice that lightning is not always associated with thunder. Heat lightning may not produce audible thunder, or the lightning may be too far away for the thunder to be heard. Lightning is not sufficient in and of itself to guarantee that our ears will subsequently always hear thunder. Conversely, it has been found that the sound of thunder does not always require lightning. Other reasons for the rapid expansion of air, such as an explosion or volcanic eruption, can also create a sound similar or identical to thunder.

The recognition of lightning as a cause of thunder came many centuries before human beings had any understanding of electricity or today's appreciation for the science of light and sounds. Similarly, cause-and-effect relationships established by epidemiological investigations do not always depend on understanding the science behind the relationships.

When a factor such as cigarettes has been demonstrated to be associated on an individual basis with an outcome such as lung cancer, we often refer to that factor as a **risk factor**.[c]

During the 1940s and early 1950s, a number of case-control studies established that individuals who developed lung cancer were far more likely to be regular smokers compared to similar individuals who did not smoke cigarettes. These case-control studies established requirement number one—the "cause" is associated with the "effect" at the individual level. They established that cigarettes are a risk factor for lung cancer.

Cohort studies are most useful for establishing requirement number two—the "cause" precedes the "effect." Those with the potential "cause" or risk factor (cigarette smoking) and those without the potential "cause" are followed over time to determine who develops the "effect" (lung cancer).[d]

Several large scale cohort studies were conducted in the late 1950s and early 1960s. One conducted by the American Cancer Society followed nearly 200,000 individuals over 3 or more years to determine the chances that smokers and nonsmokers would develop lung cancer. Those who smoked regularly at the beginning of the study had a greatly increased chance of developing lung cancer over the course of the study; thus establishing requirement number two, the "cause" precedes the "effect" in time.

Randomized controlled trials are most useful for establishing requirement number three—altering the "cause" alters the "effect." Using a chance process known as **randomization** or random assignment, individuals are assigned to be exposed or not exposed to the potential "cause" (cigarette smoking). Individuals with and without the potential "cause" are then followed over time to determine who develops the "effect."

Conducting a randomized controlled trial of cigarettes and lung cancer would require investigators to randomize individuals to smoke cigarettes or not smoke cigarettes and follow them over many years. This illustrates the obstacles that can occur in seeking to definitively establish contributory cause. Once there was a strong suspicion that cigarettes might cause lung cancer, randomized controlled trials were not practical or ethical as a method for establishing cigarette smoking as a contributory cause of lung cancer. Therefore, we need to look at additional supportive or

---

c  A risk factor, as we just discussed, usually implies that the factor is associated with the disease at the individual level. At times, it may be used to imply that the factor not only is associated with the disease at the individual level, but that it precedes the disease in time. Despite the multiple uses of the term, a risk factor does not in and of itself imply that a cause-and-effect relationship is present, though it may be considered a possible cause.

d  It may seem obvious that cigarette smoking precedes the development of lung cancer. However, the sequence of events is not always so clear. For instance, those who have recently quit smoking cigarettes have an increased chance of being diagnosed with lung cancer. This may lead to the erroneous conclusion that stopping cigarette smoking is a cause of lung cancer. It is more likely that early symptoms of lung cancer lead individuals to quit smoking. The conclusion that stopping cigarette smoking causes lung cancer is called **reverse causality**. Thus, it was important that cohort studies followed smokers and nonsmokers for several years to establish that the cigarette smoking came first.

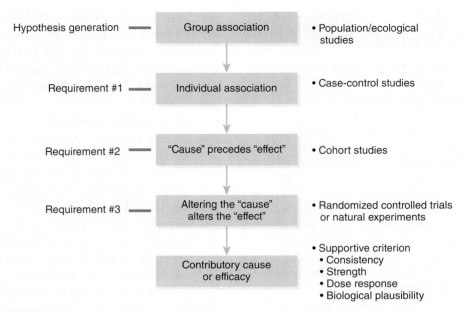

**FIGURE 2.2** Fulfilling Requirements for Establishing Contributory Cause or Efficacy

**ancillary criteria** that we can use to help us establish the existence of contributory cause.[e]

**FIGURE 2.2** illustrates the requirements for definitively establishing contributory cause and the types of studies that may be used to satisfy each of the requirements. Notice that the requirements for establishing contributory cause are the same as the requirements for establishing **efficacy**. Efficacy implies that an intervention works; that is, it increases positive outcomes or benefits in the population being investigated.

## What Can We Do If We Cannot Demonstrate All Three Requirements to Definitively Establish Contributory Cause?

When we cannot definitively establish a contributory cause, we often need to look for additional supportive evidence.[6] In evidence-based public health we often utilize what have been called supportive or ancillary criteria to make scientific judgments about cause and effect. A large number of these criteria have been used and debated. However, four of them are widely used and pose little controversy. They are:

- Strength of the relationship
- Dose-response relationship
- Consistency of the relationship
- Biological plausibility

Let us examine what we mean by each of these criteria.

The **strength of the relationship** implies that we are interested in knowing how closely related the risk factor (cigarette smoking) is to the disease (lung cancer). In other words, we want to know the probability of lung cancer among those who smoke cigarettes compared to the probability of lung cancer among those who do not smoke cigarettes. To measure the strength of the relationship, we calculate what we call the **relative risk**. The relative risk is the probability of developing the disease if the risk factor is present compared to the probability of developing the disease if the risk factor is not present. Therefore, the relative risk for cigarette smoking is calculated as:

$$\text{Relative risk} = \frac{\text{Probability of lung cancer for cigarette smokers}}{\text{Probability of lung cancer of nonsmokers}}$$

---

e  At times, a special form of a cohort study called a **natural experiment** can help establish that altering the cause alters the effect. A natural experiment implies that an investigator studies the results of a change in one group, but not in another similar group that was produced by forces outside the investigator's control. For instance, after the surgeon general's 1964 *Report on Smoking and Health* was released, approximately 100,000 physicians stopped smoking. This did not happen among other professionals. Over the next decade, the rates of lung cancer among physicians dropped dramatically, but not among other professionals. Despite the fact that natural experiments can be very useful, they are not considered as reliable as randomized controlled trials. Randomization, especially in large studies, eliminates differences between groups or potential confounding differences, even when these differences in characteristics are not recognized by the investigators.

The relative risk for cigarette smoking and lung cancer is approximately 10. A relative risk of 10 is very large. It tells us that the chances or probability of developing lung cancer are 10 times as great for the average smoker compared to the average nonsmoker.[f]

In addition to looking at the strength of the overall relationship between smoking cigarettes and lung cancer, we can ask whether smoking more cigarettes is associated with a greater chance of developing lung cancer. If it is, then we say there is a **dose-response relationship**. For instance, smoking one pack of cigarettes per day over many years increases the chances of developing lung cancer compared to smoking half a pack per day. Similarly, smoking two packs per day increases the chances of developing the disease compared to smoking one pack per day. These examples show that a dose-response relationship is present.[g]

**Consistency** implies that studies in different geographic areas and among a wide range of groups produce similar results. A very large number of studies of cigarettes and lung cancer in many countries and among those of nearly every race and socioeconomic group have consistently demonstrated a strong individual association between cigarette smoking and lung cancer.

The final supportive criterion is **biological plausibility**. This term implies that we can explain the occurrence of disease based upon known and accepted biological mechanisms. We can explain the occurrence of lung cancer by the fact that cigarette smoke contains a wide range of potentially toxic chemicals that reach the locations in the body where lung cancer occurs.

The ancillary criteria add support to the argument that cigarette smoking is a contributory cause of lung cancer. **TABLE 2.1** summarizes the use of ancillary or supportive criteria in making scientific judgments about contributory cause and illustrates these principles using the cigarette smoking and lung cancer scenario. It also cautions us to use these criteria carefully because a cause-and-effect relationship may be present even when some or all of these criteria are not fulfilled.[6]

We have now summarized the approach used in evidence-based public health to establish a contributory cause. We started with the development of group associations that generate hypotheses and moved on to look at the definitive requirements for establishing contributory cause. We also looked at the ancillary or supportive criteria that are often needed to make scientific judgments about contributory cause. **TABLE 2.2** summarizes this process and applies it to cigarette smoking and lung cancer.

## ▶ What Does Contributory Cause Imply?

Establishing a contributory cause on the basis of evidence is a complicated and often time-consuming job. In practice, our minds often too quickly jump to the conclusion that a cause-and-effect relationship exists. Our language has a large number of words that may subtly imply a cause-and-effect relationship, even in the absence of evidence. **BOX 2.5** illustrates how we often rapidly draw conclusions about cause and effect.

It is important to understand what the existence of a contributory cause implies and what it does not imply. Despite the convincing evidence that cigarette smoking is a contributory cause of lung cancer, some individuals never smoke and still develop lung cancer. Therefore, cigarettes are not what we call a **necessary cause** of lung cancer. Others smoke cigarettes all their lives and do not develop lung cancer. Thus, cigarettes are not what we call a **sufficient cause** of lung cancer.

The fact that not every smoker develops lung cancer implies that there must be factors that protect some individuals from lung cancer. The fact that some nonsmokers develop lung cancer implies that there must be additional contributory causes of lung cancer. Thus, the existence of a contributory cause implies that the "cause" increases the chances that the "effect" will develop. Its presence does not guarantee that the disease will develop. In addition, the absence of cigarette smoking does not guarantee that the disease will not develop.

Despite the fact that cigarettes have been established as a contributory cause of lung cancer, they are

---

f   A relative risk of 10 does not tell us the **absolute risk**. The absolute risk is the actual chance or probability of developing the disease (lung cancer) in the presence of the risk factor (cigarette smoking), expressed numerically—for example, as 0.03 or 3%. A relative risk of 10 might imply an increase from 1 in 1000 individuals to 1 in 100 individuals. Alternatively, it might imply an increase from 1 in 100 individuals to 1 in 10 individuals. A relative risk can be calculated whenever we have data on groups of individuals; therefore, it does not in and of itself imply that a contributory cause is present. We need to be careful not to imply that the risk factor will increase the chances of developing the disease or that reducing or eliminating the risk factor will reduce or eliminate the disease unless we have evidence of contributory cause. For case-control studies, a measure known as the **odds ratio** can be calculated and is often used as an approximation of relative risk.

g   A dose-response relationship may also imply that greater exposure to a factor is associated with reduced probability of developing the disease, such as with exercise and coronary artery disease. In this case, the factor may be called a **protective factor** rather than a risk factor.

**TABLE 2.1** Supportive or Ancillary Criteria—Cigarettes and Lung Cancer

| Criteria | Meaning of the criteria | Evidence for cigarettes and lung cancer | Cautions in using criteria |
|---|---|---|---|
| Strength of the relationship | The risk for those with the risk factor is greatly increased compared to those without the risk factor. | The relative risk is large or substantial. The relative risk is greater than 10 for the average smoker, implying that the average smoker has more than 10 times the probability of developing lung cancer compared to nonsmokers. | Even relatively modest relative risks may make important contributions to disease when the risk factor is frequently present. A relative risk of 2, for instance, implies a doubling of the probability of developing a disease. |
| Dose-response relationship | Higher levels of exposure and/or longer duration of exposure to the "cause" are associated with increased probability of the "effect." | Studies of cigarettes and lung cancer establish that smoking half a pack a day over an extended period of time increases the risk compared to not smoking. Smoking one pack per day and two packs per day further increase the risk. | No dose-response relationship may be evident between no smoking and smoking one cigarette a day or between smoking three and four packs per day. |
| Consistency of the relationship | Studies at the individual level produce similar results in multiple locations among populations of varying socioeconomic and cultural backgrounds. | Hundreds of studies in multiple locations and populations consistently establish an individual association between cigarettes and lung cancer. | Consistency requires the availability of numerous studies that may not have been conducted. |
| Biological plausibility | Known biological mechanisms can convincingly explain a cause-and-effect relationship. | Cigarette smoke directly reaches the areas where lung cancer appears. | Exactly which component(s) of cigarette smoking produce lung cancer are just beginning to be understood. |

**TABLE 2.2** Cigarettes and Lung Cancer—Establishing Cause and Effect

| Requirements for contributory cause | Meaning of the requirements | Types of studies that can establish the requirement | Evidence for cigarette smoking and lung cancer |
|---|---|---|---|
| Associated at a population level (group association) | A group relationship between a "cause" and an "effect." | Ecological study or population comparison study: a comparison of population rates between an exposure and a disease. | Men began mass consumption of cigarettes decades before women and their rates of lung cancer increased decades before those of women. |
| Individual association: "requirement one" | Individuals with a disease ("effect") also have an increased chance of having a potential risk factor ("cause"). | Case-control studies: cases with the disease are compared to similar controls without the disease to see who had the exposure. | Lung cancer patients were found to have 10 times or greater chance of smoking cigarettes regularly compared to those without lung cancer. |

| | | | |
|---|---|---|---|
| Prior association: "requirement two" | The potential risk factor precedes—in time—the outcome. | Cohort studies: exposed and similar unexposed individuals are followed over time to determine who develops the disease. | Large cohort studies found that those who smoke cigarettes regularly have a 10 times or greater chance of subsequently developing lung cancer. |
| Altering the "cause" alters the "effect": "requirement three" | Active intervention to expose one group to the risk factor results in a greater chance of the outcome. | Randomized controlled trials allocating individuals by chance to be exposed or not exposed are needed to definitively establish contributory cause. Note: these studies are not always ethical or practical. | Alternatives to randomized controlled trials, such as "natural experiments," established that those who quit smoking have greatly reduced chances of developing lung cancer. In addition, the four supportive criteria also suggest contributory cause. |

## BOX 2.5  Words that Imply Causation

Often when reading the newspaper or other media, you will find that conclusions about cause and effect are made based upon far less rigorous examination of the data than we have indicated are needed to definitively establish cause and effect. In fact, we often draw conclusions about cause and effect without even consciously recognizing we have done so. Our language has a large number of words that imply a cause-and-effect relationship, some of which we use rather casually.

Let us take a look at the many ways that a hypothetical newspaper article might imply the existence of a cause-and-effect relationship or a contributory cause even when the evidence is based only upon a group association or upon speculation about the possible relationships.

Over several decades, the mortality rates from breast cancer in the United States were observed to increase each year. This trend was due to and can be blamed on a variety of factors, including the increased use of estrogens and exposure to estrogens in food. The recent reduction in breast cancer resulted from and can be attributed to the declining use of estrogens for menopausal and postmenopausal women. The declining mortality rate was also produced by the increased use of screening tests for breast cancer that were responsible for early detection and treatment. These trends demonstrate that reduced use of estrogens and increased use of screening tests have contributed to and explain the reduction in breast cancer.

While these conclusions sound reasonable and may well be cause-and-effect relationships, note that they rely heavily on assertions for which there is no direct evidence provided. For instance, the following words are often used to imply a cause-and-effect relationship when evidence is not or cannot be presented to support the relationship:

- due to
- blamed on
- result from
- attributable to
- produced by
- responsible for
- contributed to
- explained by

It is important to be aware of conscious or unconscious efforts to imply cause-and-effect relationships when the data suggests only group associations and does not meet our more stringent criteria establishing cause and effect.

not a necessary or a sufficient cause of lung cancer. In fact, the use of the concept of necessary and sufficient cause is not considered useful in the evidence-based public health approach because so few, if any, diseases fulfill the definitions of necessary and sufficient cause. These criteria are too demanding to be used as standards of proof in public health or medicine.

By 1964, the evidence that cigarette smoking was a contributory cause of lung cancer was persuasive enough for the surgeon general of the United States to produce the first surgeon general's *Report on Smoking and Health*. The report concluded that cigarettes are an important cause of lung cancer. Over the following decades, the surgeon general's reports documented the evidence that cigarette smoking causes not only lung cancer, but also other cancers—including cancer of the throat and larynx. Cigarette smoking is also a contributory cause of chronic obstructive pulmonary disease (COPD) and coronary artery disease. Smoking during pregnancy poses risks to the unborn child, and passive or secondhand smoke creates increased risks to those exposed—especially children.[7] Based on the surgeon general's findings, there is clearly overwhelming evidence that cigarette smoking is a contributory cause of lung cancer and a growing list of other diseases. Thus, let us turn our attention to the third component of the P.E.R.I.E. process: recommendations.

## ▶ Recommendations: What Works to Reduce the Health Impact?

The evidence for cigarette smoking as a cause of lung cancer, as well as other diseases, was so strong that it cried out for action. In evidence-based public health, however, action should be grounded in **recommendations** that incorporate evidence. That is, evidence serves not only to establish contributory cause, but is also central to determining whether or not specific interventions work.[8,9]

Evidence-based recommendations are built upon the evidence from studies of interventions. Thus, recommendations are summaries of the evidence about which interventions work to improve health outcomes. They indicate whether action should be taken. Evidence-based recommendations utilize the same types of investigations we discussed for contributory cause. In fact, the requirements of contributory cause are the same as those for establishing that an intervention works or has efficacy for the particular population that was studied. Evidence-based recommendations, however, go beyond efficacy or benefits and also take into account harms or safety.

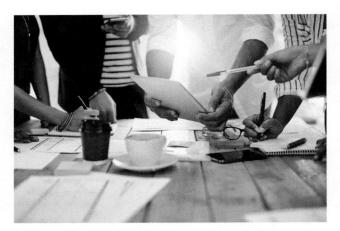

In the decades since the surgeon general's initial report, a long list of interventions has been implemented and evaluated. The term "intervention" is a very broad term in public health. Interventions range from individual counseling and prescription of pharmaceutical drugs that aid smoking cessation; to group efforts, such as peer support groups; to social interventions, such as cigarette taxes and legal restrictions on smoking in restaurants.

Recommendations for action have been part of public health and medicine for many years. Evidence-based recommendations, however, are relatively new. They have been contrasted with the traditional eminence-based recommendation, which uses the opinion of a respected authority as its foundation. Evidence-based recommendations ask about the research evidence supporting the benefits and harms of potential interventions. In evidence-based recommendations, the opinions of experts are most important when research evidence does not or cannot provide answers.

Before looking at the evidence-based recommendations on cigarette smoking made by the Centers for Disease Control and Prevention (CDC), let us look at how they are developed and graded. Evidence-based recommendations are based upon two types of criteria: the quality of the evidence and the magnitude of the impact. Each of these criteria is given what is called a **score**.[8,9] The quality of the evidence is scored based in large part upon the types of investigations and how well the investigation was conducted. Well-conducted randomized controlled trials that fully address the health problem are considered the highest quality evidence. Often, however, cohort and case-control studies are needed and are used as part of an evidence-based recommendation.

Expert opinion, though lowest on the hierarchy of evidence, is often essential to fill in the holes in the research evidence.[8,9] The quality of the evidence also determines whether the data collected during an intervention are relevant to its use in a particular population or setting. Data from young adults may not be relevant to children or the elderly. Data from severely ill patients may not be relevant to mildly ill patients. Thus, high-quality evidence needs to be based not only on the research, which can establish efficacy in one particular population, but also on the **effectiveness** of the intervention in the specific population in which it will be used.

In evidence-based public health, the quality of the evidence is often scored as good, fair, or poor. Good quality implies that the evidence fulfills all the criteria for quality. Poor quality evidence implies that there are fatal flaws in the evidence and recommendations cannot be made. Fair quality lies in between having no fatal flaws and fulfilling all the criteria for quality.[h]

In addition to looking at the quality of the evidence, it is also important to look at the magnitude of the impact of the intervention. The magnitude of the impact asks the question: How much of the disability and/or death due to the disease can be potentially removed by the intervention? In measuring the magnitude of the impact, evidence-based recommendations take into account the potential benefits of an intervention, as well as the potential harms. Therefore, we can regard the magnitude of the impact as the benefits minus the harms, or the "net benefits."[i]

The magnitude of the impact, like the quality of the evidence, is scored based upon a limited number of potential categories. In one commonly used system, the magnitude of the impact is scored as substantial, moderate, small, and zero/negative.[8] A substantial impact may imply that the intervention works extremely well for a small number of people, such as a drug treatment for cigarette cessation. These are the types of interventions that are often the focus of individual clinical care. A substantial impact may also imply that the intervention has a modest net benefit for any one individual, but can be applied to large numbers of people, such as through media advertising or taxes on cigarettes. These are the types of interventions that are most often the focus of traditional public health and social policy.

Evidence-based recommendations combine the score for the quality of the evidence with the score for the impact of the intervention.[9] **TABLE 2.3** summarizes how these aspects can be combined to produce a classification of the strength of the recommendation, graded as A, B, C, D, and I.

It may be useful to think of these grades as indicating the following:

A = Must—A strong recommendation.

**TABLE 2.3** Classification of Recommendations

| Magnitude of the impact | | | | |
| --- | --- | --- | --- | --- |
| Quality of the evidence | Net benefit: substantial | Net benefit: moderate | Net benefit: small | Net benefit: zero/negative |
| Good | A | B | C | D |
| Fair | B | B | C | D |
| Poor (insufficient evidence) | I | I | I | I |

Data from Agency for Healthcare Research and Quality, U.S. Preventive Services Task Force Guide to Clinical Preventive Services Vol 1, AHRQ Pub. No.02-500.

h  To fulfill the criteria for good quality data, evidence is also needed to show that the outcome being measured is a clinically important outcome. Short-term outcomes called **surrogate endpoints**, or surrogate outcomes, such as changes in laboratory tests, may not reliably indicate longer term or clinically important outcomes.

i  The magnitude of the impact can be measured using the relative risk calculation. When dealing with interventions, the people who receive the intervention are often placed in the numerator. Thus, an intervention that reduces the bad outcomes by half would have a relative risk of 0.5. The smaller the relative risk is, the greater the measured impact of the intervention. If the relative risk is 0.20, then those with the intervention have only 20% of the risk remaining. Their risk of a bad outcome has been reduced by 80%. The reduction in a bad outcome is called the **attributable risk percentage** or, if a contributory cause is present, the percent efficacy. The intervention can only be expected to accomplish this potential reduction in risk when a contributory cause is present and the impact of the "cause" can be immediately and completely eliminated.

B = Should—In general, the intervention should be used unless there are good reasons or contraindications for not doing so.

C = May—The use of judgment is often needed on an individual-by-individual basis. Individual recommendations depend on the specifics of an individual's situation, risk-taking attitudes, and values.

D = Don't—There is enough evidence to recommend against using the intervention.

I = Indeterminant, insufficient, or "I don't know"—The evidence is inadequate to make a recommendation for or against the use of the intervention at the present time.

Notice that evidence-based public health and medicine rely primarily on considerations of benefits and harms. However, recently issues of financial cost have begun to be integrated into evidence-based recommendations. At this point, however, cost considerations are generally only taken into account for "close calls." Close calls are often situations where the net benefits are small to moderate and the costs are large.

The evidence-based public health approach increasingly relies on the use of evidence-based recommendations that are graded based on the quality of the evidence and the expected impact of the intervention. The recommendations are made by a wide array of organizations, as discussed in **BOX 2.6**. It is important to appreciate the source of the recommendations, as well as the methods used to develop them.[6]

Let us take a look at some examples of how interventions to prevent smoking, detect lung cancer early, or cure lung cancer have been graded. The CDC publishes "The Guide to Community Prevention Services," commonly referred to as "The Community Guide."[9] This guide indicates that the following interventions are recommended, implying a grade of A or B:

- Clean indoor air legislation, prohibiting tobacco use in indoor public and private workplaces
- Federal, state, and local efforts to increase taxes on tobacco products as an effective public health intervention to promote tobacco use cessation and to reduce the initiation of tobacco use among youths
- The funding and implementation of long-term, high-intensity mass media campaigns using paid broadcast times and media messages developed through formative research
- Proactive telephone cessation support services (quit lines)
- Reduced or eliminated copayments for effective cessation therapies
- Reminder systems for healthcare providers (encouraging them to reinforce the importance of cigarette cessation)
- Efforts to mobilize communities to identify and reduce the commercial availability of tobacco products to youths

Additional recommendations encourage clinicians to specifically counsel patients against smoking,

---

## BOX 2.6 Who Develops Evidence-Based Recommendations?

Evidence-based recommendations may be developed by a range of groups, including the government, practitioner-oriented organizations, consumer-oriented organizations, organized healthcare systems, and even for-profit organizations. Organizations developing evidence-based recommendations, however, are expected to acknowledge their authorship and identify the individuals who participated in the process, as well as their potential conflicts of interest. In addition, regardless of the organization, the evidence-based recommendations should include a description of the process used to collect the data and make the recommendations.

For-profit organizations may make evidence-based recommendations. However, their obvious conflicts of interest often lead them to fund other groups to make recommendations. Thus, the funding source(s) supporting the development of evidence-based recommendations should also be acknowledged as part of the report.

One well-regarded model for the development of evidence-based recommendations is the task force model used by the United States Preventive Services Task Force of the Agency for Healthcare Research and Quality (AHRQ), as well as by the Task Force on Community Preventive Services of the CDC.[8,9] The task force model aims to balance potential conflicts of interest and ensures a range of expertise by selecting a variety of experts, as well as community participants, based upon a public nomination process. Once the task force members are appointed, their recommendations are made by a vote of the task force and do not require approval by the government agency.

As a reader of evidence-based recommendations, it is important that you begin by looking at which group developed the recommendations, whether they have disclosed their membership, including potential conflicts of interest, and the groups' procedures for developing the recommendations.

prescribe medications for adults, encourage support groups for smoking cessation, and treat lung cancer with the best available treatments when detected.

Of interest is the grade of D for recommending against screening for early detection of lung cancer using traditional chest X-rays. The evidence strongly suggests that screening using this method may detect cancer at a slightly earlier stage, but not early enough to alter the course of the disease. Therefore, early detection does not alter the outcome of the disease. Research continues to search for and identify better screening methods to detect lung cancer in time to make a difference.

Evidence-based recommendations are not the end of the process. There may be a large number of recommendations among which we may need to choose. In addition, we need to decide the best way(s) to put the recommendations into practice. Thus, implementation is not an automatic process. Issues of ethics, culture, politics, and risk-taking attitudes can and should have major impacts on implementation. A fourth step in the evidence-based public health approach requires us to look at the options for implementation and to develop a strategy for getting the job done.

## ▶ Implementation: How Do We Get the Job Done?

Strong recommendations based upon the evidence are ideally the basis of implementation. At times, however, it may not be practical or ethical to obtain the evidence needed to establish contributory cause and develop evidence-based recommendations. The process of implementation itself may be part of the process of establishing causation, as it was for cigarette smoking in the 1960s when 100,000 physicians stopped smoking and their rates of lung cancer declined rapidly, as compared to other similar professionals who did not stop smoking.

Today, there are often a large number of interventions with adequate data to consider implementation.

Many of the interventions have potential harms, as well as potential benefits. The large and growing array of possible interventions means that health decisions require a systematic method for deciding which interventions to use and how to combine them in the most effective and efficient ways. One method for examining the options for implementation uses a structure we will call the "When-Who-How" approach.

"When" asks about the timing in the course of disease in which an intervention occurs. This timing allows us to categorize interventions as primary, secondary, and tertiary. **Primary interventions** take place before the onset of the disease. They aim to prevent the disease from occurring. **Secondary interventions** occur after the development of a disease or risk factor, but before symptoms appear. They are aimed at early detection of disease or reducing risk factors while the individual is asymptomatic. **Tertiary interventions** occur after the initial occurrence of symptoms, but before irreversible disability. They aim to prevent irreversible consequences of the disease. In the cigarette smoking and lung cancer scenario, primary interventions aim to prevent cigarette smoking. Secondary interventions aim to reverse the course of disease by smoking cessation efforts or screening to detect early disease. Tertiary interventions diagnose and treat diseases caused by smoking in order to prevent permanent disability and death.

"Who" asks: At whom should we direct the intervention? Should it be directed at individuals one at a time as part of clinical care? Alternatively, should it be directed at groups of people, such as vulnerable populations, or should it be directed at everyone in a community or population?[j]

Finally, we need to ask: How should we implement interventions? There are three basic types of interventions when addressing the need for behavioral change. These interventions can be classified as information (education), motivation (incentives), and obligation (requirements).[k]

---

j  The CDC defines four levels of intervention: the individual, the relationship (for example, the family), the community, and society or the population as a whole. This framework has the advantage of separating immediate family interventions from community interventions. The group or at-risk group relationship used here may at times refer to the family unit or geographic communities. It may also refer to institutions or at-risk vulnerable groups within the community. The use of group or at-risk group relationship provides greater flexibility, allowing application to a wider range of situations. In addition, the three levels used here correlate with the measurements of relative risk, attributable risk percentage, and population attributable percentage, which are the fundamental epidemiological measurements applied to the magnitude of the impact of an intervention.

k  An additional option is innovation. Innovation implies a technical or engineering solution. A distinct advantage of technical or engineering solutions is that they often require far less behavior change. Changing human behavior is frequently difficult. Nonetheless, it is an essential component of most, if not all, successful public health interventions. Certainly, that is the case with cigarette smoking.

An information or education strategy aims to change behavior through individual encounters, group interactions, or the mass media. Motivation implies use of incentives for changing or maintaining behavior. It implies more than strong or enthusiastic encouragement—it implies tangible reward. Obligation relies on laws and regulations requiring specific behaviors. **TABLE 2.4** illustrates how options for implementation for cigarette smoking might be organized using the "When-Who-How" approach. To better understand the "who" and "how" of the options for intervention when behavior change is needed, refer to **TABLE 2.5**, which outlines nine different options.

Deciding when, who, and how to intervene depends in large part upon the available options and the evidence that they work. It also depends in part on our attitudes toward different types of interventions. In U.S. society, we prefer to rely on informational or educational strategies. These approaches preserve freedom of choice, which we value in public, as well as private, decisions. Use of mass media informational strategies may be quite economical and efficient relative to the large number of individuals they reach though messages, but they often need to be tailored to different audiences. However, information is often ineffective in accomplishing behavioral change—at least on its own.

Strategies based upon motivation, such as taxation and other incentives, may at times be more effective than information alone, though educational strategies are still critical to justify and reinforce motivational

---

**TABLE 2.4** Framework of Options for Implementation

| | When | Who | How |
|---|---|---|---|
| Levels | 1. Primary—Prior to disease or condition<br>2. Secondary—Prior to symptoms<br>3. Tertiary—Prior to irreversible complications | 1. Individual<br>2. At-risk group<br>3. General population/community | 1. Information (education)<br>2. Motivation (incentives)<br>3. Obligation (requirement) |
| Meaning of levels | 1. Primary—Remove underlying cause, increase resistance, or reduce exposure<br>2. Secondary—Postexposure intervention, identify and treat risk factors or screen for asymptomatic disease<br>3. Tertiary—Reverse the course of disease (cure), prevent complications, restore function | 1. Individual often equals patient care<br>2. At-risk implies groups with common risk factors<br>3. General population includes defined populations with and without the risk factor | 1. Information—Efforts to communicate information and change behavior on basis of information<br>2. Motivation—Rewards to encourage or discourage without legal requirement<br>3. Obligation—Required by law or institutional sanction |
| Cigarette smoking example | 1. Primary—Prevention of smoking, reduction in secondhand exposure<br>2. Secondary—Assistance in quitting, screening for cancer if recommended<br>3. Tertiary—Health care to minimize disease impact | 1. Individual smoker<br>2. At-risk—Groups at risk of smoking or disease caused by smoking (e.g., adolescents as well as current and ex-smokers)<br>3. Population—Entire population, including those who never have or never will smoke | 1. Information—Stop smoking campaigns, advertising, warning on package, clinician advice<br>2. Motivation—Taxes on cigarettes, increased cost of insurance<br>3. Obligation—Prohibition on sales to minors, exclusion from athletic eligibility, legal restrictions on indoor public smoking |

**TABLE 2.5** Examples of "Who" and "How" Related to Cigarette Smoking

| | Information | Motivation | Obligation |
|---|---|---|---|
| Individual | Clinician provides patient with information explaining reasons for changing behavior | Clinician encourages patient to change behavior in order to qualify for a service or gain a benefit (e.g., status or financial) | Clinician denies patient a service unless patient changes behavior |
| | Example: Clinician distributes educational packet to a smoker and discusses his or her own smoking habit | Example: Clinician suggests that the financial savings from not buying cigarettes be used to buy a luxury item | Example: Clinician implements recommendation to refuse birth control pills to women over 35 who smoke cigarettes |
| High-risk group | Information is made available to all those who engage in a behavior | Those who engage in a behavior are required to pay a higher price | Those who engage in a behavior are barred from an activity or job |
| | Example: Warning labels on cigarette packages | Examples: Taxes on cigarettes | Example: Smokers banned from jobs that will expose them to fumes that may damage their lungs |
| Population | Information is made available to the entire population, including those who do not engage in the behavior | Incentives are provided for those not at risk to discourage the behavior in those at risk | An activity is required or prohibited for those at risk and also for those not at risk of the condition |
| | Example: Media information on the dangers of smoking | Example: Lower healthcare costs for everyone results from reduced percentage of smokers | Example: Cigarette sales banned for those under 18 |

interventions. Motivational interventions should be carefully constructed and judiciously used, or they may result in what has been called **victim blaming**. For example, victim blaming in the case of cigarette smoking implies that we regard the consequences of smoking as the smokers' own fault.

The use of obligation or legally required action can be quite effective if clear-cut behavior and relatively simple enforcement, such as restrictions on indoor public smoking, are used. These types of efforts may be regarded by some as a last resort, but others may see them as a key to effective use of other strategies. Obligation inevitably removes freedom of choice and if not effectively implemented with regard for individual rights, the strategy may undermine respect for the law. Enforcement may become invasive and expensive, thus obligation requires careful consideration before use as a strategy.

Understanding the advantages and disadvantages of each type of approach is key to deciphering many of the controversies we face in deciding how to

implement programs to address public health problems; however, implementation is not the end of the evidence-based public health process. It is important to evaluate the success of an intervention in practice. Evaluation is the fifth and final component of the P.E.R.I.E. approach.

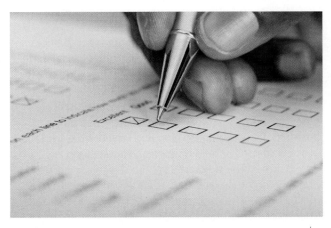

© Andrey_Popov/Shutterstock

# ▶ Evaluation: How Do We Evaluate Results?

Public health problems are rarely completely eliminated with one intervention—there are few magic bullets in this field. Therefore, it is important to evaluate whether an intervention or combination of interventions has been successful in reducing the problem. It is also critical to measure how much of the problem has been eliminated by the intervention(s) and what is the nature of the problem that remains.

Traditionally, evaluation has asked before and after questions. For instance, studies of cigarette smoking between the mid-1960s, when cigarettes were first declared a cause of lung cancer, and the late 1990s demonstrated that there was nearly a 50% reduction in cigarette smoking in the United States and that the rates of lung cancer were beginning to fall—at least among males. However, much of the problem still existed because the rates among adolescent males and females remained high and smoking among adults was preceded by smoking as adolescents nearly 90% of the time. Thus, an evaluation of the success of cigarette smoking interventions led to a new cycle of the process. It focused on how to address the issue of adolescent smoking and nicotine addiction among adults.

Many of the interventions being used today grew out of this effort to cycle once again through the evidence-based public health process and look for a new understanding of the problem, its etiology, evidence-based recommendations, and options for implementation.

The advent of e-cigarettes is again requiring us to utilize the P.E.R.I.E. framework to better understand their benefits and harms. E-cigarette research illustrates how public health research is being broadened to include not only traditional quantitative research but new methods of qualitative research. Roles of qualitative methods in public health research using e-cigarettes as an example is discussed in **BOX 2.7**.

In recent years, this process of evaluation has been extended to attempt to address how well specific interventions work and are accepted in practice. A new framework, called the **RE-AIM** framework, is increasingly being used to evaluate these factors.[11] RE-AIM is a mnemonic that stands for **r**each, **e**ffectiveness, **a**doption, **i**mplementation, and **m**aintenance. You can think of the "RE" factors as evaluating the potential of the intervention for those it is designed to include or reach as well as those it has the potential to reach in practice. It is important to recognize that interventions are often applied far beyond the groups for whom they have been designed or investigated.

The "AIM" factors examine the acceptance of the intervention in clinical or public health practice in the short and long term. **TABLE 2.6** defines the meaning of each of these components and illustrates how a new

---

**BOX 2.7** Qualitative Data and Its Importance to Public Health

Qualitative data can serve a variety of functions in public health. It can generate ideas or hypotheses for further study, provide key information on the reasons for success or failure of an intervention, and provide explanations for findings of quantitative research.

Quantitative research often includes a large sample and focuses on numbers, whereas qualitative research often looks in depth at a small sample, producing descriptions and allowing for a thorough exploration of the phenomenon of interest. Qualitative research on e-cigarettes may provide examples of the range of uses of qualitative research.

Focus groups and interviews are increasingly important forms of qualitative research that are being used to gain insight into how and why people come to conclusions or hold opinions on issues such as e-cigarettes. The opinions examined increasingly go beyond commercial products and politicians and include issues such as perceptions of the benefits and harms of e-cigarettes, access to e-cigarettes, and what

interventions would be effective in controlling use of e-cigarettes in children.

Qualitative research may also help explain quantitative research findings. For instance quantitative research might conclude that e-cigarette use is growing among 16–18 year olds but not among 12–16 year olds. The insights provided by individuals of these ages may help explain these findings.

The ideas put forward by these types of qualitative research may generate new hypotheses to be examined using quantitative studies. They may also help assess barriers to implementation and suggest new approaches.

These and other approaches to qualitative research help generate new ideas or hypotheses, predict responses to new interventions, and help us better understand the reasons for the observed results of quantitative research. Qualitative and quantitative research should be seen as complementary, not competitive, as they can work together to provide greater insight and understanding.

**TABLE 2.6** Evaluation: RE-AIM Framework

| RE-AIM component | Meaning | Example |
|---|---|---|
| **How well does the intervention work in practice?** | | |
| Reach | Asks: Who is the intervention being applied to in practice? May be groups or populations that are different than those on which it was investigated or intended for (i.e., the target population). | New prescription smoking cessation drug along with behavioral intervention approved by FDA and given evidence-based rating of A for long-standing adult smokers. Adverse events include depression and liver disease that is reversible with cessation of medication. Should not be used in teenagers who experience increased incidence of suicidal ideas. |
| Effectiveness | Asks: What is the impact in practice on the intended or target population, including beneficial outcomes as well as harm? | When used for long-term adult smokers, follow-up studies demonstrate substantial long-term quit rates similar to those observed in randomized controlled trials with no serious adverse events not identified in preapproval studies. Benefits exceed harms when used on intended target population. |
| **How well is the intervention accepted in practice?** | | |
| Adoption | Asks: How well is the intervention accepted by individuals and providers of services? | The drug is being widely used for long-term adult smokers. The drug is also being widely used for teenagers. |
| Implementation | Asks: How should the intervention be modified to reach target population and providers of services, but not those for whom the benefits do not exceed the harms? | A "black box" warning is placed on the prescribing information, warning clinicians of the potential suicide risk when used for teenagers. |
| Maintenance | Asks: How can we ensure long-term continuation of use and success of intervention among individuals and providers of services? | Long-term use of smoking cessation drug and behavioral change interventions are needed and are encouraged by coverage by health insurance plans. |

Data from Virginia Tech. RE-AIM. Available at http://www.re-aim.org/. Accessed July 14, 2017.

hypothetical intervention for cigarette cessation might be evaluated using the RE-AIM framework.

Notice that the RE-AIM framework implies that successful interventions have been widely disseminated. That is, there has been widespread circulation of information often aimed at integration into public health and/or clinical practice. **Dissemination**, while not a separate component of the P.E.R.I.E. framework, is an expected and essential component of successful interventions.

Deciding the best combination of approaches to address a public health problem remains an important part of the judgment needed for the practice of public health. In general, multiple approaches are often needed to effectively address a complex problem like cigarette smoking. Population and high-risk group approaches, often used by public health professionals, and individual approaches, often used as part of health care, should be seen as complementary. Often using both types of interventions is more effective than either approach alone. Social interventions, such as cigarette taxes and restrictions on public smoking, are also important interventions to consider.

Today, an enormous body of evidence exists on the relationship between tobacco and health. Understanding the nature of the problems, the etiology or cause-and-effect relationships, the evidence-based recommendations, and the approaches for implementing and evaluating the options for interventions remains key to the public health approach to smoking and health.[4] **FIGURE 2.3** diagrams the full P.E.R.I.E. approach.

**TABLE 2.7** summarizes the questions to ask in the evidence-based public health approach.

The P.E.R.I.E. process summarizes the steps in evidence-based public health. It emphasizes the need to understand the nature of the problem and its underlying causes. It also helps structure the use of evidence to make recommendations and decide on which options to put into practice. Finally, the circular nature of the P.E.R.I.E. process reminds us that the job of improving health goes on, often requiring multiple efforts to understand and address the problem.[10] Now that we have an understanding of the basic approach of evidence-based public health, let us turn our attention to the fundamental tools at our disposal for addressing public health problems.

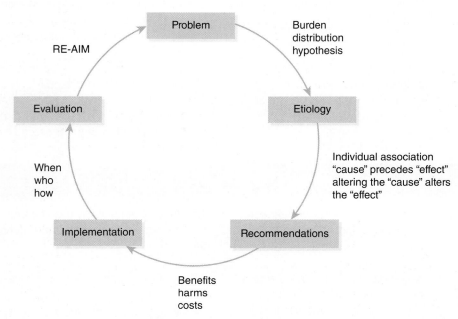

**FIGURE 2.3** Evidence-Based Public Health: The Complete P.E.R.I.E. Approach

---

**TABLE 2.7** Questions to Ask—Evidence-Based Public Health Approach

Problem—What is the health problem?

What is the burden of a disease or other health problem? What is the course of a disease or other health problem? Does the distribution of the health problem help generate hypotheses?

Etiology—What are the contributory causes?

Has an association been established at the individual level? Does the "cause" precede the "effect"? Has altering the "cause" been shown to alter the "effect"? (If not, use ancillary criteria.)

Recommendations—What works to reduce the health impacts?

What is the quality of the evidence for the intervention? What is the impact of the intervention in terms of benefits and harms? What grade should be given to indicate the strength of the recommendation?

Implementations—How can we get the job done?

When should the implementation occur? At whom should the implementation be directed? How should the intervention(s) be implemented?

Evaluation—How well does the intervention work in practice?

How well does the intervention work in practice on the intended or target population? How well does the intervention work in practice as actually used? How well is the intervention accepted in practice?

## Key Words

| | | |
|---|---|---|
| Absolute risk | Dose-response relationship | Randomization |
| Age adjustment | Effectiveness | Randomized controlled trials |
| Age distribution | Efficacy | Rate |
| Ancillary criteria | Epidemiologists | RE-AIM |
| Artifactual | Etiology | Recommendations |
| Associations | Evidence | Relative risk |
| At-risk population | Group associations | Reverse causality |
| Attributable risk percentage | Incidence | Risk factor |
| Biological plausibility | Morbidity | Risk indicators |
| Burden of disease | Mortality | Score |
| Case-control studies | Natural experiment | Secondary interventions |
| Case-fatality | Necessary cause | Standard population |
| Cohort studies | Odds ratio | Strength of the relationship |
| Confounding variable | P.E.R.I.E. process | Sufficient cause |
| Consistency | Population comparisons | Surrogate endpoints |
| Contributory cause | Prevalence | Tertiary interventions |
| Course of a disease | Primary interventions | True rate |
| Dissemination | Proportion | Victim blaming |
| Distribution of disease | Protective factor | |

## Discussion Questions

1. Use the P.E.R.I.E. framework and the list of questions to outline how each step in the P.E.R.I.E. process was accomplished for cigarette smoking.
2. How would you use the P.E.R.I.E. process to address the remaining problem of cigarette smoking in the United States?

## References

1. Cable News Network. A brief history of tobacco. http://edition.cnn.com/US/9705/tobacco/history. Accessed July 14, 2017.
2. Proctor RN. The history of the discovery of the cigarette–lung cancer link: evidentiary traditions, corporate denial, global toll. *Tobacco Control.* 2012;21:87–91.
3. Centers for Disease Control and Prevention. The public health approach to violence prevention. http://www.cdc.gov/violenceprevention/overview/publichealthapproach.html. Accessed July 14, 2017.
4. Gordis L. *Epidemiology.* 5th ed. Philadelphia, PA: Elsevier Saunders; 2014.
5. Friis RH, Sellers TA. *Epidemiology for Public Health Practice.* 5th ed. Burlington, MA: Jones & Bartlett Learning; 2013.
6. Riegelman RK. *Studying a Study and Testing a Test: Reading Evidence-based Health Research.* 6th ed. Philadelphia, PA: Lippincott, Williams & Wilkins; 2013.
7. U.S. Department of Health and Human Services. History of the surgeon general's reports on smoking and tobacco use. https://www.cdc.gov/tobacco/data_statistics/sgr/history/index.htm. Accessed July 14, 2017.
8. Agency for Healthcare Research and Quality, U.S. Preventive Services Task Force Guide to Clinical Preventive Services. 2002;1 and 2. AHRQ Pub. No. 02-500.
9. Centers for Disease Control and Prevention. The guide to community preventive services. The community guide. http://www.thecommunityguide.org. Accessed July 14, 2017.
10. Centers for Disease Control and Prevention. The social-ecological model: a framework for prevention. http://www.cdc.gov/violenceprevention/overview/social-ecologicalmodel.html. Accessed July 14, 2017.
11. Virginia Tech. RE-AIM. http://www.re-aim.org. Accessed July 14, 2017.

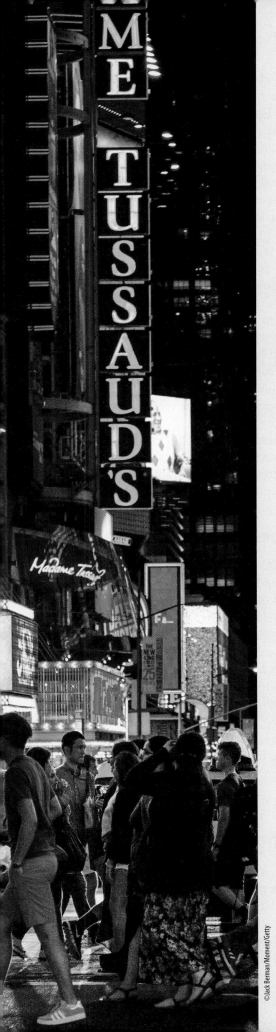

# SECTION I
# Cases and Discussion Questions

# HIV/AIDS Determinants and Control of the Epidemic

A report appeared in the CDC's "Morbidity and Mortality Weekly Report" (MMWR) on June 5, 1981, describing a previously unknown deadly disease in five young homosexual males, all in Los Angeles. The disease was characterized by dramatically reduced immunity, allowing otherwise innocuous organisms to become "opportunistic infections," rapidly producing fatal infections or cancer. Thus, acquired immune deficiency syndrome (AIDS) first became known to the public health and medical communities. It was soon traced to rectal intercourse, blood transfusions, and reuse of injection needles as methods of transmission. Reuse of needles was a common practice in poor nations. It was also widespread among intravenous drug abusers. Within several years, the disease was traced to a previously unknown retrovirus, which came to be called the human immunodeficiency virus (HIV).

A test was developed to detect the disease and was first used in testing blood for transfusion. Within a short period of time, the blood supply was protected by testing all donated blood, and transmission of HIV by blood transfusion became a rare event. Diagnostic tests for HIV/AIDS soon became available for testing individuals. For many years, these were used by clinicians only for high-risk individuals. In recent years, HIV testing has become more widely used, as the testing no longer requires blood drawing and the results are rapidly available. The CDC has put increasing emphasis on testing as part of routine health care.

In subsequent years, much has been learned about HIV/AIDS. Today, it is primarily a heterosexually transmitted disease with greater risk of transmission from male to females than females to males. In the United States, African Americans are at the greatest risk. Condoms have been demonstrated to reduce the risk of transmission. Abstinence and monogamous sexual relationships likewise eliminate or greatly reduce the risk. Even serial monogamy reduces the risk compared to multiple simultaneous partners. Male circumcision has been shown to reduce the potential to acquire HIV infection by approximately 50%.

In major U.S. cities, the frequency of HIV is often greater than 1% of the population, fulfilling the CDC definition of "high risk." In these geographic areas, the risk of unprotected intercourse is substantially greater than in most suburban or rural areas. Nearly everyone is susceptible to HIV infection, despite the fact that a small number of people have well documented protection on a genetic basis.

Maternal-to-child transmission is quite frequent and has been shown to be largely preventable by treatments during pregnancy and at the time of delivery. CDC recommendations for universal testing of pregnant women and intervention for all HIV-positive patients have been widely implemented by clinicians and hospitals and have resulted in greatly reduced frequency of maternal-to-child transmissions in the developed countries and in developing countries in recent years.

Medication is now available that greatly reduces the load of HIV present in the blood. These medications delay the progression of HIV and also reduce the ease of spread of the disease. These treatments were rapidly applied to HIV/AIDS patients in developed countries, but it required about a decade before they were widely used in most developing countries. Inadequate funding from developed countries and controversies over patent protection for HIV/AIDS drugs delayed widespread use of these treatments in developing countries.

New and emerging approaches to HIV prevention include use of antiviral medications during breastfeeding, postcoital treatments, and rapid diagnosis and follow-up to detect and treat those recently exposed.

## Discussion Questions

1. Use the BIG GEMS framework to examine the factors in addition to infection that have affected the spread of HIV and the control or failure to control the HIV/AIDS epidemic.
2. What roles has health care played in controlling or failing to control the HIV/AIDS epidemic?
3. What roles has traditional public health played in controlling or failing to control the HIV/AIDS epidemic?
4. What roles have social factors (beyond the sphere of health care or public health) played in controlling or failing to control the HIV/AIDS epidemic?

# The Aging Society

George Harwick, a middle-class American from what he calls the "heartland" was just turning 65 and was in good health. His good health, however, depended on daily treatment for high blood pressure, diabetes, and high cholesterol as well as regular check-ups for his declining kidney function. He was planning to retire when he reached what Social Security called full retirement age, which is gradually increasing, but because Medicare begins at age 65 he was going to sign up now.

George's mother Harriet turned 90 last month, but all was not so well. On the day before her birthday she found herself lying on the bathroom floor in pain after slipping getting out of the shower. Her bones were not as strong as they used to be and she was soon on her way to the operating room to replace her hip. She was told that 25 years ago she would most likely have died from the fracture but now she was faced with months of rehabilitation and a long stay in a rehabilitative facility. She wondered what would come next.

The United States is increasingly faced with what might be regarded as the price of its success. New technology is keeping the elderly like Harriet alive longer and the costs of health care for people like George is creating a financial crisis in Medicare.

The population of those over age 85 is growing faster than those of any other age group with those ages 65 to 85 trailing right behind. Those over 85 have been called the "frail elderly" because they are far more vulnerable to a range of diseases from strokes and heart disease, to falls and fractures, to Alzheimer's and Parkinson's disease. In the second decade of the 21st century there are less than 10 million people over 85 in the United States. By 2050 that number is expected to exceed 20 million.

In part because of the services provided through Medicare plus the health innovations stimulated by NIH research, the baby boomer generation, now rapidly turning 65, is expected to live longer. The life expectancy of those turning 65 today has grown to an average of approximately 20 years compared to less than 10 years when Medicare was begun in the mid-1960s. That means that about half those turning 65 today will be alive at age 85 and many will live well into their 90s. Despite gradual increases in the Social Security retirement age from 65 to 67, with debate about still higher ages, the age for eligibility for Medicare has remained at 65.

The Harwicks were fortunate since their family did not have a history of Alzheimer's disease and Harriet's mind was quite clear despite her frailty. She was glad to take advantage of new systems of caring for the frail elderly ranging from "aging in place" to senior day care, to family respite services, to efforts encouraging the elderly to remain active in their communities.

The burdens of taking care of the frail elderly are increasingly falling on family members as society seeks to limit costs. Family leave policies and tax benefits for caring for the elderly are policies which may help relieve this burden. Living alone can lead to loneliness, which is increasingly being recognized as a risk factor for deteriorating physical and mental status. Social interactions are key to good health in the elderly as well as their enjoyment of life.

Prevention takes on a different meaning for the frail elderly. Many traditional screening programs, such as routine PAP smears or routine testing for colon or breast cancer, no longer are being applied to the elderly, especially those over 85,. Control of LDL cholesterol, blood sugar, high blood pressure, and smoking cessation remain high priorities.

Efforts to prevent falls and respond quickly when they do occur have become a high priority for prevention in the frail elderly. Keeping physically active helps to prevent blood clots and worsening osteoporosis. As with Harriet, emergency treatment of these conditions when they do occur is now high on the list of common clinical procedures.

The healthcare system is gradually adjusting to the need to provide special services for the frail elderly who are often unable to navigate the increasingly complex world of community services, health care, and health insurance. Health Navigators, sometimes called community health workers, patient navigators, or health insurance navigators, are becoming an important part of the health care and community health systems. Providing health services in the home or residence is increasingly recognized as an effective and efficient method for caring for the frail elderly.

What should we do about the cost of Medicare? Some have argued that coverage under Medicare should be limited to those procedures that are considered cost-effective; by which they usually mean the extra cost is worth the extra expenses. Cost effectiveness, however, is a tricky business with ethical considerations. For instance should the cost of feeding, housing and taking care of the elderly who receive extra years of life be considered in calculating the cost? Is it cost-effective to prevent lung cancer knowing that a rapid death from lung cancer avoids the high costs for care of future chronic illnesses which will surely occur in those who no longer die of lung cancer?

Many countries have tried rationing care as an approach to limiting the healthcare costs of the elderly. Rationing is the rule in many European countries where advancing age is in-and-of itself a contraindication or disqualification for expensive medical interventions ranging from kidney dialysis to heart transplants, and even weight loss surgery. Overt rationing has been politically taboo in the United States where even the mention of treating older patients differently has resulted in the accusation of "death panels."

Some say economic growth is the way out of our bind. They argue that a larger economy means more tax revenue to pay for Medicare and other problems of the elderly. Taxing those who can afford to pay to ensure health care for those who can't afford the costs is the answer according to others. Still others say better, more efficient healthcare delivery is what we need.

George listens to these debates. Yes, he says, there's a crisis in Medicare coming but that's not my problem, I paid into the system for over 40 years and now my mother and I deserve to get what we are entitled to. I'll fight and vote for those benefits until the day I die.

## Discussion Questions

1. What makes the frail elderly different from other older individuals? Explain.
2. What health professionals and non health professional are needed to care for the frail elderly? Explain.
3. What types of costs should we consider when deciding whether a health service is "cost-effective"? Explain.
4. Would raising the Medicare eligibility age help or would it just leave large number of retirees without healthcare coverage? Explain.
5. Do you favor economic growth, taxing those who can afford to pay, or a more efficient healthcare system as the primary means to pay for the future Medicare system? Explain.

## ▶ Smoking and Adolescents— The Continuing Problem

The rate of smoking in the United States has been reduced by approximately one-half since the 1960s. However, the rate of smoking among teenagers increased in the 1980s and 1990s, especially among teenage females. This raised concerns that young women would continue smoking during pregnancy. In addition, it was found that nearly 90% of adults who smoked started before the age of 18, and in many cases at a considerably younger age.

In the 1980s and most of the 1990s, cigarette smoking was advertised to teenagers and even preteens, or "tweens," through campaigns such as Joe Camel. In recent years, a series of interventions directed at teenagers and tweens was put into effect. These included elimination of cigarette vending machines, penalties for those who sell cigarettes to those under 18, and elimination of most cigarette advertising aimed at those under 18. In addition, the Truth® campaign aimed to convince adolescents, who often see smoking as a sign of independence from their parents, that not smoking is actually a sign of independence from the tobacco companies who

seek to control their behavior. Evaluation studies concluded that these interventions have worked to reduce adolescent smoking by about one-third.

Despite the successes of the early years of the 2000s in lowering the rates of cigarette smoking among adolescents, the rates have now stabilized at over 20%. Evidence indicates that adolescents who smoke generally do not participate in athletics, more often live in rural areas, and are more often white and less often African American. Males and females smoke about the same amount overall, but white females smoke more and Asian females smoke less than their male counterparts.

New drugs taken as pills have recently been shown to increase the rates of success in smoking cessation among adults despite side effects. This is not the situation in adolescents because of increased potential for adverse effects, including suicide. A series of interventions has been suggested for addressing the continuing problem of adolescent smoking. These include:

- Expulsion from school for cigarette smoking
- Focus on adolescents in tobacco warning labels
- Selective use of nicotine gum and patches to help with withdrawal
- No smoking rules for sporting events, music concerts, and other adolescent-oriented events
- Fines for adolescents who falsify their age and purchase cigarettes
- Higher taxes on tobacco products
- Rewards to students in schools with the lowest smoking rates in a geographic area
- Higher auto insurance premiums for adolescents who smoke
- Application of technology to reduce the quantity of nicotine allowed in tobacco products to reduce the potential for addiction
- Testing of athletes for nicotine and exclusion from competition if they test positive
- Provision of tobacco counseling as part of medical care covered through insurance

The National Academy of Medicine has recommended that the age for purchase of cigarettes be raised from 18 to 21 years.[a]

## Discussion Questions

1. How does this case illustrate the P.E.R.I.E. process?
2. Which of these interventions do you think would be most successful? Explain.
3. How would you classify each of these potential interventions as education (information),

---

a The National Academy of Medicine was previously known as the Institute of Medicine.

motivation (incentives), obligation (required), or innovation (technological change)?

4. What other interventions can you suggest to reduce adolescent smoking?

# Reye's Syndrome: A Public Health Success Story

Reye's Syndrome is a potentially fatal disease of childhood that typically occurs in the winter months at the end of an episode of influenza, chicken pox, or other acute viral infection. It is characterized by progressive stages of nausea and vomiting, liver dysfunction, and mental impairment that progress over hours to days and result in a range of symptoms, from irritability to confusion to deepening stages of loss of consciousness. Reye's Syndrome is diagnosed by putting together a pattern of signs and symptoms. There is no definitive diagnostic test for the disease.

Reye's Syndrome was first defined as a distinct condition in the early 1960s. By the 1980s, over 500 cases per year were being diagnosed in the United States. When Reye's Syndrome was first diagnosed, there was over a 30% case-fatality rate. Early diagnosis and aggressive efforts to prevent brain damage were shown to reduce the deaths and limit the mental complications, but there is no cure for Reye's Syndrome.

In the late 1970s and early 1980s, a series of case-control studies compared Reye's Syndrome children with similar children who also had an acute viral infection, but did not develop the syndrome. These studies suggested that use of aspirin, then called "baby aspirin," was strongly associated with Reye's Syndrome, with over 90% of those children afflicted with the syndrome having recently used aspirin.

Cohort studies were not practical because they would require observing very large numbers of children who might be given or not given aspirin by their caretakers. Randomized controlled trials were neither feasible nor ethical. Fortunately, it was considered safe and acceptable to reduce or eliminate aspirin use in children because there was a widely used alternative—acetaminophen (often sold under the brand name Tylenol)—that was not implicated in the studies of Reye's Syndrome.

As early as 1980, the CDC cautioned physicians and parents about the potential dangers of aspirin. In 1982, the U.S. surgeon general issued an advisory on the danger of aspirin for use in children. By 1986, the U.S. Food and Drug Administration required a Reye's Syndrome warning be placed on all aspirin-containing medications. These efforts were coupled with public

service announcements, informational brochures, and patient education by pediatricians and other health professionals who cared for children. The use of the term "baby aspirin" was strongly discouraged.

In the early 1980s, there were over 500 cases of Reye's Syndrome per year in the United States. In recent years, there have often been fewer than 5 per year. The success of the efforts to reduce or eliminate the use of "baby aspirin" and the subsequent dramatic reduction in the frequency of Reye's Syndrome provided convincing evidence that aspirin was a contributory cause of the condition and its removal from use was an effective intervention.

## Discussion Questions

1. How does the Reye's Syndrome history illustrate the use of each of the steps in the P.E.R.I.E. process?

2. What unique aspects of Reye's Syndrome made it necessary and feasible to rely on case-control studies to provide the evidence to help reduce the frequency of the syndrome?

3. What types of methods for implementation were utilized as part of the implementation process? Can you classify them in terms of when, who, and how?

4. How does the Reye's Syndrome history illustrate the use of evaluation to demonstrate whether the implementation process was successful?

# Sudden Infant Death Syndrome (SIDS)

Sudden infant death syndrome, or SIDS, was first recognized as a distinct public health problem in the late 1960s when over 7000 infants each year were found to die suddenly and unexpectedly. "Crib deaths" have been recognized for centuries, but until they were formally recorded and investigated, little was known about their cause, leading some to conclude that intentional or unintentional suffocation by parents or caregivers played an important role.

Data from the investigations of SIDS indicated that the syndrome was very rare before babies' first month of life, increased during the second month, and peaked during the third month, before rapidly declining in frequency to again become rare after the fourth month of life. The timing of SIDS suggested that the condition occurs after infants begin to sleep for extended periods but prior to the time in which children can raise themselves up and roll over on their own. Additional evidence suggested a seasonal trend, with more cases of SIDS occurring during cold weather months than during warm weather months.

In the 1980s, several case-control studies of SIDS cases and similar infants without SIDS established that infants who slept on their stomachs were at substantially increased risk of dying from SIDS. The studies indicated that the chances increased 4–7 times, suggesting that if a cause-and-effect relationship exists, a clear majority of SIDS cases could be prevented if infants slept on their back. Many parents and clinicians remained skeptical because the traditional teaching emphasized sleeping prone, or on the stomach, to reduce the possibility of choking on regurgitation and vomit. Despite the lack of evidence for this hazard, generations had been raised on this practice and belief.

Additional evidence of the effectiveness of a "back-to-sleep" intervention was provided by the experience of New Zealand, which was the first country to begin a program to encourage caretakers to put infants to sleep on their backs. The rates of SIDS in New Zealand declined rapidly in parallel with the increased rate at which infants were put to sleep on their back. Similar declines in SIDS did not occur in other countries that had not yet instituted similar back-to-sleep programs.

In 1992, the American Academy of Pediatrics made a recommendation that infants be placed on their back to sleep. The initial recommendations also endorsed side sleeping. In 1994, with the support of the American Academy of Pediatrics, the National Institutes of Health (NIH), and the U.S. Public Health Service, the Back-to-Sleep campaign was launched. The educational campaign included public service announcements, brochures and other publications, including information accompanying new cribs, plus efforts for pediatricians and others who care for infants to educate parents and caretakers about the importance of having infants sleep on their backs.

The frequency of infants sleeping prone in the United States was found by survey data to be reduced from approximately 70% to less than 15% during the years immediately following the initiation of the Back-to-Sleep campaign. During these years, the rates of SIDS fell by approximately 50%, an impressive change

but less than expected by the initial data. The rate of prone sleeping among African Americans was found to be over twice as high as the rate among whites, and African American infants continued to have higher rates of SIDS than whites.

Continuing studies suggested that the side position was being commonly used. It was found that many infants moved from the side to the prone position, and movement from the side to the prone position carried a high risk of SIDS. Additional case-control studies suggested that soft objects and loose bedding as well as overheating were associated with SIDS. These relationships are consistent with the initial finding of an increase of SIDS in colder weather months.

Studies of the infants who slept on their back indicated an increasing in flattening of the head, or plagiocephaly. These changes were shown to be reduced by increasing the amount of "tummy time," or play periods in which infants are placed prone under supervision. Guidelines for tummy time are now part of the evidence-based recommendations. SIDS continues to be an important cause of infant mortality, and new contributory causes continue to be investigated. SIDS reflects the use of evidence-based public health and the importance of continuing to study and develop new approaches to public health problems.

## Discussion Questions

1.  Discuss how the problem description component of the evidence-based public health approach suggested hypotheses for the etiology of SIDS.
2.  Discuss the types of evidence used to support the relationship between sleeping prone and SIDS as well as the limitations of the evidence.
3.  Discuss how the evidence-based recommendations incorporated potential benefits and harms.
4.  Discuss how implementation and evaluation worked to establish sleeping on the back as a standard intervention to prevent SIDS.
5.  Discuss how the continuing presence of the problem of SIDS produced a new round of use of the evidence-based public health approach.

SECTION II

# Tools of Population Health

In order to protect and promote health and prevent disease, disability, and death, public health uses an array of tools. In this section, we will examine three of the basic tools of public health: public health data and communications; social and behavioral sciences; and health law, policy, and ethics. **FIGURE S02.1** provides a framework for thinking about the tools used in the population health approach and indicates where they are addressed in this text.

In Chapter 3, we will explore how health information is collected, compiled, and presented, as well as how it is perceived, combined, and used to make decisions in the arena of health communications. Chapter 4 will examine the contributions of the social and behavioral sciences in helping us to understand the sources of health and disease and the strategies available to reduce disease, disability, and death. To do this, we will explore how

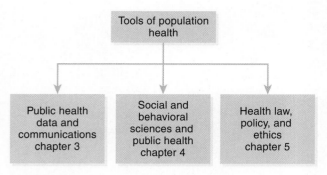

**FIGURE S02.1** Tools of Population Health Framework

social and economic factors, or social determinants, affect health. We will also examine how individual and group behavior can be changed to improve health. Finally, in Chapter 5, we will learn how health policies and laws can be used to improve health, as well as how ethical and philosophical issues limit their use.

# CHAPTER 3

# Public Health Data and Communications

You read that the rate of use of cocaine among teenagers has fallen by 50% in the last decade. You wonder where that information might come from.

You hear that life expectancy in the United States is now approximately 80 years. You wonder what that implies about how long you will live and what that means for your grandmother, who is 82 and in good health.

You hear on the news the gruesome description of a shark attack on a young boy from another state and decide to keep your son away from the beach. While playing at a friend's house, your son nearly drowns after falling into the backyard pool.

You ask why so many people think that drowning in a backyard pool is unusual when it is far more common than shark attacks.

"Balancing the harms and benefits is essential to making decisions," your clinician says. The treatment you are considering has an 80% chance of working, but there is also a 20% chance of side effects. "What do I need to consider when balancing the harms and the benefits?" you ask.

You are faced with a decision to have a medical procedure. One physician tells you there is no other choice and you must undergo the procedure, another tells you about the harms and benefits and advises you to go ahead, and the third lays out the options and tells you it is your decision. Why are there such different approaches to making decisions these days?

These are the types of issues and questions that we will address as we look at health data and communications.

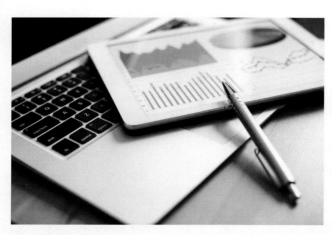

© leungchopan/Shutterstock

## What Is the Scope of Health Communications?

The term **health communications** deals with the methods for collecting, compiling, and presenting health information. It also addresses how we perceive, combine, and use information to make decisions. Thus, health communication is about information, from its collection to its use. **FIGURE 3.1** displays how these parts of the process fit into a continuous flow of information.

The field of health communications has been growing at the speed of the Internet. This field has implications for most, if not all, aspects of public

health, as well as health care. Therefore, we will focus on key issues in each of the previously mentioned components of this burgeoning field. We will look at the following aspects of health communications and ask the following questions:

- *Collecting data*: Where does public health data come from?
- *Compiling information*: How is public health information compiled or put together to measure the health of a population?
- *Presenting information*: How can we evaluate the quality of the display and presentation of public health information?
- *Perceiving information*: What factors affect how we perceive public health information?
- *Combining information*: What types of information need to be combined to make health decisions?
- *Decision-making*: How do we utilize information to make health decisions?

We can only highlight key issues in this complex and evolving field of health communications. To do this, we will use these questions and provide frameworks and approaches to explore possible answers.

## Where Does Public Health Data Come From?

Public health **data** is collected in a wide variety of ways.[a] These methods are often referred to as **public health surveillance.** Data from public health surveillance is collected, published, and distributed without identifying specific individuals. Data of this type come from a growing variety of sources. It is helpful, however, to classify these sources according to the way they are collected. **TABLE 3.1** outlines common types of quantitative public health data, provides examples

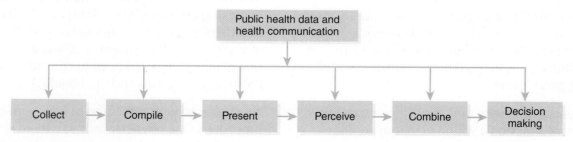

**FIGURE 3.1** Public Health Data, Health Communication, and the Flow of Information

---

a "Data" is usually defined as facts or a representation of facts, while "information" implies that the data is compiled and/or presented in a way designed for a range of uses. Thus, the term "data" is used here only in the context of collection.

**TABLE 3.1** The 7 S's of Quantitative Sources of Public Health Surveillance Data

| Type | Examples | Uses | Advantages/Disadvantages |
|---|---|---|---|
| Single case or small series | Case reports of one or a small number of cases, such as SARS, anthrax, mad cow, disease and new diseases (e.g., first report of AIDS) | Alert to new disease or resistant disease; alert to potential spread beyond initial area | Useful for dramatic, unusual, and new conditions; requires alert clinicians and rapid ability to disseminate information |
| Statistics ("Vital Statistics") and reportable diseases | Vital statistics: birth, death, marriage, divorce; reporting of key communicable and specially selected noncommunicable-diseases (e.g., elevated lead levels, child and spouse abuse, etc.)  Also may include other public government records such as accident and police reports | Required by law—sometimes penalties imposed for noncompliance; births and deaths key to defining leading causes of disease; reportable disease may be helpful in identifying changes over time | Vital statistics very complete because of social and financial consequences; reportable disease often relies on institutional reporting rather than individual clinicians; frequent delays in reporting data |
| Surveys—sampling | National Health and Nutrition Examination Survey (NHANES); Behavioral Risk Factor Surveillance System (BRFSS)  Also includes disease specific registries (e.g., Surveillance, Epidemiology End Results (SEER) cancer registry) | Drawing conclusions about overall population and subgroups from representative samples  Registries attempt to include all those with a disease in order to be representative of the population | Well-conducted surveys allow inferences to be drawn about larger populations; frequent delays in reporting data  Difficult to include all potential patients in disease registries |
| Self-reporting | Adverse effect monitoring of drugs and vaccines as reported by those affected | May help identify unrecognized or unusual events | Useful when dramatic unusual events closely follow initial use of drug or vaccine; tends to be incomplete; difficult to evaluate meaning because of selective process of reporting |
| Sentinel monitoring | Influenza monitoring to identify start of outbreak and changes in virus type | Early warnings or warning of previously unrecognized events | Can be used for "real-time" monitoring; requires considerable knowledge of patterns of disease and use of services to develop |
| Syndromic surveillance | Use of symptom patterns (e.g., headaches, cough/fever, or gastrointestinal symptoms, plus increased sales of over-the-counter drugs) to raise alert of possible new or increased disease | May be able to detect unexpected and subtle changes, such as bioterrorism or new epidemic producing commonly occurring symptoms | May be used for early warning even when no disease is diagnosed; does not provide a diagnosis and may have false positives |
| Social media | Data on outbreaks using key words from social media | Detect and monitor course of influenza epidemic | Potential for immediate data obtained from a large number of individuals  Accuracy and precision of the data for early and ongoing surveillance needs to be established |

of each type, and indicates important uses, as well as the advantages and disadvantages of each type of data.

Data from different sources is increasingly being combined to create integrated health data systems or **databases** that can be rapidly and flexibly accessed by computers to address a wide range of questions. These systems have great potential to provide useful information to contribute to evidence-based public health. This information can help describe problems, examine etiology, assist with evidence-based recommendations, and examine the options for implementation, as well as help evaluate the outcomes. Despite their great potential, integrated databases also create the potential for abuse of the most intimate health information. Thus, protecting the privacy of data and ensuring its anonymous collection and distribution is now of great concern as part of the development of integrated databases.

Data can be used for a wide range of purposes in public health and health care. One particularly important use is the compilation of data to generate summary measurements of the health of a group or population. Let us take a look at how we compile this data.

## ▶ How Is Public Health Information Compiled to Measure the Health of a Population?

Measurements that summarize the health of populations are called **population health status measures**. For over a century, public health professionals have focused on how to summarize the health status of large populations, such as countries and large groups within countries—for example, males and females or large racial groups of a particular nation. In the 1900s, two measurements became standard for summarizing the health status of populations: the **infant mortality rate** and **life expectancy**. These measurements rely on death and birth certificate data, as well as census data. Toward the latter part of the 1900s, these sources of data became widely available and quite accurate in most parts of the world.

The infant mortality rate estimates the rate of death in the first year of life. For many years, it has been used as the primary measurement of child health. Life expectancy has been used to measure the overall death experience of the population, incorporating the probability of dying at each year of life.[1,2] These measures were the mainstay of 20th-century population health measurements. Let us look at each of these measures and see why additional health status measurements are needed for the 21st century.

In the early years of the 20th century, infant mortality rates were high even in today's developed countries, such as the United States. It was not unusual for over 100 of every 1000 newborns to die in the first year of life. In many parts of the world, infant mortality far exceeded the death rate in any later years of childhood. For this reason, the infant mortality rate was often used as a surrogate or substitute measure for overall rates of childhood death. In the first half of the 20th century, however, great improvements in infant mortality occurred in what are today's developed countries. During the second half of the century, many developing countries also saw greatly reduced infant mortality rates. Today, many countries have achieved infant mortality rates below 10 per 1000, and a growing number of nations have achieved rates below 5 per 1000.[b]

The degree of success in reducing mortality among children aged 2 to 5 has not been as great.[3] Malnutrition and old and new infectious diseases continue to kill young children. In addition, improvements in the care of severely ill newborns have extended the lives of many children—only to have them die after the first year of life. Children with HIV/AIDS often die not in the first year of life, but in the second, third, or fourth year. Once a child survives to age 5, he or she has a very high probability of surviving into adulthood in most countries. Thus, a new measurement known as **under-5 mortality** has now become the standard health status measure used by the World Health Organization (WHO) to summarize the health of children.

Let us take a look at the second traditional measure of population health status—life expectancy. Life expectancy is a snapshot of a population incorporating the probability of dying at each age of life in a particular year. Life expectancy tells us how well a country is doing in terms of deaths in a particular year. As an example, life expectancy at birth in a developed country may be 80 years. Perhaps in 1900, life expectancy at

---

b  The infant mortality rate is measured using the number of deaths among those ages 0–1 in a particular year divided by the total number of live births in the same year. If the number of live births is stable from year to year, then the infant mortality rate is a measure of the rate of deaths. Health status measurements of child health have not sought to incorporate disability on the less-than-completely-accurate assumption that disability is not a major factor among children.

birth in that same country was only 50 years. In a few countries life-expectancy at birth for women already exceeds 85 years. Thus, life-expectancy allows us to make comparisons between countries, compare large groups such as males and females within a country, and to measure changes over time.

Life expectancy can be calculated at any age so we may speak of life-expectancy at age 65 or age 85. Despite its name, life expectancy cannot be used to accurately predict future life spans, especially for newborns. Accurate prediction requires assuming that nothing will change. That is, accurate prediction requires the death rates at all ages to remain the same in future years. We have seen increases in life expectancy in most countries over the last century, but declines occurred in sub-Saharan Africa and countries of the former Soviet Union in the late 1900s.[c] A substantial decline in life-expectancy could occur in the United States in the coming years as a result of the obesity and opioid epidemics.

Life expectancy tells us only part of what we want to know. It reflects the impact of dying, but not the impact of disabilities. When considering the health status of a population in the 21st century, we need to consider disability, as well as death.

Today, the WHO uses a measurement known as the **health-adjusted life expectancy (HALE)** to summarize the health of populations.[4] The HALE measurement starts with life expectancy and then incorporates measurements of the quality of health. The WHO utilizes survey data to obtain a country's overall measurement of quality of health. This measurement incorporates key components, including:[d]

- Mobility—the ability to walk without assistance
- Cognition—mental function, including memory
- Self-care—activities of daily living, including dressing, eating, bathing, and use of the toilet
- Pain—regular pain that limits function

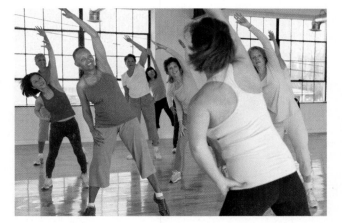
© Ariel Skelley/DigitalVision/Getty Images

- Mood—alteration in mood that limits function
- Sensory organ function—impairment in vision or hearing that impairs function

From these measurements, an overall quality of health score is obtained. A quality of health measurement of 90% indicates that the average person in the country loses 10% of his or her full health over his or her lifetime to one or more disabilities. In most countries, the quality of health ranges from 85% to 90%. We might consider a score of less than 85% as poor and greater than 90% as very good.

The quality of health measurement is multiplied by the life expectancy at birth to obtain the HALE. Thus, a country that has achieved a life expectancy at birth of 80 years and an overall quality of health score of 90% can claim a HALE of 80.00 × 0.90 = 72.00. **TABLE 3.2** displays WHO data on life expectancy at birth and HALEs[4] for a variety of large countries.[e]

Today, the under-5 mortality and HALEs are used by the WHO as the standard measures reflecting child health and the overall health of a population. An additional measure, known as the

c  Life expectancy is greater than you may expect at older ages. For instance, in a country with a life expectancy of 80 years, a 60-year-old may still have a life expectancy of 25 years, not 20 years, because he or she escaped the risks of death during the early years of life. At age 80, the chances of death are very dependent on an individual's state of health because life expectancy combines the probability of death of those in good health and those in poor health. Healthy 80-year-olds have a very high probability of living to 90 and beyond.

d  It can be argued that use of these measurements associates disability primarily with the elderly. Note that these qualities of health do not specifically include measures of the ability to work, engage in social interactions, or have satisfying sexual relationships, all of which may be especially important to younger populations.

e  Not all countries accept the HALE as the method for expressing disabilities. A measurement known as the **health-related quality of life (HRQOL)** has been developed and used in the United States. The HRQOL incorporates a measure of unhealthy days. Unhealthy days are measured by asking a representative sample of individuals the number of days in the last 30 during which the status of either their mental or physical health kept them from their usual activities. It then calculates a measure of the quality of health by adding together the number of unhealthy days due to mental plus physical health. The quality of health is obtained by dividing the number of healthy days by 30. This measurement is relatively easy to collect and calculate, but unlike the HALE, it does not reflect objective measures of disability and cannot be directly combined with life expectancy to produce an overall measure of health. That is, it does not include the impact of mortality.

**TABLE 3.2** Life Expectancy and Health-Adjusted Life Expectancy for a Range of Large Countries

| Country | Life expectancy | Health-adjusted life expectancy (HALE) |
|---|---|---|
| Nigeria | 54.5 | 47.4 |
| India | 68.3 | 59.5 |
| Russian Federation | 70.5 | 63.3 |
| Brazil | 75.0 | 65.5 |
| China | 76.1 | 68.5 |
| United States | 79.3 | 69.1 |
| United Kingdom | 81.2 | 71.4 |
| Canada | 82.2 | 72.3 |
| Japan | 83.7 | 74.9 |

Data from World Health Organization. World Health Statistics 2016. Available at http://www.who.int/whosis/whostat/EN_WHS09_Full.pdf. Accessed July 16, 2017.

**disability-adjusted life year (DALY)**, has been developed and used by the WHO to allow for comparisons and changes based on categories of diseases and conditions.[5] **BOX 3.1** describes DALYs and some of the data and conclusions that have come from using this measurement. **TABLE 3.3** displays DALYs according to these categories of diseases and conditions for the same large countries for which HALEs are displayed in Table 3.2.

The Global Burden of Disease (GBD) project has produced a number of important conclusions using DALYs, including:

Depression is a major contributor to most nations' DALYs and may become the number one contributor in the next few decades in developing, as well as developed, countries.

Chronic disabling diseases, including hookworm, malaria, and HIV, affect the young and working-age population and are the greatest contributors to the burden of disease in many developing countries.

Cancers, such as breast cancer, hepatomas (primary liver cancer), and colon cancer—which affect the working-age population and are common in

**BOX 3.1** DALYs

Disability-adjusted life years (DALYs) are designed to examine the impacts that specific diseases and risk factors have on populations, as well as provide an overall measure of population health status. They allow comparisons between countries or within countries over time, based not only on overall summary numbers, such as life expectancy and HALEs, but also on specific diseases and risk factors.

The DALY compares a country's performance to the country with the longest life expectancy, which is currently Japan. Japan has a life expectancy that is approximately 83 years. In a country with zero DALYs, the average person would live approximately 83 years without any disability and would then die suddenly. Of course, this does not occur even in Japan, so all countries have DALYs of greater than zero. The measurement is usually presented as DALYs per 1000 population in a particular country.[a]

Calculations of DALYs require much more data on specific diseases and disabilities than other measurements, such as life expectancy or HALEs. However, the WHO's Global Burden of Disease (GBD) project has made considerable progress in obtaining worldwide data collected using a consistent approach.[5] Data is often not available on the disability produced by a disease. The WHO then uses expert opinion to estimate the impact.

The GBD project presents data on DALYs divided into the following categories:

- Communicable disease; maternal, neonatal, and nutritional conditions
- Noncommunicable diseases
- Injuries

Data is also available on specific diseases and risk factors, such as the impact of cigarette smoking, alcohol use, or depression.

---

a  The newest version of the WHO DALY measurement differs from the previous versions and the numbers should not be compared. Prevalence and not incidence is used in the current version. In addition, WHO no longer discounts DALYs. Interpretation of DALYs can be confusing. If, in a country with 0 DALYs, 1000 newborns suddenly died, there would be a loss of as much as 83,000 DALYs from the death of these 1000 newborns. Thus, the total DALYs a country can lose in a particular year can range from 0 to approximately 83,000 per 1,000 persons. It is possible for a country to have more than 1000 DALYs lost per 1000 population. For instance, WHO reports that Angola has 1046 DALYs per 1000 population. If a country loses 1000 DALYs per 1000 population, it implies that one year of healthy life is lost for every year of life lived; that is, half the years of healthy life are lost. Those years of life lost mostly occur in future years since they are based on death and disability over the future life span.

| **TABLE 3.3** DALYs Lost by Disease Categories and Total of All Categories per 1000 Population | | | |
|---|---|---|---|
| **Country** | **DALYs lost due to communicable diseases; maternal, neonatal, and nutritional conditions** | **DALYs lost due to noncommunicable diseases** | **DALYs lost due to injuries (unintentional + intentional)** | **Total DALYs lost** |
| Nigeria | 583 | 189 | 75 | 847 |
| India | 137 | 208 | 46 | 391 |
| Russian Federation | 50 | 363 | 59 | 472 |
| Brazil | 44 | 202 | 45 | 291 |
| China | 20 | 217 | 25 | 262 |
| United States | 18 | 244 | 27 | 289 |
| United Kingdom | 16 | 224 | 17 | 257 |
| Canada | 15 | 201 | 20 | 236 |
| Japan | 22 | 218 | 20 | 260 |

Data from World Health Organization. Burden of Disease 2015. Available at: http://www.who.int/topics/global_burden_of_disease/en/. Accessed July 16, 2017.

many developing countries—have an important impact on the burden of disease as expressed in DALYs.

Motor vehicle, occupational, and other forms of unintentional injuries have a disproportionate impact on the burden of disease compared to merely measuring deaths because these injuries produce long-term disabilities, as well as death at young ages.

Obesity is rapidly overtaking malnutrition as a burden of disease in developing countries as early onset diabetes, heart disease, and strokes become major causes of death and disability among younger populations.

We have now looked at important sources of public health data and examined one key way that data is compiled to generate population health status measurements. Now, let us look at a third issue: the presentation of public health information.

# How Can We Evaluate the Display and Quality of the Presentation of Health Information?

Having information is not enough. A key role and essential tool of public health is to effectively present the information in ways that serve as a basis for understanding and decision-making. Issues of information presentation are increasingly important and increasingly complex. They require the study of a range of disciplines, from mass media, to computer graphics, to statistics.[f] Public health information is often presented as graphics. Graphics create a picture in our mind of what is going on, and a picture is truly worth a thousand words. Graphical presentations can accurately inform, but they can also mislead us in a wide variety of ways. The accurate presentation of visual

---

f   The use of statistics is one approach to data presentation. It asks questions, such as: What are the strengths of the relationships between risk factors and diseases? This is known as **estimation**. Statistical analysis also draws conclusions from data on small groups (samples) about larger groups or populations—this is called **inference** or statistical significance testing.

information has become an art as well as a science that deserves attention from all those who use information.[6] **BOX 3.2** takes a look at the uses and misuses of graphics.

Issues of quality are key to the presentation of information. The Internet is increasingly the primary source of public health information for the user. Thus, when we address issues of quality, we need to have a

---

## BOX 3.2 Displaying Health Information[7]

Graphics are used primarily to display and examine possible relationships or associations. The wide array of graphical displays of data that are now available means that you need to have an understanding how graphics can help inform the user but also how they can mislead the user.

Let us briefly look at the uses and abuses of the three basic forms of graphical presentation: X–Y graphics, geometric graphics, and pie charts.

### X–Y Graphics

X–Y graphics, or what are often called *line graphs*, are a popular and attractive method for presenting large amounts of information in a single figure. X–Y graphs use a horizontal scale called an *X-axis* and a vertical scale called a *Y-axis*. They are very useful for displaying possible associations, or what are often called *correlations*, when both measurements have a large number of potential levels.

**FIGURE 3.2** provides data on a hypothetical country Z illustrating the way X–Y graphs should be used. This same data will be used for all of the graphics in this box.

The figures (diamond, square, triangle, and X) represent the point when death rates are actually measured. Straight lines are then drawn to connect these points. Notice that the lines do not extend beyond the

points in which actual data or information is available. Also notice that both the X-axis and the Y-axis go all the way to zero even though there is no data close to zero.

When X–Y graphics do not strictly follow this approach, they may produce misleading results. For instance X–Y graphs may be drawn with lines that extend far beyond the data. This is known as *extrapolation beyond the data*. It assumes that events will continue to increase (or decrease) at the same pace beyond the information provided. Here, if one extrapolates the rate of cancer, it might be concluded that in the future cancer will far exceed coronary heart disease. This may or may not turn out to be true. Predicting the future is always a difficult job and requires far more than expecting current trends to continue.

It is tempting when little or no data exist near the zero point on the X-axis or Y-axis to stop the data at a higher point. **FIGURE 3.3** illustrates how this type of display of health information can be misleading. Here, it looks like the rate of cancer deaths is increasing very rapidly, far more rapidly than in Figure 3.2. Yet, both figures come from the same data. By "cutting-off" the death rates at 350 per 100,000 instead of at zero (as in Figure 3.2), the apparent increase in cancer rates is magnified.

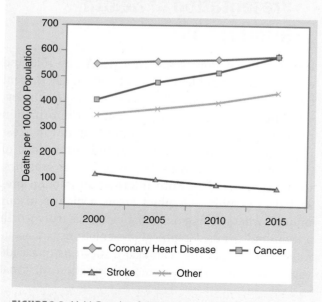

**FIGURE 3.2** X–Y Graph of the Deaths in Country Z per 100,000 Population

Reproduced from Perrin KM. *Principles of Health Navigation: Understanding Roles and Career Options.* Burlington, MA: Jones & Bartlett Learning; 2017.

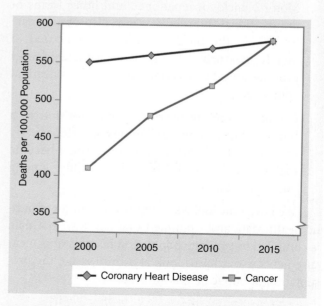

**FIGURE 3.3** X–Y Graph of the Deaths in Country Z with Rates "Cut-Off" at 350

Reproduced from Perrin KM. *Principles of Health Navigation: Understanding Roles and Career Options.* Burlington, MA: Jones & Bartlett Learning; 2017.

Notice the use of the symbol "~" on the Y-axis in Figure 3.3. It alerts the viewer that levels have been left out of the Y-axis. When not displaying the full scale on the X-axis or Y-axis, it is expected that a "~" will be inserted to alert the reader to this omission to try to avoid misinterpretation.

## Geometric Graphics

Traditional geometric graphics are often called *column charts* or *bar charts* because they display data using rectangular columns or bars, as indicated in **FIGURE 3.4**. Once again Figure 3.4 comes from the same data used in the previous figures.

Column graphics are very good ways to display information, especially when there are only a limited number of potential categories of information such as coronary artery disease, cancer, stroke, and other. Column charts help avoid extrapolation beyond the data. In addition, they do not require drawing lines between points where data is actually measured. Therefore, column graphics are often the best presentation of the data because they are the least likely to be misleading.

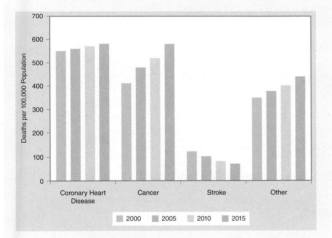

**FIGURE 3.4** Column Chart of Deaths in Country Z per 100,000 Population

Reproduced from Perrin KM. *Principles of Health Navigation: Understanding Roles and Career Options*. Burlington, MA: Jones & Bartlett Learning; 2017.

As shown in Figure 3.4, a column chart allows side-by-side comparison between different groups. However, Figure 3.4 may look more complicated than Figure 3.2, despite the fact that it includes exactly the same data. Therefore, people may prefer X–Y graphics.

## Pie Charts

Pie charts or percentage charts display the percentage of the total that is associated with each of the components that make up the whole at one point in time. **FIGURE 3.5** shows the same 2018 data that were used earlier. However, this time only the percentage of people who die from coronary artery disease, cancer, stroke, and other can be seen in Figure 3.5. Pie charts from different populations are often presented using the same size pie despite the fact that the actual rates may be very different in the two populations. Therefore, comparisons between these pies should talk about the "percentage of the pie" and not the "size of the piece of pie."

Graphics can be a very useful way to display and examine associations, literally providing a picture of what is happening. It is important, however, to be sure that the graphic does not mislead the user.

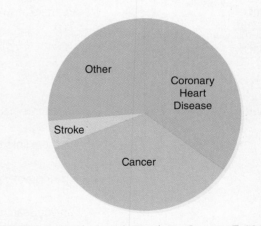

**FIGURE 3.5** Pie Chart with Deaths in Country Z, 2018

Reproduced from Perrin KM. *Principles of Health Navigation: Understanding Roles and Career Options*. Burlington, MA: Jones & Bartlett Learning; 2017.

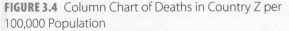

set of criteria for judging the quality of information presented on the Internet. Before relying on a website for health information, you should ask yourself key questions.[8] These questions are summarized in **TABLE 3.4**. Try these out the next time that you view a health information website.

The presentation of health information also requires taking into account the audience who will be using the material. Understanding the degree of **health literacy** of the intended audience is so important that a national movement has developed

to address these issues. Health literacy is more than the ability to read. It refers to the degree to which individuals have the capacity to obtain, process, and understand basic health information and services needed to make appropriate health decisions.[9]

Even the most accurate data presentation does not tell us how the user will perceive the data. Let us take a look at the rapidly growing component of health communications that deals with how we perceive information.

| **TABLE 3.4** Quality Standards for Health Information on the Internet | |
|---|---|
| **Criteria** | **Questions to ask** |
| Overall site quality | Is the purpose of the site clear? |
| | Is the site easy to navigate? |
| | Are the site's sponsors clearly identified? |
| | Are advertising and sales separated from health information? |
| Authors | Are the authors of the information clearly identified? |
| | Do the authors have health credentials? |
| | Is contact information provided? |
| Information | Does the site get its information from reliable sources? |
| | Is the information useful and easy to understand? |
| | Is it easy to tell the difference between fact and opinion? |
| Relevance | Are there answers to your specific questions? |
| Timeliness | Can you tell when the information was written? |
| | Is it current? |
| Links | Do the internal links work? |
| | Are there links to related sites for more information? |
| Privacy | Is your privacy protected? |
| | Can you search for information without providing information about yourself? |

Data from American Public Health Association. Criteria for Assessing the Quality of Health Information on the Internet. *American Journal of Public Health*. 2001;91(3):513–514.

## ▶ What Factors Affect How We Perceive Public Health Information?

Regardless of how accurately information is presented, communication also needs to consider how the recipient perceives the information. Therefore, we also need to look at factors known to affect the perception of information or the subjective interpretation of what the information means for an individual.

At least three types of effects can greatly influence our perceptions of potential harms and benefits.[10] We will call them the **dread effect**, the **unfamiliarity effect**, and the **uncontrollability effect**. The dread effect is present with hazards that easily produce very visual and feared consequences. It explains why we often fear shark attacks more than drowning in a swimming pool. The dread effect may also be elicited by the potential for catastrophic events, ranging from nuclear meltdowns to a poisoning of the water supply.

Our degree of familiarity with a potential harm or a potential benefit can greatly influence how we perceive data and translate it for our own situation. Knowing a friend or relative who died of lung cancer may influence how we perceive the information on the

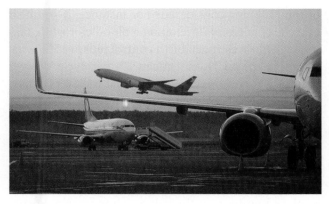

© Kichigin/Shutterstock

hazards of smoking or the presence of radon. It also may explain why we often see the danger of sun exposure as low and food irradiation as high, despite the fact that the data indicate that the degree of harm is the other way around.

Finally, the uncontrollability effect may have a major impact on our perceptions and actions. We often consider hazards that we perceive as in our control as less threatening than ones that we perceive as out of our control. Automobile collisions, for instance, are often seen as less hazardous than commercial airplane crashes, despite the fact that statistics show that commercial air travel is far safer than travel by automobile.

Perception of bad outcomes (or harms) and good outcomes (or benefits) needs to be considered along with the numbers if we are going to understand the ways information is used to make decisions. Not everyone perceives harms and benefits the same way. The selection of accurate and effective methods for conveying data is key to health communications.[g]

Understanding how we perceive information can help us design effective health messages. **BOX 3.3** discusses the SUCCESs approach to developing messages that stick.

One approach to addressing differing perceptions of information is the use of a method known as **decision analysis**. Decision analysis relies on the vast information-processing ability of computers to formally combine information on benefits and harms to reach quantitative decisions. It provides us with insight into the types of information that need to be combined. Let us look at how we combine information—the next question in our flow of health information.

---

**BOX 3.3** SUCCESs in Public Health Communications

Effective health communications starts with understanding how information is perceived. In their book *Made to Stick: Why Some Ideas Survive and Others Die*,[11] Chip and Dan Heath have come up with a memory technique they call SUCCESs, which focuses on the perception of ideas and identifies six principles of highly successful communications. SUCCESs stands for:

*Simplicity*: This first principle requires a short, memorable statement that captures the core of the message. The golden rule, the authors write, "is the ultimate model of simplicity: a one-sentence statement so profound that an individual could spend a lifetime learning to follow it."[12] While public health messages cannot be expected to rival the golden rule, some public health messages say it all. The Back-to-Sleep campaign, for instance, was able to convey the core of its message in just three words.

*Unexpectedness*: Getting and holding people's attention is often achieved by presenting unexpected facts that are counterintuitive, at least to your audience. Challenging common myths or conventional wisdom may be a good place to start when engaging an audience.

*Concreteness*: Proverbs often provide specific examples that can be remembered and generalized. For instance, "an apple a day keeps the doctor away" has become a memorable way of conveying the importance of diet in health. Providing concrete, easily visualized examples is key. Bad breath and brown teeth may be more convincing reasons for stopping cigarette smoking than the long-term consequences, which are not immediately obvious.

*Credibility*: Credibility relies not so much on numbers but rather on the source of the information. For instance, news of an epidemic may start with, "Today, the CDC announced…" Credibility is enhanced if people can test out the ideas from their own experience. "Think about the last time you texted while driving. Could it have waited until you stopped?"

*Emotions*: Connecting with people's emotions is key not only in getting their attention but also for ensuring they will retain the ideas. Emotions connect people with ideas. For instance, the Heaths write, "It's difficult to get teenagers to quit smoking by instilling in them a fear of the

---

g  For instance, we generally have difficulty distinguishing between small and very small numbers. The difference between 1 in 10,000 and 1 in 100,000 is difficult for most of us to grasp and incorporate into our decisions. When comparing these types of probabilities, it is tempting to compare the outcomes to ones that are better known, such as those with similar emotional impacts. We may compare the chances of dying from a motorcycle crash with the chances of dying from a truck or automobile crash. Comparison of different types of outcomes, such as between being struck by lightning compared to dying from a chronic exposure to chemicals or radiation, is far less informative.

consequences, but it's easier to get them to quit by tapping into their resentment of the duplicity of Big Tobacco."[13]

*Stories*: We remember and relate to stories about real or realistic people. Sharing "war stories" is a classic example of how people relate to the events in each other's lives. Short vignettes and stories help to make the issues real. Hopefully, the vignettes at the beginning of each chapter of *Public Health 101* accomplish this for you.

Putting the SUCCESs principles together as a coherent message is a real but important challenge. As the ideal example, the Heaths cite John F. Kennedy's famous challenge to "put a man on the moon and return him safely by the end of the decade."[14] They conclude that the message is simple, unexpected, amazingly concrete, and credible because it is from the president of the United States, full of emotion, and a story in miniature.

It is not so easy to put together such memorable messages, but focusing on how information is perceived and using the SUCCESs principles is a good way to start.

Data from Heath C and Heath D. *Made to Stick: Why Some Ideas Survive and Others Die.* New York: Random House; 2007.

## ▶ What Type of Information Needs to Be Combined to Make Health Decisions?

Decision analysis focuses on three key types of information that need to be combined as the basis for making decisions. We can better understand these types of information by asking the following questions:

- *How likely?*—What is the probability or chance that the particular outcome will occur?
- *How important?*—What is the value or importance we place on a good or a bad outcome?

When expressing the chances that an outcome will occur, we often express the results as a percentage from 0 to 100. Probabilities, on the other hand, range from 0 to 1. Percentages and probabilities are often used interchangeably—the probability of 0.10 can be converted to 10% and vice versa. When faced with a percentage or probability, we need to ask: What period of time is being considered? For instance, if you hear that the chances of developing a blood clot while taking high-dose estrogen birth control pills are 5%, what does that mean? Does it mean 5% per cycle, 5% per year, or 5% over the time period that the average user is on the pill?

Outcomes vary from death to disabilities. Some outcomes greatly affect our function and limit our future, while we can learn to live with other outcomes despite the limitations they impose. When dealing with a quantitative approach, we are forced to place numbers on the value or importance of specific outcomes. A scale known as a **utility scale** is one method to measure and compare the value or importance that different people place on different outcomes. This scale is intended to parallel the scale of probabilities; that is, it extends from 1 to 0 or from 100% to 0%. It defines 1% or 100% as the state of health in which there are no health-related limitations. Zero is defined as immediate death. On the utility scale, there is nothing worse than immediate death. **FIGURE 3.6** displays the utility scale.[h] **BOX 3.4** illustrates how we can use the utility scale to assign numbers to specific outcomes.

Utilities are important, especially when we need to combine potential harms with potential benefits. Probabilities alone often do not give us the answers we need when addressing issues of hazards ranging from environmental toxins to unhealthy behaviors. Utilities are also critical when looking at particular interventions, such as prevention or treatment options that include positive benefits, but also involve side effects or harms. Thus, whenever we need to combine or balance benefits and harms, we need to consider the utility of the outcomes along with the chances or probabilities of the outcomes. Probabilities and utilities (both on a scale of 0 to 1) are often combined by multiplying the probability by the utility to obtain a probability that takes into account the utility or what is called **expected utility.** Expected utilities are often displayed using graphical methods called **decision trees.**[15] **BOX 3.5** discusses the use of decision trees based on expected utilities.

100%                                          0%
|——————————————————————————|
Full Health                          Immediate Death

**FIGURE 3.6** Scale Used to Measure Utilities

---

h Many people consider prolonged incapacity or vegetative states as worse than death. The utility scale does not generally take this into account. This is a specific example of the more general limitation of quantitative decision-making—that it focuses on the outcome and not on the process of getting there.

## BOX 3.4 Obtaining a Utility Score

Let us see how we can use the utility scale to put numbers on a specific outcome: complete and permanent blindness. Using the scale in Figure 3.6, place a number on the importance or value that you give to complete and permanent blindness.

In large groups of individuals, the average utility placed on blindness is quite predictable—about 50%. However, the range of values among a group is generally quite wide ranging, from 20% to 80% and sometimes even wider. Predicting an individual's utility is quite difficult because gender, socioeconomic group, and other predictors have little impact.[a]

Individuals who place a high utility on complete and permanent blindness usually indicate that they can learn to live with blindness and it will not greatly affect their enjoyment of life. Those who place a low utility on blindness generally say just the opposite. Thus, we need to understand that a utility of 50% is an average, including some with a much higher and some with a much lower utility. Therefore, the best way to know the value or utility that an individual places on a particular outcome such as blindness is to ask him or her.

a There are at least two predictors that are of some value. Those who have experienced an outcome usually find that they can adapt to it to a certain extent and usually rate its utility as somewhat higher than those who have not experienced the outcome. Second, age does have an impact on the scoring of utility. Younger people generally rate the utility of an outcome as somewhat worse or lower than older people, perhaps due to the longer-term impact the disability has on their future options. The average utility placed on blindness by college students, for instance, is often closer to 40%. Neither of these impacts is large on average, nor can they be used to successfully predict the utility of any one individual.

## BOX 3.5 Using Decision Trees to Compare Interventions

Decision trees are a visual method for displaying the benefits and harms of two or more options for intervention. They allow us to directly compare the outcomes, incorporating the probability and the utility of each outcome in a process known as decision analysis. Decision trees are made up of two types of nodes, which reflect points in which decisions are made or events occur by chance. Therefore, we speak of **choice nodes** and **chance nodes**. As indicated in **FIGURE 3.7**, choice nodes are presented using a square box, while chance nodes are represented using a circle.

Let us see how choice nodes and chance nodes can be put together to develop a decision tree. **FIGURE 3.8**

represents a simple decision tree. For each of the outcomes, a probability is included.

Note that the probability of each of the potential outcomes adds to 1% or 100%. For intervention #1, the potential outcomes are cure and die. For intervention #2,

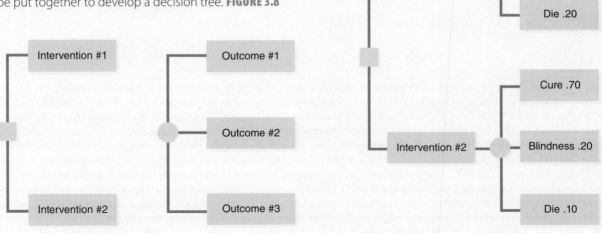

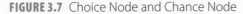

**FIGURE 3.7** Choice Node and Chance Node

**FIGURE 3.8** Decision Tree

there is a third potential outcome: blindness. To compare intervention #1 and intervention #2, we need to know more than the probabilities of each outcome—we need to know the utility of blindness.

To compare intervention #1 and intervention #2, we will need to assume that die has a utility of 0 and cure has a utility of 1. Blindness is a more subjective utility. As we have seen, on average, it has been found that people regard blindness as having a utility of about 0.5. However, many people will have a utility that is as high as 0.8 or as low as 0.2. Let us start by using a utility of 0.5. In **FIGURE 3.9**, the probabilities and utilities of each intervention have been filled in, and the probability has been multiplied by the utility to produce what is called an expected utility, or a probability that takes into account the utility of the outcomes. We can add together the expected utilities of each potential outcome to produce an overall expected utility. The overall expected utilities allow us to compare one intervention to another.

Notice that when we use a utility of 0.5, the overall expected utilities for the two interventions are the

same. At least by decision analysis, these two potential interventions are considered a toss-up.

Now let us see what happens when we change the utility of blindness first to 0.8 and then to 0.2. **FIGURE 3.10** displays the decision tree and expected utilities when blindness's utility is set at 0.8. **FIGURE 3.11** displays the decision tree and expected utilities when blindness's utility is set at 0.2.

Notice that when the utility is set at 0.8 in Figure 3.10, the overall expected utility for intervention #2 is greatest. That is, the decision analysis recommends intervention #2 over intervention #1. However, in Figure 3.11, when the utility of blindness is set at 0.2, the overall utility for intervention #1 is greater than intervention #2. That is, the decision analysis recommends intervention #1 over intervention #2. When a factor, such as the utility we place on blindness, produces a change in the recommended choice of intervention, we say that the decision analysis is **sensitive** to the factor, such as blindness.[a]

Decision trees and decision analysis are increasingly being used to display the options for intervention and

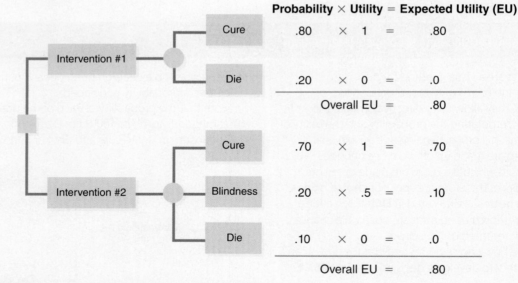

**FIGURE 3.9** Decision Analysis with Utility of Blindness Equal to 0.5

a  Decision trees assume that an outcome is measured by its probability multiplied by its utility. Thus, expected utility focuses on outcomes, not on the process of getting there. Therefore, this approach considers an outcome such as death or blindness to be the same whether it occurs suddenly or after a complicated hospitalization with multiple unsuccessful interventions. Also note that the example used does not take into account the timing of the outcome. It is possible in decision analysis to take into account the timing of outcomes through the process of discounting. Decision analysis assumes that when two chance nodes appear one after another, the probability of the second outcome is not affected by the outcome of the first node; that is, the chances of a good or bad outcome after the first and second chance nodes are independent of each other. The decision trees used in this box are also simplified in that only one choice node is presented. It is possible to introduce choice nodes even after a chance node. Decision trees may become very complex and may need to become so in order to realistically reflect the choice and chance situations faced in practice. However, the more complex the decision tree, the more data is needed to utilize it to make recommendations.

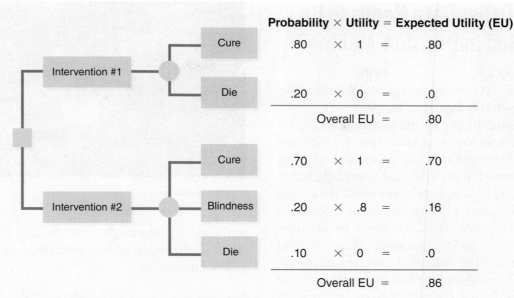

**Probability × Utility = Expected Utility (EU)**

|  |  |  |
|---|---|---|
| .80 × 1 = | .80 |  |
| .20 × 0 = | .0 |  |
| Overall EU = | .80 |  |

|  |  |  |
|---|---|---|
| .70 × 1 = | .70 |  |
| .20 × .8 = | .16 |  |
| .10 × 0 = | .0 |  |
| Overall EU = | .86 |  |

**FIGURE 3.10** Decision Analysis with Utility of Blindness Equal to 0.8

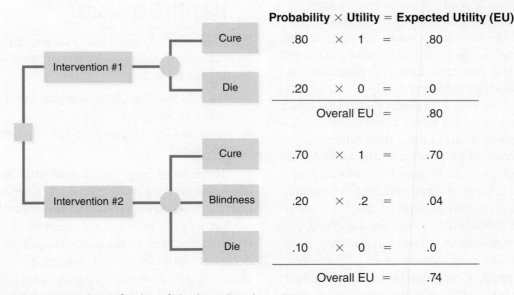

**Probability × Utility = Expected Utility (EU)**

|  |  |  |
|---|---|---|
| .80 × 1 = | .80 |  |
| .20 × 0 = | .0 |  |
| Overall EU = | .80 |  |

|  |  |  |
|---|---|---|
| .70 × 1 = | .70 |  |
| .20 × .2 = | .04 |  |
| .10 × 0 = | .0 |  |
| Overall EU = | .74 |  |

**FIGURE 3.11** Decision Analysis of Utility of Blindness Equal to 0.2

to compare them based on probabilities and utilities. Decision trees are increasingly used as part of public health decision-making for populations and for health policy decisions that affect large groups. Decision trees are often far more complex in an effort to reflect the realities of decision-making. Decision analysis can help us compare interventions and help us recognize why individuals or organizations may come to different conclusions about their preferred intervention.[b]

---

b  Decision analysis, which compares interventions for two or more conditions, frequently utilizes a measure of outcome known as **quality adjusted life-years**, or QALYs. QALYs incorporate the increase or decrease in life-expectancy as well as the probabilities and utilities of each outcome. QALYs may be used in decision analysis, but they are expected for cost-effectiveness analysis.

# What Other Data Needs to Be Included in Decision-Making?

We also need to ask:

*How soon?*—When, on average, will the particular outcome happen if it is going to happen?

The expected timing of the occurrence of good and bad outcomes can also affect how we view the outcome. Most people view the occurrence of a bad outcome as worse if it occurs in the immediate future compared to years from now. Conversely, we usually view a good outcome as more valuable if it occurs in the immediate future. Thus, whenever we consider harms and benefits and try to combine them, we need to ask: When are the outcomes expected to occur? When both the good and the bad outcomes occur in the immediate future, the timing is not an issue. In public health and medicine, however, this is rarely the case. When dealing with many treatments, the benefits come first, while the harms may occur at a later time. When dealing with vaccines and surgery, the pain and side effects often precede the potential gain. The timing of the benefits is rarely the same as the timing of the harms. Thus, we need to take the timing into account. This process is known as **discounting**. Discounting is a quantitative process in which we give greater emphasis or weight to events that are expected to occur in the immediate future compared to events that are expected to occur in the distant future.[i]

We have seen that probabilities, utilities, and timing are key components of health communications that need to be combined when making public health and healthcare decisions.[j] However, there are other factors that are characteristic not of the data itself, but of the **decision maker**. A decision maker may be an individual; a health professional; or an organization, such as a nonprofit, a corporation, or a government agency. Let us turn our attention to decision makers

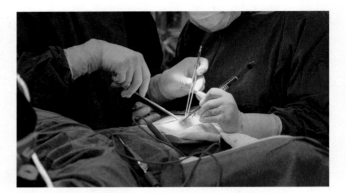

© Samrith Na Lumpoon/Shutterstock

and ask how we can go about making decisions. To do this, we need to address issues beyond probability, utility, and timing.

# How Do We Utilize Information to Make Health Decisions?

There are two key questions that we can ask to gain an understanding of how we use information to make health decisions:

- How do our risk-taking attitudes affect the way we make decisions?
- How do we incorporate information into our decisions?

There are a large number of attitudes that can affect the way we make decisions. One of the most important is known as our **risk-taking attitudes**.

Let us examine what we mean by this term and see what type of risk-taking attitude you use in making decisions. Attitudes toward risk greatly influence the choices that we all make in the prevention and treatment of disease.[9] **BOX 3.6** illustrates how you can understand

---

i The exact amount of discounting that should occur is controversial, but there is agreement that we should place less importance on outcomes that occur in the distant future than those that occur in the immediate future. There is also agreement that the rate of discounting for harms and for benefits should be the same. The concept of discounting comes from economics and can be most easily understood with a financial example. Let us imagine that we want to discount at 5% per year. A discount rate of 5% implies that I am willing to give you $95 today if you are willing to give me $100 1 year from now. Discounting is above and beyond inflation, so the actual return may be $100 plus the rate of inflation. Note that economists try to set the rate based on the average real return on money invested over a large number of years. In the past, this has been about 3% in most developed countries. When making decisions on a subjective basis, we often discount the future at a much higher rate. This is especially true of those who are very sick and are often focused heavily on the immediate future.

j Decision analysis is not the usual method used to combine information. Because the task of combining information is so complex and the ability of our minds to handle large quantities of information is so limited, we often use rules of thumb known as **heuristics**. Heuristics allow us to make decisions more rapidly and often with less information. For instance, we often prefer to structure decisions to allow only one of two choices, rather than choosing from a large number of options presented to us at the same time. Thus, we often narrow the field of candidates in primary elections to allow side-by-side comparisons in the general elections. The one-on-one comparisons allow manipulation of the results by getting rid of candidates in the primaries who might have fared better in the general election.

## BOX 3.6 Risk-Taking Attitudes

Review the following situations and write down your decisions.

### Situation A

Imagine that you have coronary artery disease and have a reduced quality of life with a utility of 0.80, compared to your previous state of full health with a utility of 1.00. You are offered the following pair of options. You can select only one option. Which of the following options do you prefer?

OPTION #1: A treatment with the following possible outcomes:

50% chance of raising the quality of your health (your utility) from 0.80 to 1.00
50% chance of reducing the quality of your health (your utility) from 0.80 to 0.60

OPTION #2: Refuse the treatment described in Option #1 and accept a quality of your health (your utility) of 0.80

### Situation B

Imagine that you have coronary artery disease and have a reduced quality of life that has a utility of 0.20, compared to your previous state of full health that had a utility of 1.00. You are offered the following pair of options. You can select only one option. Which of the following options do you prefer?

OPTION #1: A treatment with the following possible outcomes:

10% chance of raising the quality of your health (your utility) from 0.20 to 1.00
90% chance of reducing the quality of your health (your utility) from 0.20 to 0.11

OPTION #2: Refuse the treatment in Option #1 and accept a quality of your health (your utility) of 0.20

What was your answer in situation A? Situation B? To understand the meaning of your answers, you need to appreciate that in terms of the probabilities and utilities presented in each situation, these options are a toss-up.

That is, taking into account the probabilities and the utilities, there is no difference between these options. To convince yourself of this, draw a decision tree including the two options in situation A and the two options in situation B. You will find that they produce the same overall expected utilities.[a]

The information does not determine your choice; it must be your attitude toward taking chances, which is your attitude toward risk taking.

Did you choose option #2 in situation A and option #1 in situation B? Most, but not all, people make these choices. In situation A, we begin with a utility of 0.80. For many people, this is a tolerable situation and they do not want to take any chances of being reduced to a lower, perhaps intolerable utility. Thus, they want to guarantee a tolerable level of health. We can call this the **certainty effect**. In situation B, we begin with a utility of 0.20. For many people, this is an intolerable situation. Thus, people are usually willing to take their chances of getting even worse in the hopes of a major improvement in their health. When the quality of life is bad enough, most, if not all, people are willing to take their chances and go for it. This risk-taking behavior can be called the **long-shot effect**. Thus, risk-taking and risk-avoiding choices are both common, defensible, and reasonably predictable. Most of us are **risk takers** when conditions are intolerable and **risk avoiders** when conditions are tolerable.

A few people will choose option #1 in both situations A and B. These individuals are willing to take their chances in a range of situations in order to improve their outcome. We call them risk takers. Are you one of them? The only way to know is to ask yourself. Similarly, a few people will choose option #2 in both situations. These individuals seek to avoid taking chances in a range of situations in order to preserve their current state of health. We call them risk avoiders. Are you one of them? Only you can answer that question.[b]

---

a  Notice that the outcomes occur in the immediate future so there is no issue of timing or need to discount the benefits or the harms.
b  There is a fourth option, which is to choose option #2 in situation A and option #1 in situation B. The small number of individuals who make this choice usually have a very different perception of what utilities mean to them. For instance, they might perceive little difference between a 0.80 and a 0.20 utility.

---

your own attitudes toward risk taking by making some choices. We will assume that you understand what we mean by "utilities" and that you have thought through what a wide range of utilities means to you personally.

Understanding attitudes toward risk is important for analyzing how individuals make decisions about their own lives. It is also key when trying to understand how

group decisions are made that require society to balance harms and benefits. Perhaps the most common health decisions that you will make are the decisions related to your health care and that of your family. Therefore, let us complete our examination of health communications by looking at three different approaches that can be used to make clinical healthcare decisions.

# How Can We Use Health Information to Make Healthcare Decisions?

There are three basic approaches to using health information to make healthcare decisions. We will call these approaches **inform of decision**, **informed consent**, and **shared decision-making**. Preferences for these types of approaches have changed over time, yet all three are currently part of clinical practice.

The inform of decision approach implies that the clinician has all the essential information and can make decisions that are in the patient's best interest. The role of the clinician is then merely to inform the patient of what needs to be done and to prescribe the treatment, or write the orders. At one point in time, this type of decision-making approach was standard for practicing clinicians. In the not-too-distant past, clinicians rarely told patients that they had cancer, justifying their silence by arguments that the knowledge might make the patient depressed, which could interfere with their response to the disease and to the treatment. The decision to administer tests and prescribe a range of medications is still often done using the inform of decision approach.

A second type of decision-making approach is called informed consent. It rests on the principle that ultimately, patients need to give their permission or consent before major interventions, such as surgery, radiation, or chemotherapy, can be undertaken. Informed consent may be written, spoken, or implied. Clinically, informed consent implies that individuals have the right to know what will be done, why it will be done, and what the known benefits and harms are. Patients have the right to ask questions, including inquiring about the availability of other options. Informed consent does not mean that all possible options are presented to the patient, but it does imply that a clinician has made a recommendation for a specific intervention.

The third type of decision-making is called shared decision-making. In this approach, the clinician's job is to provide information to the patient with which he or she can make a decision. This might include directly giving information to the patient; providing consultations; or referring patients to sources of information, often on the Internet. Shared decision-making places a far greater burden on the patient to seek out, understand, and use information. Using this approach, clinicians are not required to provide recommendations on specific interventions, though patients are free to ask for a clinician's opinion.[16]

All three types of decision-making approaches are currently in use today. **TABLE 3.5** outlines the process and roles implied by each of these approaches, as well

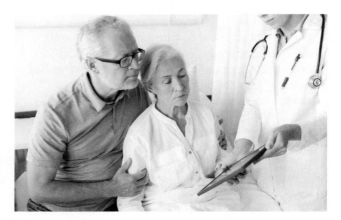

© Syda Productions/Shutterstock

| **TABLE 3.5** Types of Individual Decision-Making | | | |
|---|---|---|---|
| **Type of decision-making** | **Process/roles** | **Advantages** | **Disadvantages** |
| Inform of decision | Clinician has all the essential information to make a decision that is in the patient's best interest | May be efficient and effective when patients seek clear direction provided by an authoritative and trusted source | Patient may not gain information and understanding of the nature of the problem or the nature of the treatment |
| | Clinician aims to convey his or her decision as a clear and unambiguous action or order | Patients may favor if they do not seek out or feel they can handle independent decision-making responsibilities | Patient may not be prepared to participate in the implementation of the decision |

| | | | |
|---|---|---|---|
| | Patients accept the clinician's recommendation without necessarily understanding or agreeing with the underlying reasoning | | Patient may not accept responsibility for the outcome of the treatment |
| Informed consent | Clinician has the responsibility to convey a recommendation to the patient. The patient must decide whether to accept or reject the recommendation | Patient gains information and understanding of the nature of the problem or the nature of the treatment | Time consuming compared to informing of the decision |
| | Harms and benefits of treatment are weighed by the clinician in making a recommendation | Patient may be prepared to participate in the implementation of the decision | May require elaborate paperwork to implement formal informed consent process |
| | Clinician has a responsibility to provide information on the aim of the recommendation, the potential benefits, the known harms, and the process that will occur; the patient has the right to ask additional questions about the treatment and the availability of other alternatives | Patient may accept responsibility for the outcome of the treatment | May increase emphasis on legal documents and malpractice law |
| Shared decision-making | Clinicians serve as a source of information for patients, including providing it directly or identifying means of obtaining information | May increase the control of the patients over their own lives | May be time consuming for patients and clinicians |
| | Patients can expect to be informed of the existence of a range of accepted options and be assisted in their efforts to obtain information | May increase the types of information considered in decision-making | May increase the costs of health care |
| | Patients may seek information on experimental or alternative approaches and can discuss the advantages and disadvantages of these approaches with a clinician | May reduce the adversarial nature of the relationship between clinicians and patients | May increase the stress/anxiety for patients |
| | Considerations besides benefits and harms are part of the decision-making process, including such considerations as cost, risk-taking attitudes, and the distress/discomforts associated with the treatment | May improve the outcome of care by increasing the patient's understanding and commitment to the chosen course of care | May shift the responsibility for bad outcomes from the clinician to the patient (i.e., takes the clinician off the hook/clinician does not need to do the hard work of thinking through the decision and making a recommendation) |
| | Patients are often directly involved in the implementation of care | | |

as some of the potential advantages and disadvantages of each approach.

Health communications provides key tools for population health. We have taken a look at important issues related to each of them. We have asked questions about how public health data and information is collected, compiled, presented, perceived, combined, and used in decision-making. Data and information are key public health tools for guiding our decision-making. We will find ourselves coming back again and again to these principles as we study the population health approach. Now, let us turn our attention to the utilization of the social and behavioral sciences as key tools of public health.

## Key Words

Certainty effect
Chance nodes
Choice nodes
Data
Databases
Decision analysis
Decision maker
Decision trees
Disability-adjusted life year (DALY)
Discounting
Dread effect
Estimation
Expected utility

Health communications
Health literacy
Health-adjusted life expectancy (HALE)
Health-related quality of life (HRQOL)
Heuristics
Infant mortality rate
Inference
Inform of decision
Informed consent
Life expectancy
Long-shot effect
Population health status measures

Public health surveillance
Quality adjusted life-years (QALYs)
Risk avoiders
Risk takers
Risk-taking attitudes
Sensitive
Shared decision-making
Uncontrollability effect
Under-5 mortality
Unfamiliarity effect
Utility scale

## Discussion Questions

Take a look at the questions posed in the following scenarios, which were presented at the beginning of this chapter. See whether you can now answer these questions.

1. You read that the rate of use of cocaine among teenagers has fallen by 50% in the last decade. You wonder where that information might come from.

2. You hear that life expectancy in the United States is now approximately 80 years. You wonder what that implies about how long you will live and what that means for your grandmother, who is 82 and in good health.

3. You hear on the news the gruesome description of a shark attack on a young boy from another state and decide to keep your son away from the beach. While playing at a friend's house, your son nearly drowns after falling into the backyard pool. You ask why so many people think that drowning in a backyard pool is unusual when it is far more common than shark attacks.

4. "Balancing the harms and benefits is essential to making decisions," your clinician says. The treatment you are considering has an 80% chance of working, but there is also a 20% chance of side effects. "What do I need to consider when balancing the harms and the benefits?" you ask.

5. You are faced with a decision to have a medical procedure. One physician tells you there is no other choice and you must undergo the procedure, another tells you about the harms and benefits and advises you to go ahead, and the third lays out the options and tells you it is your decision. Why are there such different approaches to making decisions these days?

## References

1. Gordis L. *Epidemiology*. 5th ed. Philadelphia, PA: Elsevier Saunders; 2014.
2. Friis RH, Sellers TA. *Epidemiology for Public Health Practice*. 5th ed. Burlington, MA: Jones & Bartlett Learning; 2013.
3. Skolnik R. *Global Health 101*. 3rd ed. Burlington, MA: Jones & Bartlett Learning; 2016.
4. World Health Organization. Healthy life expectancy (HLE) at birth (years). World Health Statistics 2016. http://www.who.int/gho/publications/world_health_statistics/2016/en/. Accessed July 18, 2017.
5. World Health Organization. Global burden of disease. http://www.who.int/topics/global_burden_of_disease/en/. Accessed July 16, 2017.

6. Tufte ER. *The Visual Display of Quantitative Information*. 2nd ed. Cheshire, CT: Graphics Press; 2001.

7. Perrin KM. *Principles of Health Navigation: Understanding Roles and Career Options*. Burlington, MA: Jones & Bartlett Learning; 2017.

8. American Public Health Association. Criteria for assessing the quality of health information on the internet. *American Journal of Public Health*. 2001;91(3): 513–514.

9. National Network of Libraries of Medicine. Health literacy. http://nnlm.gov/outreach/consumer/hlthlit.html. Accessed July 18, 2017.

10. Dawes RM, Hastie R. *Rational Choice in an Uncertain World*. Thousand Oaks, CA: Sage Publications; 2001.

11. Heath C, Heath D. *Made to Stick: Why Some Ideas Survive and Others Die*. New York: Random House; 2007.

12. Heath C, Heath D. *Made to Stick: Why Some Ideas Survive and Others Die*. New York: Random House; 2007:16.

13. Heath C, Heath D. *Made to Stick: Why Some Ideas Survive and Others Die*. New York: Random House; 2007:18.

14. Heath C, Heath D. *Made to Stick: Why Some Ideas Survive and Others Die*. New York: Random House; 2007:21.

15. Riegelman RK. *Studying a Study and Testing a Test: Reading Evidence-Based Health Research*. Philadelphia, PA: Lippincott, Williams and Wilkins; 2013.

16. Riegelman RK. *Measures of Medicine: Benefits, Harms and Costs*. Cambridge, MA: Blackwell Science; 1995.

# CHAPTER 4

# Social and Behavioral Sciences and Public Health

## LEARNING OBJECTIVES

By the end of this chapter, the student will be able to:

- explain relationships between the social and behavioral sciences and public health.
- illustrate how socioeconomic status affects health.
- illustrate how culture and religion affect health.
- describe the relationship between income and socioeconomic status and health.
- describe key categories of social determinants of health.
- describe the role of theory in changing health behavior.
- identify the three levels of influence in which theories and models are categorized and provide examples of theories and models corresponding to these three levels.
- explain the principles of social marketing.
- identify the steps of the PRECEDE-PROCEED planning framework.

You travel to a country in Asia and find that this nation's culture affects most parts of life. From the food the people eat and their method of cooking, to their attitudes toward medical care, to their beliefs about the cause of disease and the ability to alter it through public health and medical interventions, this country is profoundly different from the United States. You ask: How does culture affect health?

You are working in a community in the United States with strict Islamic practices and find that religion, like culture, can have major impacts on health. Religious practices differ widely—from beliefs about food and alcohol; to sexual practices, such as male circumcision and female sexual behavior; to acceptance or rejection of interventions aimed at women's health. You ask: How does religion affect health?

You are trying to help your spouse quit smoking cigarettes and prevent your kids from starting. You know that gentle encouragement and support on a one-on-one basis are essential, but often not enough because cigarette smoking is an addiction that produces withdrawal and long-term cravings. You wonder what other factors in the social system influence behavior and how they can be addressed.

Your efforts to convince your friends to avoid smoking (or stop smoking) focus on giving them the facts about how cigarettes cause lung cancer, throat cancer, and serious heart disease. You are frustrated by how little impact you have on your friends. You wonder what tools are available to better explain and predict health behavior.

Your classmate, who is the first in her family to attend college, received word that her father lost his job at the local factory and she needs to take a leave from school because her family can no longer afford tuition. You wonder how this will affect her and her family.

Your town board just approved extending public transportation services to a wider geographic area. Although there are several opponents to the plan, you learn that a group of public health professionals supports this extension of services. You wonder what this transportation plan has to do with health.

You are in the checkout line at the grocery store, and a pregnant mother is ahead of you. You glance at the sugary cereals, snacks, and sodas she is purchasing and happen to notice that she is using an EBT card from the Supplemental Nutrition Assistance Program (SNAP), formerly known as the Food Stamp program. You wonder what could be done to encourage the consumption of healthy food options.

Every day on your way to work, you pass the same homeless man on the same corner. He does not look very old—you guess he is about 25 years of age. You notice that over the past few weeks, he has been coughing, and you figure he must have a cold. Today when you walk by his usual place on the corner, he is not there, but someone has left a sign that reads, "Rest in peace, Ramón." You are surprised, especially because he was so young. You wonder whether there was anything that could have been done to prevent his death.

As a new parent, you hear from your pediatrician, nurses in the hospital, and even the makers of your brand of diapers that babies should sleep on their backs. They call it "Back-to-Sleep." You are surprised to find that it is part of the class on baby-sitting given by the local community center and a required part of the training for those who work in registered day care centers. You find out that it is all part of a Back-to-Sleep social marketing campaign that has halved the number of deaths

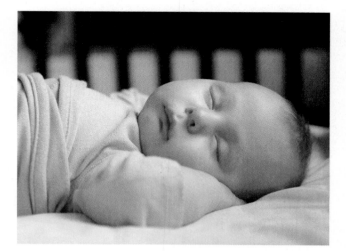

© Christin Lola/Shutterstock

from sudden infant death syndrome. You ask: Why has the Back-to-Sleep campaign been so successful?

Each of these cases illustrates ways that an understanding of social and behavioral sciences can contribute to an understanding of public health. Let us explore these connections.

## ▶ How Is Public Health Related to the Social and Behavioral Sciences?

The development of social and behavioral sciences in the 1800s and 1900s is closely connected with the development of public health. These subject areas share a fundamental belief that understanding the organization and motivation behind social forces, along with a better understanding of the behavior of individuals, can be used to improve the lives of individuals, as well as society as a whole.[1]

The 19th-century development of social and behavioral sciences, as well as public health, grew out of the Industrial Revolution in Europe, and later in the United States. It was grounded in efforts to address the social and economic inequalities that developed during this period and provided an intellectual and institutional structure for what was and is now called **social justice**. Social justice implies a society that provides fair treatment and a fair share of the rewards of society to individuals and groups of individuals. Early public health reformers advocated for social justice and saw public health as an integral aspect of it.

The intellectual link between social and behavioral sciences and public health is so basic and so deep that it

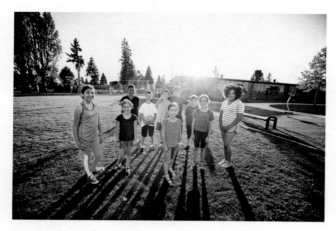

© Thomas Barwick/Digital Vision/Getty Images

is often taken for granted. For students with opportunities to learn about both social sciences and public health, it is important to understand the key contributions that social sciences make to public health. It is not an exaggeration to view public health as an application of the social sciences, or in other words, as an applied social science. **TABLE 4.1** summarizes many of the contributions that the social sciences make to public health.

## How Are Social Systems Related to Health?

### Complex Interactions

As humans, we are constantly interacting with our surroundings. Those surroundings include social systems comprised of interactions we have with other people, institutions, communities, and policies. The relationship between individuals and social systems is reciprocal, meaning we influence our social systems and our social systems influence us.

Due to our constant interaction with our surroundings, efforts aimed at improving population health require an understanding of the complex relationship between social systems and health. Medical care is only a piece of the puzzle, with a focus on treating disease without addressing the conditions in the social system that contributed to the illness in the first place.

To assist in pulling apart the complex social characteristics that impact health, it is useful to consider different levels of influence within the social system.

**TABLE 4.1** Examples of Contributions of Social and Behavioral Sciences to Public Health

| Social science discipline[a] | Examples of disciplinary contributions to public health |
| --- | --- |
| Psychology | Theories of the origins of behavior and risk-taking tendencies and methods for altering individual and social behaviors |
| Sociology | Theories of social development, organizational behavior, and systems thinking; social impacts on individual and group behaviors |
| Anthropology | Social and cultural influences on individual and population decision-making for health with a global perspective |
| Political science/public policy | Approaches to government and policy making related to public health; structures for policy analysis and the impact of government on public health decision-making |
| Economics | Understanding the micro- and macroeconomic impact on public health and healthcare systems |
| Communications | Theory and practice of mass and personalized communication and the role of media in communicating health information and health risks |
| Demography | Understanding demographic changes in populations globally due to aging, migration, and differences in birth rates, plus their impact on health and society |
| Geography | Understanding the impacts of geography on disease and determinants of disease, as well as methods for displaying and tracking the location of disease occurrence |

[a] A similar list of contributions of the humanities could be developed including the contributions of literature, the arts, history, philosophy, and ethics. These contributions of the social sciences are in addition to contributions of the sciences, mathematics, and humanities. Biology, chemistry, and statistics underpin much of epidemiology and environmental health. Languages and culture, history, and the arts provide key contributions to health communications and health policy. Thus, a broad arts and sciences education is often considered a key part of preparation for public health.

Social science models are often employed to gain an understanding of the various social influences on health as well as to assist in identifying points at which to intervene. In general, the levels of influence include:

- Individual lifestyle factors: Characteristics of the individual, including knowledge, attitudes, beliefs, and personality traits, as well as age, sex, and hereditary factors.
- Social and community networks: Points at which interaction with other individuals occurs. This sphere of influence can further be divided into the following levels:
  - Interpersonal: Family, friends, and peers who shape social identity, support, and roles.
  - Institutional/organizational: Rules and regulations of institutions, such as schools and places of employment, which may limit or promote healthy behavior.
  - Community: Comprises informal and formal social networks and norms formed among individuals, groups, and organizations, including cultural and religious practices.
- General socioeconomic, cultural, and environmental conditions: Components of the surroundings external to individuals that comprise living and working conditions, such as education, housing, work environment, and healthcare services. These conditions are shaped by public policy and laws at the local, state, and federal levels.

## Influencing Behavior

The complex relationship between social systems and individuals affects health through individual behavior. Berkman and Kawachi argue that social systems influence behavior by[2]:

1. Shaping norms: Certain behaviors may become generally accepted among social groups. An attitude of "everyone else is doing it" can have a strong influence on an individual's decision to partake in the activity. For example, in some communities, perhaps it is rare for anyone to wear a helmet while biking. So an individual who has always used a bicycle helmet in the past may decide to forego it because nobody else wears one in his new community.

2. Enforcing patterns of social control: Having rules and regulations in place creates structure for society, which can affect health. For instance, having a curfew for teenagers to be off the streets by midnight unless accompanied by an adult may assist in preventing violence.

3. Providing opportunities to engage in healthy behaviors: The opportunities, or lack thereof, in our surroundings can have a strong influence on our health. For instance, having access to a community pool can encourage individuals to learn to swim, thus preventing drowning, while also serving as a form of physical exercise and social cohesion.

4. Encouraging selection of healthy behaviors as a coping strategy: For example, college students often go through stressful periods throughout their academic career, particularly around exam time. Some students may decide to cope with this stress by "blowing off steam." This can take many forms, from binge drinking to going for a run, each selection having a different effect on health.

Having introduced the complex relationship between social systems and individuals, let us now look at three key components of the social system and their relationship to health: socioeconomic status, culture, and religion.

## ▶ How Do Socioeconomic Status, Culture, and Religion Affect Health?

### Socioeconomic Status

Beginning in the 1800s, social scientists developed the concept of **socioeconomic status**. They also developed elaborate systems to operationalize the definition of "socioeconomic status" and classify individuals. In the United States, the definition has generally included measures that are strongly related to income including:[a]

- family income
- educational level or parents' educational level
- professional status or parents' professional status

In developed countries such as the United States, health status, at least as measured by life expectancy, is strongly associated with socioeconomic status.[3,4] Greater longevity is associated with higher social status, with a gradient of increasing longevity from lowest to highest on the socioeconomic scale. **BOX 4.1** provides greater detail on this important relationship.

---

a A more formal social hierarchy has traditionally existed in Europe. European social scientists utilized the concept of social class when categorizing individuals by socioeconomic status. In Europe, economics alone was not thought to be adequate to explain socioeconomic status or categorize individuals.

**BOX 4.1**  Income and Population Health

Health status as measured by life expectancy has been found to improve with increasing average gross domestic product (GDP), up to a threshold of about $10,000 per person, which is the current level for the many successful middle income developing nations. The United States currently has an average GDP above $45,000.

Once this threshold of adequate income is reached, the health status of countries does not continue to steadily rise as income increases. At these higher levels of GDP, as seen in most developed countries, income disparities are a better predictor of life expectancy than absolute levels of average GDP. Developed countries with lower levels of income disparity, such as Japan, Canada, Sweden, and France, have longer life expectancies than countries such as the United States and the United Kingdom, which have greater income disparities.

Even in countries with modest levels of income disparities, a **socioeconomic gradient** of health status exists such that individuals with a higher socioeconomic status tend to have better health outcomes compared to those with a lower socioeconomic status. This gradient can be viewed as a ladder in that moving down the socioeconomic ladder, more ill health and shorter life expectancy are experienced at each rung. Therefore, socioeconomic determinants of health do not solely affect the very poorest or those in the lowest socioeconomic levels but are rather an issue throughout all income levels.

An argument has been made that poorer health leads to lower income and not the other way around. There is little evidence that this phenomenon explains the socioeconomic factors that affect health. Education level is an even stronger predictor of life expectancy than income, and education levels are usually well established before poor health develops.

Education level, income level, and professional status are three key components of socioeconomic status as measured in the United States. Therefore, it may be more accurate to say that disparities in

socioeconomic status are associated with poorer population health status.

A measure that has been adapted to calculate economic inequity across populations is the **Gini index**, also known as the Gini coefficient. This is a commonly used measure of income distribution, with an index ranging from 0 to 1, with higher values indicating greater inequality. A Gini index of 0 indicates complete income equality (everyone has the same income), and 1 indicates complete inequality in income (one individual receives all the income). Oftentimes, for ease of reporting and drawing comparisons, the index is multiplied by 100 so that the values range from 0 to 100. The index measures the extent of deviation between an economy's distribution of income among individuals or households and that of perfectly equal distribution.

Among developed countries, income inequality is strongly associated with higher rates of mortality. Countries with a wider gap between the poorest of the poor and richest of the rich (a Gini index closer to 1) experience poorer population health outcomes on measures such as infant mortality and life expectancy, compared to countries with a narrow gap between rich and poor (a Gini index closer to 0).[5,6]

The United States has the highest Gini index of major developed countries. The U.S. Gini index is approximately 41 compared to 33 in France and Canada, 32 in Japan, and 30 in Germany.[6]

Place matters. Some Americans will die 20 years earlier than others who live just a short distance away because of differences in education, income, race, ethnicity, and where and how they live. One classical study revealed dramatic disparities in life expectancy across U.S. counties overall, and particularly when racial or ethnic differences were also considered. For example, black men in the county with the shortest life expectancy for blacks lived approximately 60 years, while white men in the county with the longest life expectancy for whites could expect to live two decades longer.[7,8,a]

a  The association between socioeconomic status and longevity is most strongly associated with an individual's socioeconomic status as an adult. The socioeconomic status of an individual's parents has a much weaker association. This suggests that genetic factors have little to do with the association between socioeconomic status and life expectancy. Education has a stronger association with health status than income or professional status. Lower socioeconomic status leads to poor health rather than poor health leading to lower socioeconomic status. Socioeconomic factors are associated with an increase in relative risk of death of 1.5 to 2.0 when comparing the lowest and highest socioeconomic groups. This means that those in the lowest group have more than a 50% increase in the death rate compared to the highest group. This relative risk steadily increases as the socioeconomic level decreases. The relationship has a dose-response relationship; that is, there is an increase in longevity with every increase in socioeconomic status. Thus, the impact is not limited to those with the lowest status. The largest contributors to the differences in the death rate are cardiovascular disease, violence, and, increasingly, AIDS; however, the death rate is impacted in general by a wide range of diseases—most being malignancies and infectious diseases.[9]

We understand many, but not all, of the ways that socioeconomic factors affect health. Greater economic wealth usually implies access to healthier living conditions. Improved sanitation, less crowding, greater access to health care, and safer methods for cooking and eating are all strongly associated with higher economic status in developed, as well as developing, countries.

Education is also strongly associated with better health. It may change health outcomes and increase longevity by encouraging behaviors that provide protection against disease and also reduce exposure to behaviors that put individuals at risk of disease. Higher education levels, coupled with the increased resources that greater wealth can provide, may increase access to better medical care and provide greater ability to protect against health hazards.

Individuals of lower socioeconomic status are more likely to be exposed to health hazards at work and in the physical environment through toxic exposure in the air they breathe, the water they drink, and the food they eat. **TABLE 4.2** outlines a number of mechanisms by which socioeconomic status can directly and indirectly influence health.

These factors, while important, do not explain the entire observed differences in life expectancy among individuals of different socioeconomic status. For instance, the rates of coronary heart disease are considerably higher among those of lower socioeconomic status—even after taking into account cigarette smoking, high blood pressure, cholesterol levels, and blood sugar levels.[9]

Considerable research is now being directed to better understand these and other effects of socioeconomic status. One theory suggests that social control and social participation may help explain these substantial differences in health. It contends that control over individual and group decision-making is much greater among individuals of higher socioeconomic status. The theory holds that the ability to control one's

**TABLE 4.2** Examples of Ways that Socioeconomic Status May Affect Health

| Ways | Examples |
| --- | --- |
| Living conditions | Increases in sanitation, reductions in crowding, methods of heating and cooking |
| Overall educational opportunities | Education has the strongest association with health behaviors and health outcomes<br>May be due to better appreciation of factors associated with disease and greater ability to control these factors |
| Educational opportunities for women | Education for women has an impact on the health of children and families |
| Occupational exposures | Lower socioeconomic jobs are traditionally associated with increased exposures to health risks |
| Access to goods and services | Ability to access goods, such as protective devices, and high-quality foods and services, including medical and social services to protect and promote health |
| Family size | Large family size affects health and is traditionally associated with lower socioeconomic status and lower health status |
| Exposures to high-risk behaviors | Social alienation related to poverty may be associated with violence, drugs, and other high-risk behaviors |
| Environmental | Lower socioeconomic status is associated with greater exposure to environmental pollution, "natural" disasters, and dangers of the "built environment" |

life may be associated with biological changes that affect health and disease.[9] Additional research is needed to confirm or reject this idea and/or provide an adequate explanation for these important, yet unexplained, differences in health based upon socioeconomic status.

## Culture

Culture, in a broad sense, helps people make judgments about the world and decisions about behavior. Culture defines what is good or bad, and what is healthy or unhealthy. This may relate to lifestyle patterns, beliefs about risk, and beliefs about body type—for example, a large body type in some cultures symbolizes health and well-being, not overweight or other negative conditions.

Culture directly affects the daily habits of life. Food choice and methods of food preparation and preservation are all affected by culture, as well as socioeconomic status. The Mediterranean diet, which includes olive oil, seafood, vegetables, nuts, and fruits, has been shown to have benefits for the heart even when used in countries far removed from the Mediterranean.

There are often clear-cut negative and/or positive impacts on disability related to cultural traditions as diverse as feet binding in China and female genital mutilation in some parts of Africa. Some societies reject strenuous physical activity for those who have the status and wealth to be served by others.

Culture is also related to an individual's response to symptoms and acceptance of interventions. In many cultures, medical care is exclusively for those with symptoms and is not part of prevention. Many traditional cultures have developed sophisticated systems of self-care and self-medication supported by family and traditional healers. These traditions greatly affect how individuals respond to symptoms, how they communicate the symptoms, and the types of medical and public health interventions that they will accept.

Many cultures allow and even encourage the use of traditional approaches alongside Western medical and public health approaches. In some cultures, traditional healers are considered appropriate for health problems whose causes are not thought to be biological, but instead related to spiritual and other phenomena. Recent studies of alternative, or complementary, medicine have provided evidence that specific traditional interventions, such as acupuncture and specific osteopathic and chiropractic manipulation, have measurable benefits. Thus, cultural differences should not be viewed as problems to be addressed, but rather as practices to be understood. **TABLE 4.3** summarizes a number of the ways that culture can affect health.

**TABLE 4.3** Examples of Ways that Culture Can Affect Health

| Ways that culture may affect health | Examples |
| --- | --- |
| Culture is related to behavior—social practices may put individuals and groups at increased or reduced risk | Food preferences—vegetarian, Mediterranean diet Cooking methods History of binding of feet in China Female genital mutilation Role of exercise |
| Culture is related to response to symptoms, such as the level of urgency to recognize symptoms, seek care, and communicate symptoms | Cultural differences in seeking care and self-medication Social, family, and work structures provide varying degree of social support—low degree of social support may be associated with reduced health-related quality of life |
| Culture is related to the types of interventions that are acceptable | Variations in degree of acceptance of traditional Western medicine, including reliance on self-help and traditional healers |
| Culture is related to the response to disease and to interventions | Cultural differences in follow-up, adherence to treatment, and acceptance of adverse outcome |

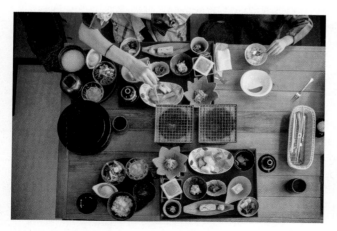

## Religion

Social factors affecting health include religion along with culture. Religion can have a major impact on health, particularly for specific practices that are encouraged or condemned by a particular religious group. For instance, we now know that male circumcision reduces susceptibility to HIV/AIDS.

Religious attitudes that condone or condemn the use of condoms, alcohol, and tobacco have direct and indirect impacts on health as well.

Some religions prohibit specific healing practices, such as blood transfusions or abortion, or totally reject medical interventions altogether, as is practiced by Christian Scientists. Religious individuals may see medical and public health interventions as complementary to religious practice or may substitute prayer for medical interventions in response to symptoms of disease. **TABLE 4.4** outlines some of the ways that religion may affect health.

**TABLE 4.4** Examples of Ways that Religion May Affect Health

| Ways that religion affects health | Examples |
|---|---|
| Religion may affect social practices that put individuals at increased or reduced risk | Sexual: circumcision, use of contraceptives Food: avoidance of seafood, pork, beef Alcohol use: part of religion versus prohibited Tobacco use: actively discouraged by Mormons and Seventh-Day Adventists as part of their religion |
| Religion may affect the response to symptoms | Christian Scientists reject medical care as a response to symptoms |
| Religion may affect the types of interventions that are acceptable | Prohibition against blood transfusions Attitudes toward stem cell research Attitudes toward abortion End-of-life treatments |
| Religion may affect the response to disease and to interventions | Role of prayer as an intervention to alter outcome |

We have examined a number of ways that the broad social influences of socioeconomic status, culture, and religion may affect health and the response to disease. Let us now explore additional social factors that determine health.

## ▶ What Are Social Determinants of Health?

A subset of all the determinants of health, **social determinants of health** refer to the conditions in which people are born, grow up, live, learn, work, play, worship, and age, as well as the systems put in place to deal with illnesses that affect health and quality of life. These conditions are shaped by a wider set of forces, including economics, social policies, and politics.[10,11]

Although there is no universally agreed upon set of social determinants, the following categories highlighted by the World Health Organization encompass many key social determinants that affect health. Each individual has his or her unique combination of influences; however, patterns have been observed and are summarized in the following sections.[12,13] Notice that these social determinants should not be viewed in isolation because they often interact with each other.

## ▶ 10 Key Categories of Social Determinants of Health

### Social Status

Societies place value on certain characteristics so that a hierarchical social structure is formed. In the United States, value tends to be placed on income, education, and occupation, which collectively form socioeconomic status. Social status interacts and influences many of the other social determinants of health.

### Social Support or Alienation

Being part of a social network has benefits to health, including emotional effects associated with feelings of inclusion and tangible benefits, such as having someone to go jogging with or having someone to provide a ride to the doctor's office. Social exclusion can occur due to racism, discrimination, and other forms of marginalization, limiting the opportunities for education, leisure activities, and other community services, either directly through discriminatory practices or as a consequence of cumulative exposure to discrimination resulting in fear, anger, distrust, or stress so that individuals do not seek out such opportunities.

## Food

An inadequate or insecure food source remains an issue for disadvantaged populations in the United States and around the world. However, excess calorie intake and the lack of a nutritious diet is a rapidly growing problem. Not only is education important in being aware of what constitutes a good diet, but having access to affordable, healthy food is also a central component of leading a healthy lifestyle. A **food desert** is a term used to describe geographic areas that lack grocery stores and other establishments in which low-income individuals are able to purchase nutritious food due to high prices or inaccessibility. Although these areas may have food available, the options easily accessible via public transportation and price to low-income families often include unhealthy food such as that offered at convenience stores and fast food establishments.

## Housing

Having affordable, stable housing influences health in a number of ways. Homelessness can lead to malnutrition, lack of medical care, drug use, and violence. Therefore, those with a home tend to have better overall health compared to those without. However, hazards can also be present in the home, including lack of clean water and sanitation, asthma triggers such as mold and dust, lead paint, cockroaches, inadequate sanitation, and unsafe structural conditions.

## Education

Even within the same overall socioeconomic status, those with more education tend to experience better health compared to those with less education. Efforts to address health should, therefore, include making quality education at all levels widely accessible to populations. In the United States, increasing the high school graduation rate is now a leading indicator of *Healthy People,* a collaborative initiative of the United States Department of Health and Human Services which guides the national prevention agenda.

## Work

Several aspects of work can affect health. Overall, being employed tends to be better for health compared to being unemployed. This is partially attributed to the connection between socioeconomic status and health. Having an income assists a person's ability to secure resources that may protect and promote health, such as safe housing, food, and education. Being employed can also assist in accessing health services if the employer provides health insurance to its employees. Type of employment can also affect health. Some jobs are more hazardous to health than others. Health effects associated with work are not restricted to physical health because work can also affect mental health. Job satisfaction and stress in the workplace contribute to health and disease. Those who are unemployed also face psychological consequences due to the anxiety and stress that can be associated with lack of job security and inability to adequately provide for their families.

## Stress

Stress is a social and psychological response with biological consequences. A variety of circumstances can create anxiety and worry, whether it is an intense work setting or the threat of losing one's home. Sustained periods of stress can negatively affect physical health due to the body's fight or flight response, which increases the heart rate and cortisol levels. Over time, stress can lead to such conditions as cardiovascular disease and depression.

## Transportation

A component of environmental health, transportation also affects health in a number of ways. By driving less and walking/cycling more and using mass transit, people increase their physical activity levels. It is becoming even more important to find ways to integrate physical activity into our lives as lifestyles in the United States grow increasingly sedentary and obesity is on the rise. Opting for walking, cycling, and mass transit also increases social contact, which can serve as a protective health factor. Relying less on cars also reduces air and noise pollution, contributing to environmental health as well. Therefore, city planning can have an impact on health.

## Place

Where you live affects your health. For example, those living in rural areas have fewer healthcare services available nearby, whereas those living in urban areas are exposed to increased air pollution from factories and vehicles. The built environment also affects health

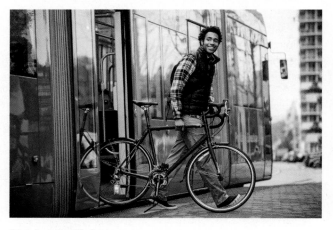

© Jordan Siemens/Digital Vision/Getty Images

in that it influences whether there are safe places to be physically active, including walking and biking trails and green spaces, as well as easy access to nutritious food.

## Access to Health Services

Having access to preventive health services and medical care contributes to overall health. Access to such services is often limited by health insurance. On a broader scale, having an appropriate number and type of healthcare professionals is instrumental to maintaining the health of individuals and populations.

## ▸ How Do Social Determinants Affect Health?

Social determinants of health contribute to a wide variety of illnesses and diseases rooted in lifestyle, environmental, and social factors. Recent increased attention on social determinants of health has been driven by their connection with **health disparities**. A health disparity is a type of difference in health that is closely linked with social or economic disadvantage. Health disparities negatively affect groups of people who have systematically experienced greater social or economic obstacles to health. These obstacles stem from characteristics historically linked to discrimination or exclusion, such as race or ethnicity, religion, socioeconomic status, gender, disability, mental health, sexual orientation, and geographic location.[b]

Disparities occur in a wide range of health conditions, including communicable and noncommunicable diseases and environmental health and safety. **TABLE 4.5** provides a few examples of conditions in which disparities occur within the U.S. population.

It is important to note that social determinants affect not only physical health, but mental health as well.

---

**TABLE 4.5** Disparities in Health, United States

**Noncommunicable Disease**

**Coronary heart disease:** Black men and women are much more likely to die of heart disease and stroke compared to white men and women.

**Colorectal cancer screening:** Disparities in colorectal cancer screening rates exist with lower rates of screening among those with lower education level and lower income.

**Environmental Health and Safety**

**Air pollution:** Local sources of air pollution, often in urban areas, can impact the health of people who live or work near these sources. Everyone in these areas, regardless of socioeconomic status, can experience the negative health effects of air pollution; however, because racial/ethnic minority groups are more likely to live in the most polluted sections of urban areas, they continue to experience a disproportionately larger impact.

**Motor vehicle crashes:** Men of all races/ethnicities are two to three times more likely to die in motor vehicle crashes than are women, and death rates are twice as high among American Indians/Alaska Natives.

**Communicable Disease**

**HIV:** Racial/ethnic minorities, with the exception of Asians/Pacific Islanders, experience disproportionately higher rates of new human immunodeficiency virus diagnoses than whites, as do men who have sex with men (MSM). In addition, rates are increasing among black and American Indian/Alaska Native males, as well as MSM, while rates hold steady or are decreasing in other groups.

**Influenza vaccination:** Whites aged 65 years and older consistently have higher rates of influenza vaccine coverage compared to all other races/ethnicities in this age group, with non-Hispanic blacks experiencing the lowest rates of flu vaccine coverage.

Data from Centers for Disease Control and Prevention. CDC Health Disparities and Inequalities Report—United States, 2011. *Morbidity and Mortality Weekly Report.* Supplement/Vol. 60. January 14, 2011.

---

b When discussing differences in health, a variety of terms are used, each with a slightly different focus. In addition to "health disparity," other terms include **healthcare disparity**, **health equity**, **health inequity**, and **health inequality**.

**Mental health** is a state of successful performance of mental function, resulting in productive activities, fulfilling relationships with other people, and the ability to adapt to change and to cope with challenges.[14] Mental illness refers to all diagnosable mental disorders, which are health conditions characterized by alterations in thinking, mood, and/or behavior associated with distress and/or impaired functioning. Examples of mental disorders are depression, anxiety, bipolar disorder, schizophrenia, and dementia. Mental disorders are the leading cause of disability in the United States, with approximately 1 in 17 U.S. adults exhibiting a debilitating mental illness in any given year.[14]

Between 1999 and 2014 the suicide rate increased by over 24% among the U.S. population, with increases of over 50% among those 45–64. These middle aged Americans have been disproportionately affected by the "great recession" as well as ongoing economic changes which may help to explain this very large increase in suicides.[15]

Mental health is not only essential to successful function in and contribution to society but it can also impact physical health. For example, depression may limit an individual's desire and motivation to exercise and seek out nutritious food, contributing to chronic conditions such as cardiovascular disease and diabetes. Therefore, understanding the factors, both internal and external to the individual, contributing to emotional, psychological, and social well-being is critical in addressing population health. National objectives, as part of *Healthy People*, have been set to improve mental health status and expand mental health screening and treatment services.

## ▶ Can Health Behavior Be Changed?

Much of the preventable disease and disability today in the United States and other developed countries is related to the behavior of individuals. From cigarette smoking to obesity, from intentional to unintentional injuries, from sexual behavior to drug abuse, health issues can be traced to the behavior of individuals.

Consider all the behaviors related to health. Some are intentional health behaviors, while others are not necessarily motivated by health concerns. Getting a mammogram could be an example of an intentional health behavior because it is a behavior most likely undertaken for health benefits—in this case, screening for breast cancer. However, driving the speed limit may be a behavior that has an effect on health but is undertaken not because the individual is concerned about the health benefits of doing so (avoiding injury

from a motor vehicle crash) but because he or she wants to avoid getting a ticket. Therefore, in order to have an impact on health, a wide range of behavioral motivations and factors needs to be addressed.

At times, we hear discouraging messages that behavior cannot be changed. However, if we take a relatively long-term view, we find that there are many examples of behavioral change that have occurred for the better. For instance:

- Cigarette smoking in the United States among males has been reduced from approximately 50% in the 1960s to approximately 20% today.
- Infants today generally are placed on their backs for sleeping and napping and not on their stomachs, as was the usual practice in the 1980s and earlier. Back-to-Sleep campaigns are believed to have reduced sudden infant death syndrome (SIDS) by nearly 50% in the United States.
- Seat belt use in the United States has increased from <25% in the 1970s to over 80% currently.
- Drunk driving in the United States has been dramatically reduced, with a resulting decline in automobile-related fatalities.
- Mammography use increased by approximately 50% during the 1990s and has been credited with beginning to reduce the previously rising mortality rates from breast cancer.

The potential to change behavior can make health worse as well. The following changes for the worse have also occurred in the United States in recent years:

- Over the last three decades, Americans have increased their caloric intake and reduced their average amount of exercise, resulting in more than doubling the obesity rate to nearly 35% of all adults.
- Between the 1960s and the 1990s, teenage girls and young adult women increased their cigarette smoking, subjecting their unborn children to additional hazards of low birthweight. Fortunately this trend has been reversed in recent years.

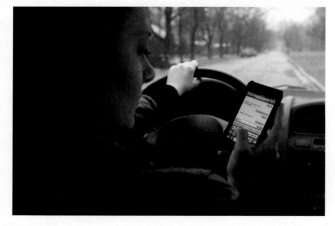

© Burlingham/Shutterstock

■ Texting and driving has increased dramatically in recent years though national educational campaigns and new technologies have begun to reverse this trend.

Behavioral change is possible for the better and for the worse. Some behaviors, however, are easier to change than others. Let's take a look at why this is.

## ▶ Why Are Some Individual Health Behaviors Easier to Change Than Others?

Some behaviors are relatively easy to change, while others are extremely difficult. Being able to recognize the difference is an important place to start when trying to alter behavior. It is relatively easy when one behavior can be substituted for a similar one and results in a potentially large payoff. In these situations, knowledge often goes a long way. For instance, the substitution of acetaminophen (Tylenol) for aspirin to prevent Reye's Syndrome was relatively easy. Similarly, the Back-to-Sleep campaign was quite successful in reducing the rate of death from SIDS. In both of these cases, an acceptable and convenient substitute was available, making the needed behavioral change much easier to accomplish.

Along with knowledge, incentives—such as reduced cost, increased availability, or improvements in ease of use—can encourage rapid acceptance and motivate behavioral change. For instance, easier-to-install child restraint systems have increased their use. Greater insurance coverage and widespread availability of modern mammography equipment has led to an increase in the number of mammograms performed.

The most difficult behaviors to change are those that have a physiological component, such as obesity, or an addictive element, such as cigarette smoking. Individual interventions aimed at smoking cessation or long-term weight control generally succeed less than 30% of the time—even among motivated individuals. Even intensive interventions with highly motivated individuals cannot be expected to be successful more than 50% of the time, as was illustrated by the Multiple Risk Factor Intervention Trial (MRFIT), which attempted intensive interventions to reduce risk factors for cardiovascular disease.

In addition, physical, social, and economic barriers can stand in the way of behavior change, even if individuals themselves are motivated. If health care is not accessible, or if survival needs require individuals to engage in risks they might not take otherwise, change in behavior may be impeded.

Successful behavioral change requires that we understand as much as we can about how behavior can be changed and what we can do to help.

## ▶ How Can Individual Behavior Be Changed?

The behavior of individuals is often the final common pathway through which disease, disability, and death can be prevented. The fact that individual behavior has a clearly observable connection with these factors does not necessarily imply that the best or only way to address the behavior of individuals is to focus exclusively on individuals. The forces at work to mold individual behaviors are sometimes referred to as **downstream factors**, **mainstream factors,** and **upstream factors**.

Downstream factors are those that directly involve an individual and can potentially be altered by individual interventions, such as an addiction to nicotine. Mainstream factors are those that result from the relationship of an individual with a larger group or population, such as peer pressure to smoke or the level of taxation on cigarettes. These factors require attention at the group or population level. Finally, upstream factors are often grounded in social structures and policies, such as government-sponsored programs that encourage tobacco production. These require us to look beyond traditional healthcare and public health interventions to the broader social and economic forces that affect health.

Changes in behavior often require more than individual motivation and determination to change. They require encouragement and support from groups ranging from friends and families to work and peer groups. Behavioral change may also require social policies and expectations that reinforce individual efforts.

## ▶ How Can Health Behavior Be Explained and Predicted?

When addressing issues affecting the health of populations, behaviors contributing to these issues must be explored and understood. But what tools do we have to understand these behaviors? A **theory** is a set of interrelated concepts that presents a systematic view of relationships among variables in order to explain and predict events and situations.

Similarly, a **model** is a combination of ideas and concepts taken from multiple theories and applied to specific problems in particular settings. Theories and models are tools commonly used by health researchers and health practitioners to gain insight into why people behave in healthy or unhealthy ways and to guide the development and evaluation of interventions aimed at changing behavior to improve health.

Because theories present a systematic way to understand events or situations, linking various factors and elements together, they provide a useful framework to study health problems, develop appropriate interventions, and evaluate the impact of the interventions. Theory serves as a road map for research and practice, exploring the "why," "what," and "how" of health issues and their solutions. In accordance with evidence-based public health principles, interventions developed based on theory and supported by evidence using these theories are more likely to succeed than those that were not.

Let us take a look at a few examples of theories and their application to health behavior.

## What Are Some Key Theories and Models Used to Address Health Behavior?

Many theories and models are used in health behavior research and practice. A few key theories and models will be highlighted here. Theories and models are categorized according to three levels of influence:

- Intrapersonal: Focusing on characteristics of the individual, including knowledge, attitudes, beliefs, motivation, self-concept, past experiences, and skills
- Interpersonal: Focusing on relationships between people, acknowledging that other people influence behavior by sharing their thoughts, advice, feelings, emotional support, and other assistance
- Population and community: Focusing on factors within social structures, such as norms, rules, regulations, policies, and laws

### Intrapersonal Level

Health promotion and health education efforts set out to raise awareness of health issues among individuals; therefore, a number of intrapersonal theories and models exist, focusing on factors within the individual

that influence behavior, such as knowledge, attitudes, beliefs, and skills.

One of the original theories of health behavior that remains among the most widely recognized today is the **Health Belief Model**. The model, developed in the 1950s by a group of U.S. Public Health Service social psychologists, originated out of a desire to understand why so few people were taking advantage of a free mobile X-ray unit to screen for tuberculosis (TB).[16] The social psychologists theorized that people's readiness to act was influenced by their beliefs about whether or not they were susceptible to TB and their perceptions of the benefits of screening for the disease.

The Health Belief Model is an intrapersonal theory, as it focuses on individuals' characteristics, including their perceptions and thought processes prior to taking health-related action. The premise of the model is that personal beliefs influence health behavior. The model proposes that people will be more likely to take action if they believe they are susceptible to the condition; they believe the condition has serious consequences; they believe taking action would benefit them, with the benefits outweighing the harms; and they are exposed to factors that prompt action and believe in their ability to successfully perform the action. **TABLE 4.6** summarizes the model's constructs and their application to osteoporosis.

Another widely used intrapersonal model is the **Stages of Change Model**, also referred to as the Transtheoretical Model. The underlying assumption of this model is that people go through a set of incremental stages when changing behavior rather than making significant changes all at once.[17c]

The first stage, called precontemplation, implies that an individual has not yet considered changing his or her behavior. At this stage, efforts to encourage change are not likely to be successful. However, efforts to educate and offer help in the future may lay the groundwork for later success.

The second phase, known as contemplation, implies that an individual is actively thinking about the benefits and barriers to change. At this stage, information focused on short- and immediate-term gains, as well as long-term benefits, can be especially useful. In addition, the contemplation stage lends itself to developing a baseline—that is, establishing the

---

c  Designing interventions based upon the Stages of Change model has not been uniformly successful. One potential reason for this may be that individuals are often in different stages of change for different types of interventions. With complex interventions, such as those required to address obesity, an individual may be in one stage of change for exercise, another for adding fruits and vegetables to his/her diet, and a different stage in terms of calorie reduction. A critique of this model is that people do not always go through the set of stages consecutively, but instead may revert back to an earlier stage before moving through the other stages.

**TABLE 4.6** Health Belief Model and Osteoporosis

| Construct | Description | Example: osteoporosis |
|---|---|---|
| Perceived susceptibility | An individual's opinion of getting a condition | "Osteoporosis only happens to old women, not me." |
| Perceived severity | An individual's opinion of how serious a condition is and its consequences | "Osteoporosis is not a big deal." |
| Perceived benefits | An individual's belief in the advised action to reduce risk and/or severity of condition | "Screening for osteoporosis will catch it early so I can continue to live an active lifestyle." |
| Perceived barriers | An individual's belief about the costs (tangible and psychological) of the advised action | "Screening for osteoporosis takes too much time." |
| Modifying variables | Individual characteristics that influence personal perceptions | "Women in my culture are viewed as strong; therefore, we do not concern ourselves with osteoporosis." |
| Cues to action | Strategies/events that encourage one's "readiness" to act | "My sister was recently diagnosed with osteoporosis, so I should get screened." |
| Self-efficacy | Belief in one's ability to take action | "If I am diagnosed with osteoporosis, I know I can manage it." |

Data from National Cancer Institute. U.S. Department of Health and Human Services. *Theory at a Glance: A Guide for Health Promotion Practice.* 2nd ed. Available at: https://cancercontrol.cancer.gov /brp/research/theories_project/theory.pdf. Accessed July 14, 2017.

current severity or extent of the problem in order to measure future progress.

The third phase is called preparation. During this phase, the individual is developing a plan of action. At this point, the individual may be especially receptive to setting goals, considering a range of strategies, and developing a timetable. Help in recognizing and preparing for unanticipated barriers can be especially useful to the individual during this phase.

The fourth phase is the action phase, when the change in behavior takes place. This is the time to bring together all possible outside support to reinforce and reward the new behavior and help with problems or setbacks that occur.

The fifth—and hopefully final—phase is the maintenance phase, in which the new behavior becomes a permanent part of an individual's lifestyle. The maintenance phase requires education on how to anticipate the long-term nature of behavioral change, especially how to resist the inevitable temptations to resume the old behavior. Using cigarette smoking as illustration again, **TABLE 4.7** summarizes the stages of behavioral change and the specific actions that can be helpful at each of the stages.

A third widely used intrapersonal theory is the **Theory of Planned Behavior**. This theory is based on the idea that intention is the main predictor of behavior. The theory proposes that behavioral intention is influenced by an individual's attitude toward performing a behavior, his or her beliefs about whether people important to him or her approve or disapprove of the behavior, and his or her beliefs about their control over performing the behavior. According to the theory, intention determines whether someone will engage in a behavior; therefore, interventions based on the Theory of Planned Behavior set out to affect individuals' intention to perform a behavior.[18] **FIGURE 4.1** illustrates the theory's constructs in relation to getting a flu vaccine.

**TABLE 4.7** Stages of Change Model and Cigarette Smoking

| Stages of change | Actions | Example: cigarette smoking |
|---|---|---|
| *Precontemplation* | *Prognosticate* | |
| Individual not considering change | Assessing readiness for change—timing is key | Determine individual's readiness to quit<br>If not ready, indicate receptivity to help in the future<br>Look for receptive timing, such as during acute respiratory symptoms<br>Social factors, such as workplace and indoor restriction on smoking and taxation, increase likelihood of entering precontemplation phase |
| *Contemplation* | *Motivate change* | |
| Individual thinks actively about the health risk and action required to reduce that risk<br>Issue of change is on the individual's agenda but no action is planned | Provide information focused on short and intermediate gains from behavioral change, as well as long-term benefits<br>Doubtful, dire, and distant impacts are less effective | Reinforce increase in exercise level, reduction in cough, financial savings, serving as example to children, protection of fetus, etc.<br>Continue to inform of longer term effects on health |
| | Establish baseline to assess severity of the problem; focus attention on the problem and provide basis for comparison | Develop log of timing, frequency, and quantity of smoking, as well as associated events |
| *Preparation* | *Plan change* | |
| Prepare for action, including developing a plan and setting a timetable | Set specific measurable and obtainable goals with deadlines | Quit date or possible tapering if heavy smoker |
| | Two or more well-chosen simultaneous interventions may maximize effectiveness | Family support, peer support, individual planning, medication, etc., may reinforce and multiply impacts |
| | Recognize habitual nature of existing behavior and remove associated activities | Remove cigarettes, ashtrays, and other associated smoking equipment<br>Remove personal and environmental impacts of past smoking, such as teeth cleaning and cleaning of drapery<br>Anticipate temptations, such as associations with food, drink, and social occasions |
| *Action* | *Reinforce change* | |
| Observable changes in behavior with potential for relapse | Provide/suggest tangible rewards | Provide rewards, such as alternative use of money, focus on personal hygiene or personal environment |

| | | |
|---|---|---|
| | Positive feedback and encouragement of new behavior<br>Anticipate adverse effects and frustrations | Focus on measurable progress toward new behavior<br>Provide receptive environment, but avoid focus on excuses<br>Take short-term, one-day-at-a-time approach<br>Recognize potential for symptoms to worsen at first before improvement occurs<br>Anticipate potential for weight gain and encourage exercise and other behaviors to reduce potential for weight gain |
| | Utilize group/peer support | Family and peer reinforcement critical during action phase |
| **Maintenance** | **Maintain change** | |
| New behavior needs to be consolidated as part of permanent lifestyle change | Practice/reinforce methods for maintaining new behavior | Avoid old associations and prepare/practice response when encountering old circumstances |
| | Recognize long-term nature of behavioral change and need for supportive peers and social reinforcement | Negative social attitudes toward smoking among peers and society along with social restrictions, such as limiting public indoor smoking, and social actions, such as taxation, help prevent smoking and reinforce maintenance of cessation |

Data from Prochaska JO, and DiClemente CC. Stages and processes of self-change of smoking: Toward an integrative model of change. *Journal of Consulting and Clinical Psychology*. 1983;51(3):390–395.

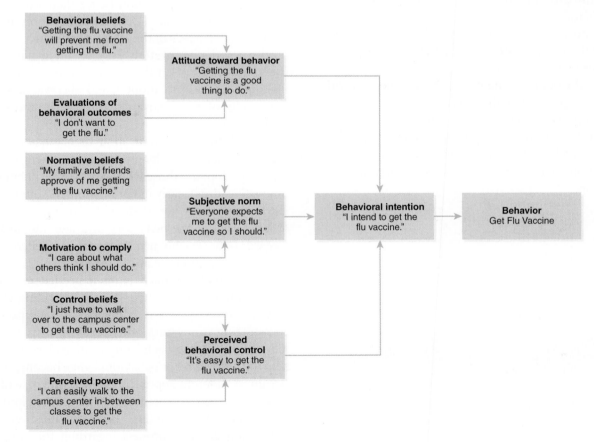

**FIGURE 4.1** Theory of Planned Behavior and Flu Vaccine

Data from Azjen I and Drive BL. Prediction of leisure participation from behavioral, normative, and control beliefs: an application of the theory of planned behavior. *Leisure Science*. 1991;13:185–204.

## Interpersonal Level

Interpersonal theories and models take into consideration the influences of other people on an individual's behavior. These other people can include family members, peers, coworkers, healthcare providers, etc., and they can influence behavior by sharing their advice, feelings, and opinions and through the support and assistance they provide.

One of the most commonly used interpersonal theories is the **Social Cognitive Theory**. The Social Cognitive Theory, originally known as the Social Learning Theory, focuses on the interaction between individuals and their social systems. According to the theory, changing behavior requires an understanding of:

- Individual characteristics, such as knowledge, skills, and beliefs
- Influences in the social and physical environment, such as peer influence, level of family support, characteristics of the neighborhood, and work and school environments that help or hinder opportunities for health
- Interaction among all these factors

A key concept of the theory is **reciprocal determinism**, the dynamic interplay among personal factors, the environment, and behavior. The theory proposes that changing one of these factors will change them all.[19] **FIGURE 4.2** illustrates the concept of reciprocal determinism.

Social Cognitive Theory can be applied to a wide variety of public health issues that encompass the complex interactions between individual characteristics, influences in the social system, and individual behavior such as drug addiction. **TABLE 4.8** illustrates application of the Social Cognitive Theory to drug addiction.

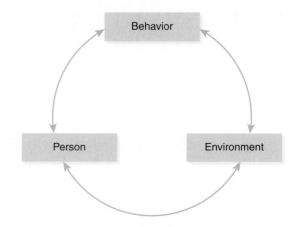

**FIGURE 4.2** Reciprocal Determinism

Data from Bandura A. *Social Foundations of Thought and Action: A Social Cognitive Theory.* Englewood Cliffs, NJ: Prentice Hall, 1986.

## Population and Community Level

Theories and models on the population, or community, level explore factors within social systems, offering strategies that can be used to alter these factors to address health issues within the population. Theories and models on the community level are typically viewed as change theories guiding strategies that change aspects within the social systems, such as norms, rules, regulations, policies, and laws. This is in contrast to theories and models on the intrapersonal and interpersonal levels, which are viewed as explanatory theories because they primarily identify and describe reasons for a problem.

A commonly used community-level theory is the **Diffusion of Innovation**. This theory focuses on how a new idea, product, or social practice (an innovation) is disseminated and adopted in a population. The theoretical constructs include the innovation itself, the time it takes to adopt the innovation, the communication channels used to transmit the innovation, and the social system in which diffusion of the innovation takes place.[20]

The theory proposes that the diffusion and adoption, or rejection, of an innovation is affected by perceived attributes of the innovation, including relative advantage (Is the innovation better than what it will replace?), compatibility (Does the innovation fit with the values and needs of the intended audience?), complexity (Is the innovation easy to understand and use?), trialability (Can the innovation be tried before making a decision to adopt?), and observability (Are the results of the innovation observable and easily measureable?).

The diffusion of innovation theory has contributed the concept of different types of adopters, including early adopters (those who seek to experiment with innovative ideas), early majority adopters (often opinion leaders whose social status frequently influences others to adopt the behavior), and late adopters (or laggards—those who need support and encouragement to make adoption as easy as possible).

A different approach is often needed to engage each of these groups. For instance, marketing efforts may initially target early adopters with an approach encouraging innovation and creativity. This may be followed by an approach to opinion leaders who can help the innovation or behavior change become mainstream. A different approach emphasizing ease of use and widespread acceptance may be most helpful for encouraging late adopters. **TABLE 4.9** illustrates the innovation-decision process regarding the adoption of the new idea to sneeze into one's elbow as a public health measure.

**TABLE 4.8** Social Cognitive Theory and Drug Addiction

| Construct | Description | Example: drug addiction |
|---|---|---|
| Self-efficacy | Belief in one's ability to take action | "I am able to stop taking drugs." |
| Observational learning (modeling) | Learning by watching others | "My best friend has been drug-free for 3 years." |
| Expectations | The likely outcome of a particular behavior | "If I quit taking drugs, I will be able to hold a job and earn income." |
| Expectancies | The value placed on the outcome of the behavior | "Being able to work and have an income is very important to me." |
| Emotional arousal | Emotional reaction to a situation | "When I take drugs, I feel like I am out of control and that is very frightening." |
| Behavioral capability | Knowledge and skills needed to engage in a behavior | "I know I need to seek professional assistance to quit my drug addiction and I know where and how to get that assistance." |
| Reinforcement | Rewards or punishments for performing a behavior | "When I take drugs, people do not want to hang out with me. But when I am not taking drugs, I am surrounded by my friends and family." |
| Locus of control | One's belief regarding one's personal power over events | "Only I can get myself drug-free." |

Data from Bandura A. *Social Foundations of Thought and Action: A Social Cognitive Theory*. Englewood Cliffs, NJ: Prentice Hall, 1986.

**TABLE 4.9** Innovation-Decision Process: Diffusion of Innovation of Sneezing into Elbow

| Stage | Description | Example |
|---|---|---|
| Knowledge | Before people can adopt an innovation, they must know it exists. Communication channels, such as media, friends, family members, and physicians, are influential in this stage. | Knowing sneezing into elbow exists as a public health measure |
| Persuasion | In the persuasion stage, people develop an opinion about the innovation. That opinion may be positive or negative. The perceived characteristics of the innovation are particularly influential in the persuasion stage. | Considering whether to begin sneezing into elbow Relative advantage: "Sneezing into your elbow is a lot better than sneezing into your hand." Compatibility: "Sneezing into my elbow is consistent with my desire to prevent the spread of disease." Complexity: "Sneezing into your elbow is easy to do." Trialability: "I can give sneezing into my elbow a try." Observability: "I have seen others sneeze into their elbows." |

*(continues)*

**TABLE 4.9** Innovation-Decision Process: Diffusion of Innovation of Sneezing into Elbow *(continued)*

| Stage | Description | Example |
|---|---|---|
| Decision | During the decision stage, people decide to either adopt or reject an innovation. | Deciding to sneeze into elbow |
| Implementation | During the implementation stage, an innovation is tried. | Sneezing into elbow |
| Confirmation | During the confirmation stage, support is sought for the decision, so that there is continued adoption, continued rejection, later adoption, or discontinuance of the innovation. | Continue to sneeze into elbow as a common practice that becomes a habit after continued use |

Data from Rogers EM. *Diffusion of Innovations*. New York: Free Press; 2003.

## ▶ How Can Theories Be Applied in Practice?

### Choosing a Theory/Model

Choosing which theory or model to use requires an understanding of the public health issue and population being addressed, but there is no set formula for which theory or model is most appropriate in every situation. Components from multiple theories and models may be used when addressing particular situations and populations. Even though there are no right and wrong theories and models to use in given situations, some guidance is helpful in selecting the theoretical framework. Hayden offers the following guidance in choosing a theory:[21]

- Identify the health issue or problem and the population affected.
- Gather information about the issue, population, or both.
- Identify possible reasons or causes for the problem.
- Identify the level of interaction (intrapersonal, interpersonal, or community) under which the reasons or causes most logically fit.
- Identify the theory or theories that best match the level of interaction and the reasons or causes.

### Planning Frameworks

Theory is useful in identifying points at which to intervene in an effort to protect and promote the health of populations. These points will vary depending on the issue and the population. For instance, assume that theory-guided research on colon cancer screening suggests that women are unlikely to get screened because they do not think they are susceptible to the disease, while men are unlikely to get screened because they are not encouraged or reminded to do so. Interventions aimed at addressing colon cancer screening would, therefore, vary for women and men. Perhaps an intervention for women would focus on raising awareness of colon cancer among women, whereas an intervention for men may focus on the role of physicians and significant others to encourage them to make an appointment.

A variety of approaches can be undertaken to apply theory to practice. Two useful approaches, social marketing and the PRECEDE-PROCEED framework, will be described.

In recent years, public health has begun to apply marketing approaches to try to better understand and change the health behaviors of groups of people—especially those who are at high risk for the health impacts of their behavior, such as cigarette smokers. **Social marketing**, a use and extension of traditional product marketing, has become a key component of a public health approach to behavioral change.[22] Social marketing campaigns were first successfully used in the developing world for promoting a range of products and behaviors, including family planning and pediatric rehydration therapy. In recent years, social marketing efforts have been widely and successfully used in developed countries, including such efforts as:

- The Truth® campaign—Developed by the American Legacy Foundation, it aims to redirect the perception of smoking being seen as a teenage rebellion to the decision to not smoke being a rebellion against the alleged behavior-controlling tobacco industry.

- The National Youth Anti-Drug campaign—It uses social marketing efforts directed at young people, including the "Parents. The Anti-Drug." campaign.
- The VERB™ campaign—It focused on 9- to 13-year-olds, or "tweens," with a goal of making exercise fun and "cool" for everyone, not just competitive athletes.

Social marketing incorporates the "4 Ps," which are widely used to structure traditional marketing efforts. These are:

- **Product**: Identifying the behavior or innovation that is being marketed
- **Price**: Identifying the benefits, the barriers, and the financial costs
- **Place**: Identifying the target audiences and how to reach them
- **Promotion**: Organizing a campaign or program to reach the target audience(s)

Social marketing, like product marketing, often relies on what marketers call **branding**. Branding includes words and symbols that help the target audience identify with the service; however, it goes deeper than just words and symbols. It can be seen as a method of implementing the fourth "P," or promotion. It also builds upon the first three "Ps":

- Branding requires a clear understanding of the product or the behavior to be changed (product).
- Successful branding puts forth strategies for reducing the financial and psychological costs (price).
- Branding identifies the audience and segments of the audience and asks how each segment can be reached (place).

Branding is the public face of social marketing, but it also needs to be integrated into the core of the marketing plan.[d]

Social marketing efforts in developing and developed countries have demonstrated that it is possible to change key health behaviors of well-defined groups of people, including adolescents, who are often regarded as the hardest to reach. An example of the use of social marketing to reach young people, the VERB™ campaign, is examined in **BOX 4.2**.[23]

---

### BOX 4.2 VERB™ Campaign

The VERB™ social marketing campaign was funded through the Centers for Disease Control and Prevention (CDC), which worked with advertising agencies to reach tweens and make exercise "cool." After a series of focus groups and other efforts to define and understand the market, it was concluded that the message should not be one of improving health, but rather of having fun with friends, exploring new activities with a sense of adventure, and being free to experiment without being judged on performance.

Marketing efforts also identified barriers, including time constraints and the attraction of other activities, from social occasions to television to computers. In addition, barriers included lack of access to facilities, as well as negative images of competition, embarrassment, and the inability to become an elite athlete.

The VERB™ campaign implied action and used the tagline "It's what you do." Initial messages used animated figures of children covered with verbs being physically active. Later, messages turned these animated verb–covered kids into real kids actively playing. Widely used logos were developed and promoted as part of the branding effort. The VERB™ campaign partnered with television channels that successfully reach tweens, sponsored outreach events, and distributed promotional materials.

During the four years of the VERB™ campaign, tweens developed widespread recognition of the program and rated it highly in terms of "saying something important to me" and "makes me want to get more active," with maximum levels of recognition of 64% and 68%, respectively.

Data from Wong F, Huhman M, Asbury L, Mueller RB, McCarthy S, Londe P, et al. VERB™—A social marketing campaign to increase physical activity among youth. *Prev Chronic Disease.* 2004;3(1):1–7.

---

d Social marketing has not only incorporated traditional product marketing approaches; it has extended them to address the special circumstances of not-for-profit and government organizations. The use of social marketing in public health has required modifications and enhancements that have been described using four more "Ps": publics, partnerships, policies, and purse strings. "Publics" refers to the need to reach not only a target audience whose behavior we seek to change, but also those people who influence the target audience—be they parents, employers, or opinion leaders. For example, a campaign to address obesity, cigarettes, or high-risk sexual behavior in schools requires support from parents. "Partnerships" refers to the need for collaborations to achieve most public health goals. The VERB™ campaign, for instance, partnered with television stations appealing to tweens and schools to help get its message out. Successful efforts to reduce adolescent smoking, increase exercise, and reduce drug use also require changing institutional policies, which means reaching adult decision makers. Finally, the "purse string" aspect is money—few public health social marketing campaigns have adequate resources to do the job. Funding issues may require public health marketing teams to incorporate a long-term approach and look for nontraditional sources of funding.

The **PRECEDE-PROCEED** planning framework provides a structure to design and evaluate health education and health promotion programs through a diagnostic planning process followed by an implementation and evaluation process. There are nine steps of the framework, divided into two phases: PRECEDE and PROCEED.[24e]

**TABLE 4.10** illustrates the nine steps of the PRECEDE-PROCEED framework. Theory is applied in each step of the PRECEDE-PROCEED framework, guiding researchers and practitioners in their decisions.

The diagnostic phase of PRECEDE consists of collecting data and information to understand societal needs (step 1: social assessment), prioritizing community needs (step 2: epidemiological assessment), identifying factors contributing to the health issue (step 3: behavioral and environmental assessment), identifying factors that must be in place to initiate and sustain behavioral change (step 4: educational and ecological assessment), and identifying policies, resources and other circumstances that may assist or hinder efforts (step 5: administrative and policy assessment).

**TABLE 4.10** PRECEDE-PROCEED Framework and Application

| Step | Description | Example: gun violence |
|---|---|---|
| *Diagnostic phase: PRECEDE* | | |
| 1: Social assessment | Assess people's perceptions of their own needs and quality of life through data collection activities such as surveys, interviews, focus groups, and observation. | Gun violence emerged as a major concern among community members through focus groups that were conducted to explore health and safety concerns in the community. |
| 2. Epidemiological assessment | Determine which health problems are most important for which groups in a community, often by analyzing data from vital statistics, state and/or national surveys, etc. This step should assist in identifying subpopulations at high risk and provide data to set measurable objectives for the program. | Data from death certificates and crime reports reveals that the majority of deaths among males aged 24 years and younger in the community are due to gunshot wounds. |
| 3. Behavioral and environmental assessment | Identify factors, internal and external to the individual, that contributes to the health issue of interest. Literature searches and theory application provide guidance during this step. | A literature search provides insight into factors contributing to gun violence among males aged 24 years and younger. Gang-related behavior is found to be frequent in populations with similar socioeconomic status as that of the target population. |
| 4. Educational and organizational assessment | Preceding and reinforcing factors that initiate and sustain behavior change are identified, such as an individual's knowledge, skills and attitudes, social support, peer influence, and availability of services. | Interventions aimed at males 16 years and younger are found to be most successful. Young males with older male role models are more likely to view gangs as negative and more likely to participate in sports and community service. |
| 5. Administrative and policy assessment | Identify policies, resources, and circumstances that may help or hinder implementation of the intervention. | Communication system recently established between school system and law enforcement to report truancy and criminal behavior among student population. May assist in identifying subgroups to target intervention. |

e PRECEDE is an acronym for predisposing, reinforcing, enabling constructs in educational/environmental diagnosis, and evaluation. PROCEED is an acronym for policy, regulatory, and organizational constructs in educational and environmental development. Combined, these two phases view health behavior as influenced by both individual and environmental factors.

| Implementation and evaluation phase: PROCEED | | |
|---|---|---|
| 6. Implementation | The intervention is implemented. | After-school program implemented that incorporates educational, service-oriented, and physical activity components, led by males from the community. The program is tailored for males 12–16 years of age. |
| 7. Process evaluation | Process evaluation assesses the extent to which the intervention was implemented as planned. | Evaluate how program activities were delivered. |
| 8. Impact evaluation | Impact evaluation assesses the change in the factors identified in steps 3 and 4. | Evaluate gang associations among participants in the after-school programming. |
| 9. Outcome evaluation | Outcome evaluation assesses the effect of the intervention on the health issue of interest. | Evaluate deaths due to gun violence in the community before and after intervention. |

Data from Green LW and Kreuter MW. *Health Promotion Planning: An Educational and Ecological Approach*. 3rd edition. New York, NY: McGraw-Hill; 1999.

The implementation and evaluation phase of PROCEED begins with implementation of the strategies developed based on the findings from the PRECEDE phase in step 6. Knowing what works and what does not work is important across all public health interventions; therefore, evaluation is a critical component embedded within this planning model. In step 7, evaluation of the intervention components takes place to determine if the program is functioning the way it was intended, reaching the target population, etc. Step 8 evaluates the impact the intervention has on the factors being targeted. In step 9, outcomes of the intervention are evaluated to determine whether the intervention has affected the overall public health issue it set out to address.

Finally, in **BOX 4.3**, let us take a look at how new understandings of human behavior are beginning to be used to improve health and health care.[25]

---

**BOX 4.3** Behavioral Economics and Improving the Outcome of Care

A new field known as **behavioral economics** seeks to utilize new understandings about human behavior to change the behavior of clinicians and patients. These new understandings include:

- *Losses loom larger than gains*—Incentive systems for behavioral changes such as weight loss and cigarette cessation are more effective when patients have a potential loss, not just a potential gain. Incentive systems that require participants to put money down initially, with the possibility of gaining it back and more as a reward for changing behavior are most likely to be effective.
- *Just-in-time reminders work well*—Desirable behavior is often reinforced by reminders that are seen just before the time of the desirable behavior. These types of reminders have been successfully used to remind clinicians to wash their hands and elevator users to walk a flight or two of stairs.
- *Default choices are usually retained*—When people need to take action to change the default choice, they usually accept the default. This principle has been shown to affect clinicians' choice of generic versus name brand drugs and patients' choices of health insurance and even end-of-life care.
- *We are more influenced by our colleagues and peers than by the evidence*—Information on colleagues' prescribing practices has been shown to have a greater impact on changing physicians' prescribing behavior than evidence of effectiveness. Other patients' data also may be effective in changing individual behavior.
- *Creating new habits is key to behavioral change*—Apps which provide reminders to take medication, exercise, or do other routine behavior may be useful for developing and reinforcing new behaviors.

New understanding from the behavioral sciences is likely to continue to improve our ability to change behavior in ways that improve outcomes.

As we have seen, understanding human behavior and applying social and behavioral theories are central to population health. Study and use of the social and behavioral sciences play an important role in improving population health.

Analyzing the factors that influence health behavior assists in developing targeted interventions to promote healthy behavior and reduce health disparities. Health behavior theories and models are important tools used to explain and predict health behavior, providing useful road maps for the development of health promotion strategies. Additional planning frameworks, such as social marketing and PRECEDE-PROCEED, are also employed throughout the development, implementation, dissemination, and evaluation processes, contributing to sound health behavior interventions aimed at preserving, promoting, and protecting the health of populations.

## Key Words

Behavioral economics
Branding
Diffusion of innovation
Downstream factors
Food desert
Gini index
Health belief model
Health disparities
Health equity
Health inequality
Health inequity

Healthcare disparity
Mainstream factors
Mental health
Model
Place
PRECEDE-PROCEED
Price
Product
Promotion
Reciprocal determinism
Social cognitive theory

Social determinants of health
Social justice
Social marketing
Socioeconimic gradient
Socioeconomic status
Stages of change model
Theory
Theory of planned behavior
Upstream factors

## Discussion Questions

Take a look at the questions posed in the following scenarios, which were presented at the beginning of this chapter. See now whether you can answer these questions.

1. You travel to a country in Asia and find that this nation's culture affects most parts of life. From the food the people eat and their method of cooking, to their attitudes toward medical care, to their beliefs about the cause of disease and the ability to alter it through public health and medical interventions, this country is profoundly different from the United States. You ask: How does culture affect health?

2. You are working in a community in the United States with strict Islamic practices and find that religion, like culture, can have major impacts on health. Religious practices differ widely— from beliefs about food and alcohol; to sexual practices, such as male circumcision and female sexual behavior; to acceptance or rejection of interventions aimed at women's health. You ask: How does religion affect health?

3. You are trying to help your spouse quit smoking cigarettes and prevent your kids from starting. You know that gentle encouragement and support on a one-on-one basis are essential, but often not enough because cigarette smoking is an addiction that produces withdrawal and long-term cravings. You wonder what other factors in the social system influence behavior and how they can be addressed.

4. Your efforts to convince your friends to avoid smoking (or stop smoking) focus on giving them the facts about how cigarettes cause lung cancer, throat cancer, and serious heart disease. You are frustrated by how little impact you have on your friends. You wonder what tools are available to better explain and predict health behavior.

5. Your classmate, who is the first in her family to attend college, received word that her father lost his job at the local factory and she needs to take a leave from school because her family can no longer afford tuition. You wonder how this will affect her and her family.

6. Your town board just approved extending public transportation services to a wider geographic area. Although there are several opponents to the plan, you learn that a group of public health professionals supports this extension of services. You wonder what this transportation plan has to do with health.

7. You are in the checkout line at the grocery store, and a pregnant mother is ahead of you. You glance at the sugary cereals, snacks, and sodas she is purchasing and happen to notice that she is using an EBT card from the Supplemental

Nutrition Assistance Program (SNAP), formerly known as the Food Stamp program. You wonder what could be done to encourage the consumption of healthy food options.

8.  Every day on your way to work, you pass the same homeless man on the same corner. He does not look very old—you guess he is about 25 years of age. You notice that over the past few weeks, he has been coughing, and you figure he must have a cold. Today when you walk by his usual place on the corner, he is not there, but someone has left a sign that reads, "Rest in peace, Ramón." You are surprised, especially because he was so young. You wonder whether there was anything that could have been done to prevent his death.

9.  As a new parent, you hear from your pediatrician, nurses in the hospital, and even the makers of your brand of diapers that babies should sleep on their backs. They call it "Back-to-Sleep." You are surprised to find that it is part of the class on baby-sitting given by the local community center and a required part of the training for those who work in registered day care centers. You find out that it is all part of a social marketing campaign that has halved the number of deaths from sudden infant death syndrome. You ask: Why has the Back-to-Sleep campaign been so successful?

## References

1.  Edberg M. *Essentials of Health Behavior: Social and Behavioral Theory in Public Health.* Burlington, MA: Jones & Bartlett Learning; 2015.

2.  Berkman LF, Kawachi I, eds. *Social Epidemiology.* New York, NY: Oxford University Press; 2000.

3.  Commission on Social Determinants of Health. Closing the gap in a generation: Health equity through action on the social determinants of health. *Final Report of the Commission on Social Determinants of Health.* Geneva, Switzerland: World Health Organization; 2008.

4.  Marmot M. *The Status Syndrome: How Social Standing Affects Our Health and Longevity.* New York, NY: Henry Holt and Company; 2004.

5.  Wilkinson R, Marmot M, eds. *Social Determinants of Health: The Solid Facts.* 2nd ed. Copenhagen, Denmark: World Health Organization; 2003.

6.  The World Bank. GINI Index. http://data.worldbank.org/indicator/SI.POV.GINI?end=2013&locations=US-DE-GB&start=1986&view=chart. Accessed July 14, 2017.

7.  Braveman P, Egerter S. *Overcoming Obstacles to Health.* Washington, DC: Robert Wood Johnson Foundation Commission to Build a Healthier America; 2008.

8.  Murray CJL, Michaud CM, McKenna M, et al. *U.S. Country Patterns of Mortality by County and Race: 1965–1994.* Cambridge, MA: Harvard Center for Population and Development Studies; 1998.

9.  Marmot M. *The Status Syndrome: How Social Standing Affects Our Health and Longevity.* New York, NY: Henry Holt and Company; 2004.

10. The World Health Organization. Social determinants of health. http://www.who.int/social_determinants/en. Accessed July 14, 2017.

11. *Healthy People 2020.* Social determinants of health. https://www.healthypeople.gov/2020/topics-objectives/topic/social-determinants-of-health. Accessed July 14, 2017.

12. Wilkinson R, Marmot M, eds. *Social Determinants of Health: The Solid Facts.* 2nd ed. Copenhagen, Denmark: World Health Organization; 2003.

13. The World Health Organization. Social determinants of health. *Themes.* http://www.who.int/social_determinants/themes/en. Accessed July 14, 2017.

14. *Healthy People 2020.* Mental health and mental disorders. https://www.healthypeople.gov/2020/topics-objectives/topic/mental-health-and-mental-disorders. Accessed July 14, 2017.

15. New York Times. U.S. Suicide Rate Surges to a 30-Year High. https://www.nytimes.com/2016/04/22/health/us-suicide-rate-surges-to-a-30-year-high.html?_r=0. Accessed July 14, 2017.

16. National Cancer Institute. U.S. Department of Health and Human Services. *Theory at a Glance: A Guide for Health Promotion Practice.* 2nd ed. https://cancercontrol.cancer.gov/brp/research/theories_project/theory.pdf. Accessed July 14, 2017.

17. Prochaska JO, DiClemente CC. Stages and processes of self-change of smoking: Toward an integrative model of change. *Journal of Consulting and Clinical Psychology.* 1983;51(3):390–395.

18. Azjen I, Drive BL. Prediction of leisure participation from behavioral, normative, and control beliefs: An application of the theory of planned behavior. *Leisure Science.* 1991;13:185–204.

19. Bandura A. *Social Foundations of Thought and Action: A Social Cognitive Theory.* Englewood Cliffs, NJ: Prentice Hall; 1986.

20. Rogers EM. *Diffusion of Innovations,* 5th ed. New York, NY: Free Press; 2003.

21. Hayden J. *Introduction to health behavior theory.* Burlington, MA: Jones & Bartlett Learning; 2019.

22. Weinreich NK. What is social marketing? http://www.social-marketing.com/Whatis.html. Accessed July 14, 2017.

23. Wong F, Huhman M, Asbury L, et al. VERB™—A social marketing campaign to increase physical activity among youth. *Preventing Chronic Disease.* 2004;3(1):1–7

24. Green LW, Kreuter MW. *Health Promotion Planning: An Educational and Ecological Approach.* 4th ed. New York, NY: McGraw-Hill; 2005.

25. New York Times. How Behavioral Economics Can Produce Better Health Care. https://www.nytimes.com/2017/04/13/upshot/answer-to-better-health-care-behavioral-economics.html?emc=eta1. Accessed July 14, 2017.

# CHAPTER 5

# Health Law, Policy, and Ethics

## LEARNING OBJECTIVES

By the end of this chapter, the student will be able to:

- explain the scope of health law, policy, and ethics.
- identify key legal principles that form the basis for public health law.
- identify four types of law.
- discuss and illustrate the concept of Health in All Policies.
- explain the differences between market and social justice.
- illustrate the potential tensions between individual rights and the needs of society using public health examples.
- discuss key principles that underlie the ethics of human research.
- identify principles of public health ethics.
- discuss policies aimed at preparing for and responding to pandemic disease.

A new statute and subsequent administrative regulations give only a temporary license to newly licensed drivers, prohibiting late night driving and the use of cell phones and limiting the number of passengers. You ask: Should elderly drivers be subject to these same types of regulations, such as being required to retake a driver's test?

You hear that a neighbor has TB and refuses treatment. You wonder: What if he has the type of TB that can't be cured with drugs? You ask: Can't they make him take his medicine or at least get him out of the neighborhood?

A friend of yours experienced a grand mal seizure in which she totally lost consciousness. Fortunately, cancer is ruled out and she is tolerating the medications without serious side effects and without another seizure. It is 2 months later and your friend tells you her driver's license was taken away by the motor vehicle administration and she does not know when she will get it back. You ask: What types of issues are involved in deciding if and when she can drive again?

You receive an email encouraging your participation in a new research study. It sounds like you are eligible, so you check into it. You are surprised to find that even if you participate, you may not receive the new drug, and you will not even be told which treatment you are receiving. Despite your willingness to take your chances, you are told that you are not eligible for the study due to conditions that put you at increased risk of developing side effects. You ask: Why am I barred from participating if I am willing to take the risks?

The latest breaking news announces that WHO has declared what it called a Public Health Emergency of International Concern because of the rapid spread of a new strain of Influenza. You wonder: What does this declaration mean? What will change as a result of this declaration?

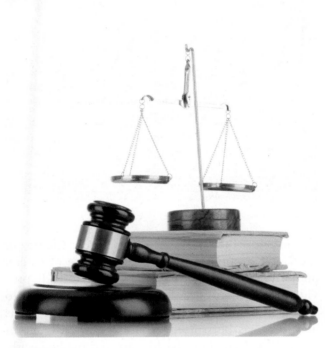

© Africa Studio/Shutterstock

These are the types of issues that are part of health law, policy, and ethics. Let us begin by examining the scope of these issues.

# What Is the Scope of Health Law, Policy, and Ethics?

Health law, policy, and ethics reflect a wide range of tools that society uses to encourage and discourage behaviors by individuals and groups. These tools apply to health care, as well as to traditional public health. In addition, in recent years, a field called **bioethics** has been defined, which includes elements of both health care and public health and focuses on applying morals or values to areas of potential conflict.[1]

Health law, policy, and ethics affect the full range of issues that confront us in population health. They address such things as the access to and the quality and cost of health care. They also address the organizational and professional structures designed to deliver health care. Health law, policy, and ethics are key tools for accomplishing the goals of traditional public health, ranging from occupational safety to drug and highway safety, and from control of communicable diseases to noncommunicable and environmental diseases. Bioethics lies at the intersection of health law and policy and attempts to apply individual and group values and morals to controversial issues, such as use of new technologies, stem cell research, and end-of-life care. **TABLE 5.1** outlines a range of issues that are addressed by health law, policy, and ethics.

The scope of health law, policy, and ethics is so vast that we will focus on first defining key principles and philosophies that underlie our society's approach to these issues. Then we will focus on three examples

| **TABLE 5.1** Components of Health Law, Policy, and Ethics | | |
|---|---|---|
| **Component** | **Scope** | **Examples of issues** |
| Health care | Access, quality, and cost of health care    Organizational and professional structures for the delivery of care | Rules governing Medicare and Medicaid, as well as laws governing private insurance    Hospital governance and professional licensure |
| Public health | Population health and safety, including governmental efforts to provide services to entire populations, as well as vulnerable groups | Food and drug laws and procedures, environmental laws and procedures, regulations for control of communicable diseases |
| Bioethics | Application of individual and group values and morals to controversial areas | End-of-life care, stem cell research, use of new technology , protection of research subjects |

that illustrate key issues confronted in the healthcare, public health, and bioethics arenas. These are:

1.  Is there a right to health care?
2.  How does public health attempt to balance the rights of individuals and the needs of society?
3.  What bioethical principles are used to address public health issues?

Finally we will take a look at an example of how global health policy is struggling to find effective ways to address new **pandemic** diseases.

Let us start by taking a look at key legal principles that underlie the approach to public health and health care in the United States.

## What Legal Principles Underlie Public Health and Health Care?

In order to better appreciate the issue of health policy and law, it is important to understand some key legal principles that underlie both public health and healthcare law in the United States.[1] First, the U.S. Constitution is a fundamental document that governs the issues of public health and healthcare law. However, the U.S. Constitution does not mention health. As a result, public health and health care are among those issues that are left primarily to the authority of the states, unless delegated by the state to local jurisdictions, such as cities or counties. The use of this authority, known as **police power**, allows states to pass legislation and take actions to protect the common good. The authority to protect the common good may justify a wide range of state actions, including the regulation of healthcare professionals and facilities; the establishment of health and safety standards in retail and other occupational settings; and the control of hazards ranging from requiring the use of car restraint systems, to vaccinations, to restricting the sale of tobacco products.[1,2]

The use of state police power is limited by the protections afforded to individuals. These protections are known as **rights** and are created either through the U.S. Constitution, through a state's constitution, or through laws passed at the federal or state levels. The U.S. Constitution allows, but does not require, governments to act to protect public health or to provide healthcare services.

This has been referred to as the **negative constitution**. Thus, while governments often have the authority to act, they are not required to do so. For instance, the Supreme Court has not found an obligation on the part of states to act to prevent child or spousal abuse even when the state is fully aware of specific circumstances or a court has issued a restraining order.[1]

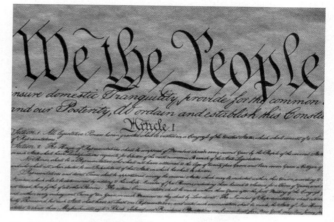

© Joseph Sohm/Shutterstock

Second, the Interstate Commerce Clause of the U.S. Constitution is the major source of federal authority in public health and health care. It provides the federal government with the authority to tax, spend, and regulate interstate commerce.[2] This authority has been used to justify a wide range of federal involvement in health care and public health. Federal authority is often exerted through incentives to the states. For instance, states may be offered federal funding or matching funding if they enact specific types of legislation, such as the rules governing Medicaid or definitions of blood-alcohol levels for driving under the influence.[3] The U.S. Constitution's supremacy clause declares that legitimate federal laws are the supreme laws of the land and they preempt or overrule state laws that conflict with them.[a] This provision has been used by federal public health agencies, such as the Food and Drug Administration and the Environmental Protection Agency, to justify national standards that overrule and limit state rules and regulations ranging from quality controls on drugs to levels of permissible exposures to toxic substances.[1,2]

Third, the U.S. Constitution grants individual rights. Some of them, such as freedom of speech, religion, and assembly and the right to bear arms, are explicit in the document. Others have been inferred by the U.S. Supreme Court, such as the right to procreation, privacy, bodily integrity, and travel. These

---

a  Another implication of constitutional law is the supremacy of the U.S. Constitution even over international law. Human rights and standards incorporated into international documents are not directly enforceable in the United States. These rights and standards are only enforceable in the United States through enactment of federal or state laws.[1]

inferred rights are often the basis for individual protections in public health and health care, including the right to utilize contraception, have an abortion, and limit the state and federal authority to use quarantine and other travel restrictions.[1,2] Unless the U.S. Constitution explicitly includes a right or one has been "found" by the Supreme Court of the United States, no right exists. However, federal and state legislatures may create rights through legislation ranging from access to education to access to medical care. The existence of a right implies that state and/or federal courts are expected to uphold and enforce the right.[b]

Health law is based upon these rules governing the authority of federal and state governments and also the rights of individuals. It is derived from four sources that are summarized in **BOX 5.1**.[1]

---

**BOX 5.1** Types of Law

To appreciate the complex relationship between the law and public health and health care, it is important to appreciate that there are four sources of law. These may be classified as **constitutional law**, **legislative statutes**, **administrative regulations**, and **judicial law** (also called case law or common law).

Constitutional law includes not only the U.S. Constitution, but also the constitutions of the 50 states. The provisions of state constitutions are important because the responsibilities for health lie with the states unless the federal Constitution grants authority to the federal government. As we have seen, the commerce clause and the due process clauses of the Constitution have been the basis for extensions of federal authority into areas of health. State constitutions are often easier to amend than the federal Constitution, and thus can and do change more frequently. Constitutions often limit the role of government and define its processes. Constitutional law, however, does not usually directly mandate roles for government in the area of health.

Legislative law, or statutes, is written by legislative bodies at local, state, and federal levels. Federal statutes preempt, or overrule, conflicting state statutes, as long as they are consistent with the limitation placed on the federal government by the U.S. Constitution. Statutes often directly address health issues. Legislative law may place requirements or prohibition on future activities. Statutes may authorize governmental regulation, such as professional or institutional licensure; require specific activities, such a restaurant inspections; prohibit other activities, such as smoking in public places; or provide funding to pay for governmental services or reimburse those who provide the services, such as health care.

Administrative law is produced by executive agencies of the federal, state, and local governments in order to implement legislative statutes, which are often written in quite general language. Executive agencies must follow legally defined processes and stay within what is called the legislative intent of the statute. Administrative law can be seen as operationalizing statutes passed by legislative bodies. These types of laws may define who is eligible for services, how these services may be provided, the levels of reimbursement received, and a large number of other important details that affect the day-to-day operations of government services and programs. Administrative law affects public health in many ways, from the regulation of septic tanks to requirements for immunization to enroll in public education. Executive agencies often set up quasi-judicial processes to review contested cases. These judicial processes usually provide for limited access to the court system to contest their decisions.

Judicial, case, or common law is law made by courts when applying constitutional, statutory, or administrative law to specific cases. In addition, common law may fill in the holes when statutory law does not provide guidance. For instance, case law may be the basis for addressing environmental health issues, which the law defines as "nuisances" ranging from excess noise to disposal of garbage. Judges' primary responsibility is to apply previous rulings or precedence to new cases that come before them; however, they may take into account existing traditions and customs of society when applying the law to specific cases. Higher courts including appellate courts, and ultimately the U.S. Supreme Court, and in some instances, state Supreme Courts may decide that a statute violates the relevant constitutions. That is, they can rule a statute unconstitutional.

---

b  Enforcement is required by law to occur based on due process. Due process includes **substantive due process**, which refers to the grounds for depriving an individual of a right, as well as **procedural due process**, which refers to the processes that must be undertaken to deprive an individual of a right. The former implies that state and federal governments must justify depriving an individual of life, liberty, and property. When fundamental rights are involved or laws are based on suspect classifications, such as gender or race, the court applies strict criteria that place difficult burdens of proof on the government to justify these types of actions. Procedural due process implies that when a right exists, governments may not deny individuals the right in an arbitrary or unfair way. This process requires that acceptable legal processes be followed before an individual can be deprived of a right. The Supreme Court has considered a fundamental right as one that is explicit in the U.S. Constitution, that has been "found" in the U.S. Constitution by the Supreme Court, or that is rooted in the nation's history and traditions.[1,2]

Health law refers to a vast array of legal issues that influence much of what goes on in public health and health care. However, the influence of health policy often extends beyond that of the formal legal system. Let us take a look at what we mean by "health policy."

## What Do We Mean by "Health Policy"?

Within the constraints set by law, there is considerable latitude for governments, as well as private groups, to develop policies that affect the ways that public health and health care are conducted. The main distinction between a law and a policy is defined by who can create each and how they can be enforced. Essentially any organization can create a policy and subsequently enforce the policy it created. A range of governmental organizations create the law that is enforced through the legal system.

Health policy is a subset of the larger arena of public policy. According to Teitelbaum and Wilensky, "when deciding on whether something is a public policy decision, the focus is not only on who is making the decision, but also on what kind of decision is being made."[4] They define individuals or groups that make public policy based on the ability of the individual or group to make an **authoritative decision**. An authoritative decision is a decision made by an individual or group that has the power to implement the decision. A range of governmental and private groups make public policy decisions in areas such as cigarette smoking. In government, authoritative decisions may be made by an executive branch official, such as the president or a governor, or administrative officials, such as federal, state, or local health officers. These may range from policies that discourage the growing of tobacco, to policies that encourage the sale of tobacco products abroad, to policies that restrict smoking in public places or tax tobacco sales. These policies may or may not be incorporated into laws or statutes.

At times, health policy may be made by private groups, including professional societies, such as the American Public Health Association, or commercial trade associations representing hospitals, the drug industry, the insurance industry, etc. Policies that affect large numbers of people, such as those that restrict smoking in hospitals, encourage clinicians to incorporate smoking prevention and cessation programs, compensate clinicians' efforts through insurance, and encourage the development of new drugs to assist with smoking cessation, are all examples of health policies that may be set by groups outside of government. Thus, the "public" in public policies does not necessarily imply that the policies were developed or implemented by government.

Health policy is a rapidly expanding field because there is growing recognition that collaboration is necessary across sectors in order to successfully address the varied and complex health issues facing our society. A **health in all policies approach** has begun to be used in which private and public entities work toward common goals to achieve improved health for all while reducing health inequities.

**BOX 5.2** takes a look at what is meant by health in all policies.

According to Teitelbaum and Wilensky, in addition to being authoritative, a public policy decision must be one that "goes beyond the individual sphere and affects the greater community."[4] Decisions to seek vaccinations or screenings, to smoke cigarettes at home, or to purchase health insurance are individual decisions. Public policy issues revolve around incentives or requirements to encourage or discourage these actions by groups of individuals or the society as a whole.

## How Are Public Health Policy Priorities Established?

The United States is faced with multiple, complex, and evolving issues that affect the health of the population. Prioritizing these issues has been the task of an initiative known as *Healthy People*. The initiative, organized by the U.S. Department of Health and Human Services, is a collaborative effort of a multitude of private and public organizations that sets evidence-based national objectives aimed at improving the health of the population. Since the decade beginning in 1980, a revised set of objectives has been established for the nation each subsequent decade. *Healthy People* tracks a large number of specific objectives. These objectives, which are supported

**BOX 5.2** Health in All Policies

*Health in All Policies is an approach to public policies across sectors that systematically takes into account the health implications of decisions, seeks synergies, and avoids harmful health impacts in order to improve population health and health equity.*[5]

Helsinki Statement on Health in All Policies; WHO (WHA67.12) 2014.

The American Public Health Association and the World Health Organization (WHO) have endorsed and are working to implement Health in All Policies. The key to Health in All Policies is the interaction between health and non health sectors of government and society. Traditionally both medicine and public health have been structurally and functionally separated from other sectors. Budgeting and decision-making have been distinct. For instance, cost effectiveness considerations have long been integrated into decisions about urban planning and construction but only recently integrated into health decisions.

The WHO has developed an example of how Health in All Policies should work which is illustrated in **FIGURE 5.1**.[6]

In order for health in all policies to be effective, policies adopted by different sectors must reinforce one another. For instance, a health in all policies approach targeting health and development in early childhood may include education policies that provide opportunities for women of childbearing age among all income-levels to attain a college education; employment policies that allow mothers to take maternity leave while maintaining their salary and health benefits; and housing policies that require landlords to maintain safe structures free of hazards for young children, such as avoiding lead poisoning and asthma triggers.

Health in all policies is an overarching framework for integrating health issues into a broad range of social and economic issues. You are likely to hear more about health in all policies as law and policy makers come to better understand the complex relationships between health and social and economic policy.

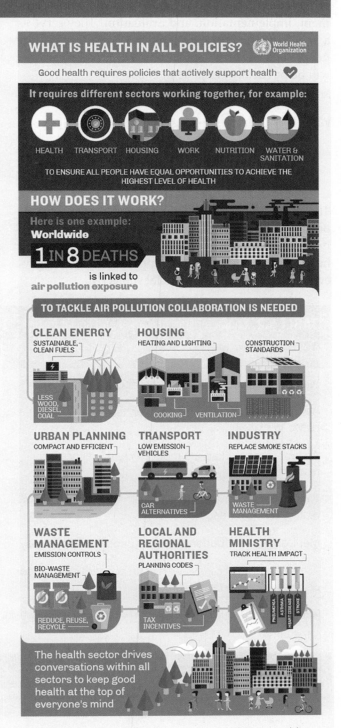

**FIGURE 5.1** World Health Organization. What is Health in All Policies?

Reproduced with permission of the World Health Organization. What is Health in All Policies? Available at: http://who.int/social_determinants/publications/health-policies-manual /HiAP_Infographic.pdf?ua=1. Accessed July 19, 2017.

with data and need to be measurable, assist in identifying issues in need of program and policy development, implementation, and evaluation. They serve as a way to monitor progress toward achieving healthy people and healthy populations[7] *Healthy People 2030* will be publically available in 2020.

## How Do Philosophies Toward the Role of Government Affect Health Policies?

The types of health policies favored depend greatly on one's philosophies about the role that public and private institutions should play in public health and health care. Specifically, the appropriate role of government is often a controversial subject.

One of the most fundamental differences within our society is the attitude or philosophy about the roles that government and the economic market should play in advancing health. To appreciate this issue, it is useful to look at two contrasting philosophies regarding the government's role in health care and public health. These philosophies are called **social justice** and **market justice**. A social justice approach views the equitable distribution of health as a social responsibility, in contrast to a market justice approach, which emphasizes individual, rather than collective, responsibility for health.

Understanding these quite different approaches is helpful because our current system of health care and public health borrows from both of these basic approaches to varying degrees. **TABLE 5.2** outlines the contrasting characteristics of market justice and social justice. **TABLE 5.3** examines many of the implications of the two different philosophies.[8]

**TABLE 5.2** Characteristics of Market and Social Justice

| Market justice | Social justice |
|---|---|
| Views health care as an economic good | Views health care as a social resource |
| Assumes free market conditions for health services delivery | Requires active government involvement in health services delivery |
| Assumes that markets are more efficient in allocating resources equitably | Assumes that the government is more efficient in allocating health resources equitably |
| Production and distribution of health care determined by market-based demand | Medical resource allocation determined by central planning |
| Medical care distribution based on people's ability to pay | Ability to pay inconsequential for receiving medical care |
| Access to medical care viewed as an economic reward for personal effort and achievement | Equal access to medical services viewed as a basic right |

Reproduced from Shi L, Singh DA. *Delivering health care in America: a systems approach.* Burlington, MA: Jones & Bartlett Learning; 2019.

**TABLE 5.3** Implications of Market and Social Justice

| Market justice | Social justice |
|---|---|
| Individual responsibility for health | Collective responsibility for health |
| Benefits based on individual purchasing power | Everyone is entitled to a basic package of services |
| Limited obligation to the collective good | Strong obligation to the collective good |
| Emphasis on individual well-being | Community well-being supersedes that of the individual |
| Private solutions to social problems | Public solutions to social problems |
| Rationing based on ability to pay | Planned rationing of health care |

Reproduced from Shi L, Singh DA. *Delivering health care in America: a systems approach.* Burlington, MA: Jones & Bartlett Learning; 2019.

We have now looked at key principles of health law and health policy that underlie our approach to health care and public health. To see how these principles operate in practice, let us review the three questions introduced earlier:

1. Is there a right to health care?
2. How does public health attempt to balance the rights of individuals and the needs of society?
3. What bioethical principles are used to address public health issues?

## ▶ Is There a Right to Health Care?

In 1948, a right to health care was incorporated into the Universal Declaration of Human Rights and the Constitution of the WHO. The former states that "everyone has the right to a standard of living adequate for the health and well-being of himself and his family, including…medical care…and the right to security in the event of…sickness…."[9] Most developed countries have incorporated a right to health care in their constitution or have created rights to health care as part of the legislative process, usually as part of a healthcare system that provides universal coverage. This internationally recognized right to health care cannot be enforced in the United States unless it is found to be recognized by the U.S. Constitution or a state constitution or has been incorporated into federal, state, or local statutes. Therefore, we need to examine what has happened within the legal system of the United States.

As we have discussed, the U.S. Constitution does not mention the word "health." Rights, however, can be "found" or created by the Supreme Court through its interpretation of the Constitution. Rights to travel and privacy, for example, have been "found" by the Supreme Court, while a right to health care has not been. State courts, such as the Supreme Court of Indiana, have addressed the meaning of a license to practice medicine (the Indiana Supreme Court tackled this in *Hurley v. Eddingfield*). In the case, a licensed physician refused services to a pregnant woman despite being offered prepayment and despite the fact that the physician knew that no other qualified physician was available. As a result, the woman did not receive medical care and both she and her unborn child died.[1] The court established what has been called the **no-duty principle**. This principle holds that healthcare providers (whether they are individuals or institutions) do not have an obligation to provide health services. A right to health care can be created within a state via its constitution. It can also be created in the United States or within a state by legislative action.[1]

Limited rights to health care have been established by legislative action. For instance, federal law includes the 1986 Treatment for Emergency Medical Conditions and Women in Labor Act, which provides a right to emergency medical care usually provided through hospital emergency departments.[c] This act establishes a right to health care by those seeking emergency services and establishes a duty on the part of hospital emergency departments to provide these services.

This right and the corresponding duty, however, are quite limited. Patients have the right to receive care and the hospital has a duty to provide an "appropriate" examination. The institution also has the duty to stabilize an emergency situation by providing as much treatment as possible within its capacity. When a hospital does not have the capacity to treat the emergency condition, it is required to transfer the patient to another facility in a medically appropriate fashion. These rights and duties are limited to emergency conditions in hospital emergency departments and do not provide more general rights to health care.[d]

A right to health care in the United States has not been generally established. As with health law

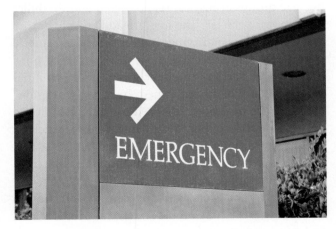

© cleanfotos/Shutterstock

---

c This act is often referred to as EMTALA, which is an acronym for the law's original name—the Emergency Medical Treatment and Active Labor Act.

d Another example of legislation that has established rights to health care is the Medicaid program. Medicaid establishes defined criteria for eligibility to enroll that are partially governed by federal law and partially by state law. During the time that an individual is qualified for Medicaid, they have certain rights to health care that can be enforced by individuals in the courts.

and policies in general, this issue has not been definitively settled. As the state and federal governments struggle with the problems of providing health care for everyone, the right to health care is again emerging as an issue for debate and consideration. Let us now take a look at another fundamental issue that is at the core of public health law and policy—the balance between the rights of the individual and the needs of society.

## How Does Public Health Attempt to Balance the Rights of Individuals and the Needs of Society?

Public health interventions often create a level of tension between the concerns of individuals and the needs of society. This is the situation even when individual rights are not involved. For instance, the courts have been clear that a driver's license is a privilege and not a right. Thus, it can be regulated by states without having to justify that individuals who are denied a driver's license are being denied a right. The regulation of driver's licenses is a state responsibility, and as such, there is enormous variation in factors such as age requirement, the length of time and requirement for learning permits, the type of examination required, the rules for suspension of a driver's license, and requirements for renewal of a driver's license.

Motor vehicle injuries remain a major cause of death and disability. It is widely accepted that there are two age groups at highest risk of death and disability from motor vehicles. The first are adolescents during their initial years of driving, and the second are elderly individuals. Until recently, most states imposed minimum or no barriers to either group once an initial driver's license had been issued. In many states, limitations have now been imposed for one or both age groups. Possible public health interventions include raising the driving age; requiring stricter standards for licensure; and placing initial limitations on new drivers, including restricting nighttime driving, the number of passengers, and the use of cell phones. Common restrictions on older drivers include vision and hearing tests and reexamination including road testing.

The type of risk also plays a role in determining how we balance individual rights and the needs of society. **Self-imposed risk** is risk an individual knowingly and willingly takes on through his or her own actions, such as choosing not to wear a motorcycle helmet while riding a motorcycle. Even though helmet laws are intended to protect motorcyclists, the laws could be viewed as infringing on an individual's desire not to wear a helmet. If a motorcyclist decides to forego wearing a helmet, he or she is putting himself or herself at risk for injury.

However, not all risks to health can be attributed to individual behavior, blurring the line between individual rights and societal needs. **Imposed risk** refers to risk to individuals and populations that is out of their direct control. An example of an imposed risk would be exposure to environmental toxins from a local factory. The imposed risk itself may therefore be viewed as infringing on an individual's desire for clean air in his or her town. Because the factory's emissions are out of the direct control of the individual, interventions aimed to address imposed risk require actions external to the individual, perhaps in the form of governmental intervention to enforce environmental emissions regulations. As can be seen, the focus of responsibility differs depending on whether the risk is self-imposed or imposed.

The tension level between the individual and society is even greater when fundamental rights are denied, as is the case with the use of quarantine. **BOX 5.3** examines the historical and current uses of quarantine.[10]

Now let us turn our attention to our third question and see how ethical and bioethical principles are being applied to public health.

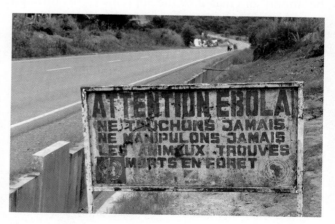

© Sergey Uryadnikov/Shutterstock

**Quarantine**, the compulsory physical separation of those with a disease—or at high risk of developing a disease—from the rest of the population goes back to ancient times, when it was used to restrict entry of ships into ports where epidemic diseases threatened. Attempts to control epidemics of yellow fever, smallpox, and other infectious disease by quarantine were very much a part of the early history of the United States.

In the 1800s, tuberculosis (TB) sanatoriums often isolated those afflicted on a voluntary basis. Laws existed and were occasionally used that allowed quarantine of patients who felt well though were thought to be carriers of TB and other contagious diseases, such as typhoid. In the early years of the 20th century, "Typhoid Mary," who was infected with typhoid but had no symptoms, was quarantined on an island in New York after she refused to voluntarily refrain from working as a food handler.

Quarantine was only occasionally used to control disease in the 1900s. However, in the early 2000s, it again became a public health issue precipitated by the recognition of SARS and the fear of rapid global spread of SARS and other communicable diseases. The spread of drug-resistant tuberculosis has again made the use of quarantine for TB an ongoing important public health issue. The Ebola epidemic drew renewed attention to the issue of quarantine of those exposed to disease.

Quarantine laws are in the process of revision. The issues of quarantine reflect many of the tensions between the right of the individual and the rights of society. For instance, a *New England Journal of Medicine* article on the use of quarantine for control of extremely resistant TB states:

> In recent decades, courts have clarified the legal rights of patients with tuberculosis who are subject to compulsory isolation. Drawing an analogy between isolation orders and civil commitment for mental illness, courts have affirmed that patients who are isolated by law have many procedural due-process rights, including the right to counsel and a hearing before an independent decision maker. States must also provide "clear and convincing" evidence that isolation is necessary to prevent a significant risk of harm to others. Most important, some courts have held that isolation must be the least restrictive alternative for preventing such a risk. If the government can protect public health without relying on involuntary detention, it must and should do so.[10]

The use of quarantine is thus likely to be restricted and used very infrequently in the future. Increasingly, the emphasis on the rights of the individual outweighs any value that quarantine may have in protecting the public's health.

# What Bioethical Principles Are Used to Address Public Health Issues?

A code of ethics has been prepared through the Public Health Leadership Society to guide public health practitioners. **TABLE 5.4** lists the Principles of the Ethical Practice of Public Health.[11]

Public health officials face the need to make decisions and take action. Therefore, a set of ethical principles to guide action is very important. Bernheim and Childress[12] have outlined a set of principles for guiding public health action as follows:

- Producing benefits
- Avoiding, preventing, and reducing harms
- Producing the maximal balance of benefits over harms and other costs
- Distributing benefits and burdens fairly and ensuring public participation, including the participation of affected parties

- Respecting autonomous choices and actions, including liberty of action
- Protecting privacy and confidentiality
- Keeping promises and commitments
- Disclosing information as well as speaking honestly and truthfully
- Building and maintaining trust

When considering whether action is justified, the following conditions should be met[12]:

- Effectiveness: Is the action likely to accomplish the public health goal?
- Necessity: Is the action necessary to override the conflicting ethical claims to achieve the public health goal?
- Least infringement: Is the action the least restrictive and least intrusive?
- Proportionality: Will the probable benefits of the action outweigh the infringed moral norms and any negative effects?
- Impartiality: Are all potentially affected stakeholders treated impartially?

---

**TABLE 5.4** Principles of the Ethical Practice of Public Health

Public health should address principally the fundamental causes of disease and requirements for health, aiming to prevent adverse health outcomes.

Public health should achieve community health in a way that respects the rights of individuals in the community.

Public health policies, programs, and priorities should be developed and evaluated through processes that ensure an opportunity for input from community members.

Public health should advocate and work for the empowerment of disenfranchised community members, aiming to ensure that the basic resources and conditions necessary for health are accessible to all.

Public health should seek the information needed to implement effective policies and programs that protect and promote health.

Public health institutions should provide communities with the information they have that is needed for decisions on policies or programs and should obtain the community's consent for their implementation.

Public health institutions should act in a timely manner on the information they have within the resources and the mandate given to them by the public.

Public health programs and policies should incorporate a variety of approaches that anticipate and respect diverse values, beliefs, and cultures in the community.

Public health programs and policies should be implemented in a manner that most enhances the physical and social environment.

Public health institutions should protect the confidentiality of information that can bring harm to an individual or community if made public. Exceptions must be justified on the basis of the high likelihood of significant harm to the individual or others.

Public health institutions should ensure the professional competence of their employees.

Public health institutions and their employees should engage in collaborations and affiliations in ways that build the public's trust and the institution's effectiveness.

Modified from Public Health Leadership Society. *Principles of the Ethical Practice of Public Health*, Version 2.2. Available at: http://phls.org/CMSuploads/Principles-of-the-Ethical-Practice-of-PH-Version-2.2-68496.pdf. Published 2002. Accessed March 25, 2017.

---

■ Public justification: Can public health officials offer public justification that citizens, and in particular those most affected, could find acceptable in principle?

In addition to applying general ethical principles to public health practice, public health is frequently involved in the development and applications of ethical principles to public health and clinical research. In fact, the modern field of bioethics grew out of the efforts to protect participants in research, while ensuring that society can benefit from the results of ethical human research. Let us look at how these standards developed and how research subjects are protected today.

# ▶ How Can Bioethical Principles Be Applied to Protecting Individuals Who Participate in Research?

Ethical issues pervade nearly every aspect of public health and medical practice. However, ethical considerations have had an especially strong impact on the conduct of research. The modern field of bioethics in general and research ethics in particular grew out of the Nuremberg trials of German physicians who performed experiments on prisoners in Nazi concentration camps. These crimes included exposure to extremes of temperature, mutilating surgery, and deliberate infection with a variety of lethal germs. The report of the Nuremberg trials established internationally accepted principles known as the Nuremberg Code shown in **BOX 5.4**.[13]

Abuse of individuals participating in research has not been limited to victims of Nazi concentration camps. In the United States from the late 1930s through the early 1970s, the Tuskegee Syphilis Study used disadvantaged, rural black men to study the untreated course of syphilis. These men were recruited to a study of "bad blood" and were misled into believing that they were receiving effective treatment; in addition, they were provided deceptive information in order to retain them in the study. These subjects were deprived of penicillin treatment in order not to interrupt the research, long after such treatment became generally available for syphilis.

The Tuskegee Study was a major reason for the creation of The National Commission for the Protection of Human Subjects of Biomedical and Behavioral Research, which produced what has come to be called the **Belmont Report**. The Belmont Report focused on the key issues of defining informed consent and the selection of participants and led to the development of **institutional review boards (IRBs)**, which now must approve most human research. The report remains a vital part of the framework for defining the rights of research subjects.[14] The following excerpts outline three basic ethical principles:

1.  **Respect for persons**—Respect for persons incorporates at least two ethical convictions: first, individuals should be treated as autonomous agents, and second, that persons with diminished autonomy are entitled to protection. The principle of respect for persons thus divides into two separate moral requirements: the requirement to acknowledge autonomy and the requirement to protect those with diminished autonomy.

2.  **Beneficence**—Persons are treated in an ethical manner not only by respecting their decisions and protecting them from harm, but also by making efforts to secure their well-being. Such treatment falls under the principle of beneficence. Two general rules have been formulated as complementary expressions of beneficent actions in this sense:

---

**BOX 5.4**  The Ten Principles Contained in the Nuremberg Code

1.  The voluntary consent of the human subject is absolutely essential.
2.  The experiment should be such as to yield fruitful results for the good of society, unprocurable by other methods or means of study, and not random and unnecessary in nature.
3.  The experiment should be so designed and based on the results of animal experimentation and knowledge of the natural history of the disease or other problem under study that the anticipated results will justify the performance of the experiment.
4.  The experiment should be so conducted as to avoid all unnecessary physical and mental suffering and injury.
5.  No experiment should be conducted where there is an a priori reason to believe that death or disabling injury will occur, except, perhaps, in those experiments where the experimental physicians also serve as subjects.
6.  The degree of risk to be taken should never exceed that determined by the humanitarian importance of the problem to be solved by the experiment.
7.  Proper preparations should be made and adequate facilities provided to protect the experimental subject against even remote possibilities of injury, disability, or death.
8.  The experiment should be conducted only by scientifically qualified persons. The highest degree of skill and care should be required through all stages of the experiment of those who conduct or engage in the experiment.
9.  During the course of the experiment, the human subject should be at liberty to bring the experiment to an end if he has reached the physical or mental state where continuation of the experiment seems to him to be impossible.
10. During the course of the experiment, the scientist in charge must be prepared to terminate the experiment at any stage, if he has probable cause to believe, in the exercise of the good faith, superior skill, and careful judgment required of him, that a continuation of the experiment is likely to result in injury, disability, or death to the experimental subject.

Reproduced from United States Government. *Trials of War Criminals before the Nuremberg Military Tribunals under Control Council Law.* No. 10, Vol. 2. Washington, DC: U.S. Government Printing Office; 1949:181–182.

(1) do no harm and (2) maximize possible benefits and minimize possible harms.

3. **Justice**—Who ought to receive the benefits of research and bear its burdens? This is a question of justice, in the sense of fairness in distribution or what is deserved. An injustice occurs when some benefit to which a person is entitled is denied without good reason or when some burden is imposed unduly. Another way of conceiving the principle of justice is that equals ought to be treated equally.

IRBs were created to ensure the ethical conduct of research. The code of federal regulations outlines the following key roles that the IRB is expected to play. In order to approve research, the IRB shall determine that all of the following requirements are satisfied:[15]

1. Risks to subjects are minimized.
2. Risks to subjects are reasonable in relation to anticipated benefits.
3. Selection of subjects is equitable.
4. Informed consent will be sought from each prospective subject or the subject's legally authorized representative.
5. The research plan makes adequate provision for monitoring the data collected to ensure the safety of subjects.
6. When appropriate, there are adequate provisions to protect the privacy of subjects and to maintain the confidentiality of data.
7. When some or all of the subjects are likely to be vulnerable to coercion or undue influence, such as children, prisoners, pregnant women, mentally disabled persons, or economically or educationally disadvantaged persons, additional safeguards have been included in the study to protect the rights and welfare of these subjects.

We have come a long way from the days when human research was conducted without informed consent on individuals who could be coerced to participate. The standards of research, however, continue to evolve and will most likely continue to change through the identification of ethical limitations of current studies.[e]

We have now examined key principles of health law, policy, and ethics and their applications to issues in health care, public health, and bioethics. These principles are basic tools, along with public health data, health communications and the social and behavioral sciences, and can be considered options for implementation when striving to achieve the goals of public health. They are especially powerful tools because they often carry with them the compulsory authority of government. The police powers of public health are increasingly being used cautiously and with careful consideration of the rights of individuals. In many ways, the use of laws is seen as a last resort when the provisions of information and incentives for change have not been successful.

To complete our examination of health policy and law, let us take a look at the development of a key set of international policies and laws, those related to the response to the threat of pandemic disease; that is disease which crosses international borders and affects a large number of people.

## ▶ What Can Be Done to Respond to the Threat of Pandemic Diseases?

Pandemic disease by definition requires more than a national response; it requires a global response. Epidemic and widespread pandemics have occurred since ancient times yet until the late 19th century there was little or no coordinated international response.

The International Sanitary Convention of 1892, the first such international effort, focused attention on a subset of diseases primarily cholera, plague, and yellow fever and the quarantine regulations necessary to prevent the shipping trade from transporting these diseases across international borders.

WHO was established as a United Nations organization in 1948. In 1951 WHO adopted the existing agreements as the International Health Regulations (IHR) which became binding on all WHO members. These regulations were limited to cholera, plague, yellow fever, and smallpox with smallpox being removed after its eradication in the late 1970s.

Public health emergencies of the 21st century were required before the international community

---

e Bioethics is continuing to evolve. Recent changes in research ethics include limitations on the use of placebos and requirements to register randomized controlled trials before they begin. Placebos are now considered ethical only when no effective active intervention is accepted as the standard of care. The requirement to register randomized controlled trials before they begin was put into effect after randomized controlled trials came to public attention that were never submitted for publication because the results were in conflict with the interests of the trial's sponsor.

succeeded in modernizing the IHR. In 2005 after the SARS epidemic the IHR were modified in a number of important ways[16,17]:

- The scope of the IHR (2005) was expanded with an aim to prevent, protect against, control, and provide a public health response to the international spread of disease.
- The IHR (2005) embraced an all-hazards strategy, covering health threats irrespective of their origin or source as opposed to the previous disease specific coverage. The intention was to include biological, chemical, and nuclear events.
- The IHR (2005) requires nations to develop "core capacities" for rapid detection, assessment, reporting, and response to potential public health emergencies of international concern, including for surveillance, laboratories, and risk communication. Core capacities were central to a public health strategy of strengthening local infrastructure and systems to detect and contain outbreaks at their source before they spread internationally.
- To be in compliance, member countries were required to promptly notify WHO of events that might constitute a public health emergency of international concern, with a continuing obligation to inform WHO of any updates.
- On the basis of information from nations (official sources) and/or from unofficial sources WHO's Director General was authorized to declare what is called a "**public health emergency of international concern**" (PHEIC). Declaration of a PHEIC allowed WHO to make unbinding disease control recommendations, provide assistance, and communicate with other nations regarding the health threat.

PHEIC were declared by the WHO Director for the Influenza Pandemic of 2009–2010 as well as the Ebola epidemic of 2014–2015, and the Zika epidemic in February 2016.

The Ebola epidemic, like the SARS epidemic, created enormous world-wide fear and eventually major international responses. One impact of the Ebola epidemic was the creation of the Commission on a Global Health Risk Framework for the Future (Commission)[f] which was developed to provide advice on how the international community should react to future public health emergencies.[18]

The Commission described the Ebola epidemic as follows:

With failures occurring at all levels, the recent Ebola outbreak in West Africa exposed significant weaknesses in the global health system and culminated in a tragic humanitarian disaster. At the national level in affected countries, there was significant delay in acknowledging the magnitude of the outbreak. And after the outbreak was recognized, the international response was slow and uncoordinated. Mechanisms for the establishment of public–private partnerships were lacking. For example, the development of lifesaving medical products was reactive, rather than proactive. An easily mobilized reserve of funds to support the response was not available. Critical financial and human resources were slow to arrive or never arrived at all. Countries were reluctant to acknowledge the severity of the outbreak and obstructed early notification. Surveillance and information systems were not in place or failed to provide early warning. (GHRF Commission, p. 9)[18]

The Commission argued that public health emergencies should be viewed in light of their potential economic costs and their impact on global security not solely as health issues. The Commission made specific recommendations with a short timeline for action in three areas. First, public health infrastructure-the Commission recommended reinforcing national public health capabilities and infrastructure as the first line of defense against potential pandemics. Second, the Commission recommended more effective global and regional capabilities led by a reenergized WHO, through a dedicated Center for Health Emergency Preparedness and Response (CHEPR) designed to coordinate effectively with the rest of the UN system, as well as the World Bank and International Monetary Fund (IMF). Finally, the Commission recommended an accelerated WHO-led research and development effort coordinated by an independent Pandemic Product Development Committee to mobilize, prioritize, allocate, and oversee research and development resources relating to infectious diseases with pandemic potential.

The Commission did not recommend changing the basic legal framework of the 2005 IHR. Rather it recommended a series of changes in IHR procedures plus new funding and authority to better position the

---

f   Commission was an independent group of 17 international experts from 12 countries overseen by "eminent and diverse leaders" from Africa, Asia, Europe and the Americas and supported by many of the world's largest private Foundations in the world including the Gates Foundation and the Wellcome Trust as well as the U.S. Agency for International development.

international and national communities to respond to future public health emergencies of international concern.

**TABLE 5.5** summarizes and compares the IHR as they existed from 1951 until 2007 when the IHR (2005) were implemented as well as the changes recommended by the Commission.

In the 21st century, the international community has begun to respond to the threat of pandemic disease by strengthening the role of the WHO and other international organizations as well as attempting to ensure local capacities. This process will require continuing modifications and enhancements if the world expects to effectively control emerging infections and prevent pandemic diseases.

Now that we have examined key tools of population health, let us turn our attention to efforts to prevent disease, disability, and death for noncommunicable diseases, communicable disease, and environmental health and safety.

| **TABLE 5.5**  International Health Regulations Changes | | | |
|---|---|---|---|
| | **1951–2007** | **2007–Present** | **"Commission" proposed** |
| Scope | Cholera, plague, yellow fever, smallpox (removed after eradication)<br><br>Control at borders/ports | Required reporting of Public Health Emergency of International concern-not limited to infectious disease<br><br>Detection and containment at source | Additional reporting of "watch list" of outbreaks with potential to become a Public Health Emergency of International Concern |
| WHO authority | WHO could not initiative an inquiry | WHO can initiate an inquiry based on "unofficial sources" and can ask for additional information from "official sources." WHO can declare a "public health emergency of international concern" | WHO would also have authority over "watch list" outbreaks |
| Expectations of member states/nations | Defined capabilities at ports | Set of minimum "core capacity" for detection, reporting, and assessment with self-reporting of capacity | Require external assessment of "core capacity" with use of "name and share" to encourage compliance |
| Consequence of non compliance with reporting requirements and implementation of "core capacities" | No formal consequences or required external assessment of capacity | No formal consequences or required external assessment of capacity | International Monetary Fund and World Bank take non compliance and pandemic preparedness into account in their economic and policy assessment of nations |
| Coordination of response | No mechanism for coordination of response | WHO expected to provide assistance in response, communicate with other nations, and recommend control measures | Release of financial resources from WHO emergency funds and World Bank resources |
| International response capabilities | Set of predetermined controls limited to borders and ports | Flexible "evidence-based" responses adapted to nature of the threat | Greater technical assistance and scientific advice including funds for research and development (PPDC) |

## Key Words

Administrative regulations
Authoritative decision
Belmont report
Beneficence
Bioethics
Constitutional law
Health in all policies approach
Imposed risk
Institutional review boards (IRBs)

Judicial law
Justice
Legislative statutes
Market justice
Negative constitution
No-duty principle
Pandemic
Police power
Procedural due process

Public health emergency of
   international concern
Quarantine
Respect for person
Rights
Self-imposed risk
Social justice
Substantive due process

## Discussion Questions

Take a look at the questions posed in the following scenarios, which were presented at the beginning of this chapter. See now whether you can answer them.

1. A new statute and subsequent administrative regulations give only a temporary license to newly licensed drivers, prohibiting late night driving and the use of cell phones and limiting the number of passengers. You ask: Should elderly drivers be subject to these same types of regulations, such as being required to retake a driver's test?

2. You hear that a neighbor has TB and refuses treatment. You wonder: What if he has the type of TB that can't be cured with drugs? You ask: Can't they make him take his medicine or at least get him out of the neighborhood?

3. A friend of yours experienced a grand mal seizure in which she totally lost consciousness. Fortunately, cancer is ruled out and she is tolerating the medications without serious side effects and without another seizure. It is 2 months later and your friend tells you her driver's license was taken away by the motor vehicle administration and she does not know when she will get it back. You ask: What types of issues are involved in deciding if and when she can drive again?

4. You receive an email encouraging your participation in a new research study. It sounds like you are eligible, so you check into it. You are surprised to find that even if you participate, you may not receive the new drug, and you will not even be told which treatment you are receiving. Despite your willingness to take your chances, you are told that you are not eligible for the study due to conditions that put you at increased risk of developing side effects. You ask: Why am I barred from participating if I am willing to take the risks?

5. The latest breaking news announces that WHO has declared what it called a Public Health Emergency of International Concern because of the rapid spread of a new strain of Influenza. You wonder: What does this declaration mean? What will change as a result of this declaration?

## References

1. Teitelbaum JB, Wilensky SE. *Essentials of Health Policy and Law*. 3rd ed. Burlington, MA: Jones & Bartlett Learning; 2017.
2. Gostin LA. *Public Health Law: Power, Duty, Restraint*. Berkeley, CA, and New York, NY: University of California Press and Milbank Memorial Fund; 2000.
3. Turnock BJ. *Public Health: What It Is and How It Works*. 4th ed. Sudbury, MA: Jones and Bartlett Publishers; 2009.
4. Teitelbaum JB, Wilensky SE. *Essentials of Health Policy and Law*. 2nd ed. Sudbury, MA: Jones and Bartlett Publishers; 2007:12.
5. World Health Organization. Helsinki statement on health in all policies 2013; WHO (WHA67.12) 2014:7. http://apps.who .int/iris/bitstream/10665/112636/1/9789241506908_eng.pdf. Accessed July 19, 2017.
6. World Health Organization. What is health in all policies? http:// who.int/social_determinants/publications/health-policies -manual/HiAP_Infographic.pdf?ua=1. Accessed July 19, 2017.
7. *Healthy People 2020*. U.S. Department of Health and Human Services. https://www.healthypeople.gov/2020/About -Healthy-People. Accessed March 25, 2017.
8. Shi L, Singh D. *Delivering Health Care in America*. 3rd ed. Sudbury, MA: Jones and Bartlett Publishers; 2004.
9. United Nations General Assembly. The universal declaration of human rights. http://www.un.org/Overview/rights.html. Accessed July 19, 2017.
10. Parmet WE. Legal power and legal rights—isolation and quarantine in the case of drug-resistant tuberculosis. *New England Journal Medicine*. 2007;357–434.
11. Public Health Leadership Society. Principles of the ethical practice of public health. Version 2.2. 2002. http://phls .org/CMSuploads/Principles-of-the-Ethical-Practice-of-PH -Version-2.2-68496.pdf. Accessed March 25, 2017.
12. Bernheim RG, Childress JF, Melnick AL, et al. *Essentials of Public Health Ethics*. Burlington, MA: Jones & Bartlett Learning; 2014.
13. U.S. Government. *Trials of War Criminals before the Nuremberg Military Tribunals under Control Council Law*. No. 10, Vol. 2. Washington, DC: U.S. Government Printing Office; 1949:181–182.
14. The National Commission for the Protection of Human Subjects of Biomedical and Behavioral Research. The belmont

report: ethical principles and guidelines for the protection of human subjects of research. http://www.hhs.gov/ohrp/humansubjects/guidance/belmont.html. Accessed July 19, 2017.

15. U.S. Department of Health and Human Services. Title 45: public welfare, Department of Health and Human Services, part 46: protection of human subjects. http://www.hhs.gov/ohrp/humansubjects/guidance/45cfr46.html. Accessed July 19, 2017.

16. Katz R, Fischer J. The revised International Health Regulations: a framework for global pandemic response. *Global Health Governance.* Vol. III, No. 2 (Spring 2010). http://blogs. shu.edu/ghg/2010/04/01/the-revised-international-health-regulations-a-framework-for-global-pandemic-response/. Accessed July 19, 2017.

17. World Health Organization. Alert, response, and capacity building under the International Health Regulations (IHR). http://www.who.int/ihr/about/10things/en/. Accessed July 19, 2017.

18. GHRF Commission (Commission on a Global Health Risk Framework for the Future). 2016. *The Neglected Dimension of Global Security: A Framework to Counter Infectious Disease Crises.* https://nam.edu/initiatives/global-health-risk-framework/. Accessed July 19, 2017.

# SECTION II

# Cases and Discussion Questions

# ▶ Don's Diabetes

Don had been a diabetic for over a decade and took his insulin pretty much as the doctor ordered. Every morning, after checking his blood sugar levels, he would adjust his insulin dose according to the written instructions. From the beginning, Don's doctor worried about the effect of the diabetes—he ordered tests, adjusted dosages and prescriptions, and sent his patient to the ophthalmologist for assessment and laser treatment to prevent blindness.

It was the amputation of his right foot that really got Don's attention. Don was not exactly athletic, but he did play a round of golf once in a while. He first noticed a little scratch on his foot after a day on the golf course. It was not until a week later that he noticed the swelling and the redness in his foot and an ulceration that was forming. He was surprised that his foot did not hurt, but the doctor informed him that diabetic foot ulcers often do not cause pain. That is part of the problem with diabetes—you lose your sensation in your feet.

After 6 months of receiving treatment on a weekly basis, a decision had to be made. "There is not any choice," his doctor said. "The foot infection is spreading, and if we do not amputate the foot, we may have to amputate to the knee or even higher." So after describing the potential benefits and harms of the surgery and asking whether there were any questions, the doctor asked Don to sign a form. The next morning, Don's leg was amputated above the ankle, leaving him with a stump in place of a foot.

The surgeon came to Don's room the day after surgery to take a look at his amputation. "Beautiful work," he said with a big smile on his face. *Maybe it is a beautiful stump,* Don thought to himself, *but it does not work like my old foot.* At first, he felt sorry for himself, thinking of what lay ahead to literally get back on his feet. The physical therapist who visited Don in the hospital told him, "You got off lucky—now, are you going to take control or let diabetes control you?" *But diabetes is already controlling me,* Don thought to himself—daily insulin; blood sugar testing; weekly trips to the doctor; and now, despite it all, an amputated foot.

"Diabetes can be a bad disease," his doctor told him. "We are doing everything we can do, and you are still experiencing complications."

Maybe the doctors were doing everything they could, but Don wondered what else was possible. He enrolled in a self-help group for diabetics. They shared stories of medical care, new advances in diabetes management, and their own frustrations with the disease and with their medical care. Don realized he had received good medical care, but he also acknowledged that good care by good doctors is not enough.

There needs to be a system that makes the pieces work together, but there also needs to be a patient who takes charge of his care.

So take charge, he did. He worked closely with the practice's physician assistant and nurse practitioner, who were experts in diabetic management. He learned how to interpret his finger stick blood sugar tests and how they were useful for day-to-day monitoring of his disease. He also learned about hemoglobin A1c blood tests, which measure how well diabetes is doing over a period of months. After several months, his clinicians taught him how to adjust his dose of insulin to accommodate for changes in his routine or during minor illnesses. They always let him know that care was available and that he did not need to make decisions all by himself. Don also learned to examine his feet and how to prevent minor injuries from turning into major problems. His sporadic eye doctor appointments turned into regular question-and-answer sessions to compare the most recent photographs of his retina to those from the past.

Don found himself keeping his own records to be sure that he had them all in one place, fearing that one doctor would not talk to another. Don's fears were well founded: when his kidney function began to deteriorate and his primary care doctor sent him to a kidney specialist, who sent him to a transplant surgeon, and then to a vascular surgeon to prepare him for dialysis, sure enough, the only records the dialysis doctors could rely upon were the ones that Don had kept on his own.

Soon the dialysis doctor told Don that he had a tough decision to make. Did he want to come into the dialysis center half a day twice a week, where they take care of everything, or did he want to learn home dialysis and take care of this treatment on his own? Don had lots of questions. He needed to understand what each dialysis option entailed and the advantages and disadvantages of each option, including the costs and discomforts. He also wanted to know about any other potential treatments. Don asked questions of his doctors, learned as much as he could about dialysis on the Internet, and outlined the pros and cons of home dialysis. After that, it was an easy decision for Don. "Sure, I will learn how to do it myself. I want to be in charge of my own care. I want to stand on my own two feet," he told the doctor without a moment's hesitation.

## Discussion Questions

1. What type of decision-making process was going on during the early stages of Don's diabetes? Explain.

2.  What type of decision-making process was used to reach the decision to have an amputation? Explain.

3.  What type of decision-making process occurred in the decision about dialysis? Explain.

4.  In Don's case, what are the advantages and disadvantages of each of these approaches to decision-making from both the patient's and the clinician's perspectives? Explain.

## ▶ A New Disease Called SADS—A Decision Analysis

Imagine that a new disease called sudden adult disability syndrome (SADS) has become the most common cause of death among previously healthy 18- to 24-year-olds. The etiology of SADS is unknown, but it is thought to be infectious. SADS is a disease of sudden onset that without treatment produces progressive weakness, slow mental deterioration, and death within a year 50% of the time. The other 50% of individuals who develop SADS make a rapid, spontaneous full recovery without any treatment.

There are three known treatments for SADS:

■ Ordinary Knowledge (O.K.)—the conventional treatment (in other words, standard treatment)
■ Live-Better
■ Live-Longer

The probabilities of cure and side effects have been extensively investigated:

■ Ordinary Knowledge (O.K.) results in an 80% probability of cure without side effects. The remaining 20% die of SADS.
■ Live-Better results in an 85% probability of cure. There are no known side effects. The remaining 15% die from SADS.
■ Live-Longer results in an 80% probability of cure. However, 10% of those who take the treatment become totally and permanently blind in both eyes. The remaining 10% die of SADS.

### Discussion Questions

1.  Prior to conducting a decision analysis, which intervention would you recommend?

2.  Draw a decision tree indicating the potential outcomes for each of the three treatments (O.K. therapy, Live-Better, and Live-Longer) and indicate the probability of occurrence of each of the potential outcomes.

3.  Assume cure brings your utility to full health; in other words, 1.0, and death's utility is 0. Use a utility of 0.5 for blindness. Can any of the possible interventions be eliminated based on the expected utilities? Explain.

4.  Now use a utility of 0.8 for blindness and recalculate the expected utilities. Which intervention is now recommended by the decision analysis?

5.  Now use a utility of 0.2 for blindness and recalculate the expected utilities. Which intervention is now recommended by the decision analysis? What can you conclude about the importance of the utility that is placed on blindness?

6.  Now use the utility for blindness that indicates the utility that you personally place on blindness. Again recalculate the expected utilities. What intervention is recommended by this decision analysis? How does this recommendation compare to the recommendation you made prior to conducting the decision analysis? If it is different, what other factors did you take into account in reaching your own recommendation?

## ▶ José and Jorge—Identical Twins Without Identical Lives

José and Jorge were identical twins separated at birth. José grew up in a large family in an impoverished slum in the middle of a crime-ridden and polluted district of a major city. Jorge grew up in an upper-middle-class professional family with one other brother in a suburban community in the same city. Despite the fact the José and Jorge were identical twins, their lives and health could not have been more different.

José had few opportunities for medical care or public health services as a child. His nutrition was always marginal and he developed several severe cases of diarrhea before he was 1 year of age. He received a polio vaccine as part of a community vaccination program, but never received vaccinations for measles, mumps, rubella, or other childhood illnesses. At age 4, he developed measles and was so sick his mother was sure he would not make it.

As a child, José also developed asthma, which seemed to worsen when he played outdoors on hot smoggy days. Dropping out of school at age 14, José went to work in a factory, but quit when he found himself panting for breath at the end of the day.

As a teenager, José was repeatedly exposed to crime and drugs. Once, he was caught in the cross fire of gangs fighting for control of drugs in his community. Experimenting with drugs with his teenage friends, José contracted HIV from use of contaminated needles. José did not know he had HIV until he was nearly 30 years old and developed tuberculosis (TB). He did receive treatment for the TB free of charge from the health department, but once he felt better, he did not follow up with treatment.

By the time the TB returned, José had lost 30 pounds and could barely make it into the emergency room of the public hospital because of his shortness of breath. He was hospitalized for the last 2 months of his life, mostly to prevent others from being exposed to what was now drug-resistant tuberculosis. No one ever knew how many people José exposed to HIV or TB.

Jorge's life as a child was far less eventful. He received "well child" care from an early age. His family hardly noticed that he rarely developed diarrhea and had few sick days from diseases of childhood. He did well in school, but like José, he developed asthma. With good treatment, Jorge was able to play on sports teams, at least until he began to smoke cigarettes at age 14.

Jorge soon began to gain weight, and by the time he graduated from college, he was rapidly becoming obese. In his 20s, he developed high blood pressure, and in his 30s he had early signs of diabetes. Jorge had a heart attack in his mid-40s and underwent bypass surgery a few years later. The treatments for diabetes, hypertension, and high cholesterol worked well and Jorge was able to lead a productive professional life into his 40s.

By the time that Jorge turned 50, his diabetes began to worsen and he developed progressive kidney disease. Jorge soon needed twice-a-week dialysis, which kept him alive as he awaited a kidney transplant.

## Discussion Questions

1. How do social determinants of health contribute to the different disease patterns of José and Jorge?
2. How do factors in the physical environment explain differences in the health of José and Jorge?
3. What role does medical care play in the differences between the health outcomes of José and Jorge?
4. What roles do public health services play in the health outcomes of José and Jorge?

## ▶ The Obesity Epidemic in the United States—The Tip of an Iceberg

Before the last half of the 20th century, obesity was often seen as a sign of prosperity. Look at the great art of 18th- and 19th-century Europe and you will find portraits of the prosperous and portly prominently displayed. In the last half of the 20th century and the early years of the 2000s, obesity has become the province of the poor and the middle class.

Obesity is defined as a BMI over 30. Overweight is defined as a BMI from 25 to 30. The BMI is calculated as the weight in kilograms/height in meters squared. A BMI of 30 for a 5 foot, 8.5 inch male or female is approximately 200 pounds. To determine whether a child aged 2–19 years is considered obese, a BMI for age is calculated, but further assessment is needed to determine fat distribution, such as measurement of skinfold thickness. The prevalence of obesity has been steadily rising in the United States over the last 50 years, increasing over 250%. Today, approximately 20% of children aged 2–19 are obese, along with approximately 35% of adults.

U.S. data confirm a strong association of obesity with lower socioeconomic levels overall and in most but not all racial and ethnic groups. Overall, children and adolescents 2–19 years in families with an income under 133% of the poverty level (a little over $30,000 for a family of 4) have almost twice the prevalence of obesity as children and adolescents in families with income over 350% of the poverty level. However, these patterns do not apply to non-Hispanic black girls or to Mexican American boys or girls, in whom high levels of obesity occur at all income and educational levels.

A number of factors play important roles in giving the portrait of obesity in the United States a far less prosperous persona. The availability of cheap, high-calorie foods has played an important role in allowing access to abundant quantities of food by lower socioeconomic individuals. Technologies using concentrated sugars, such as high fructose corn syrup, and trans fats have reinforced this tendency. Once obesity is established, exercise may be more difficult, setting in motion a vicious circle of sedentary lifestyle and increased weight. Similarly, once obesity is established, the large quantities of food required daily often necessitate the purchase of cheap high-calorie food.

Obesity is strongly associated with a constellation of other health conditions in what has been called a syndemic, or the occurrence together of two or more health conditions. Obesity is the strongest risk factor associated with type 2 diabetes. Abdominal obesity, defined as a waistline of approximately 37 inches for males and 31.5 inches for females, is central to what is called the metabolic syndrome. The metabolic syndrome requires the presence of abdominal obesity and also includes diabetes, high blood pressure, and cholesterol and triglyceride abnormalities, including low good cholesterol. Each of these conditions can and should be treated, but treatment is far more successful and carries fewer side effects if weight can be reduced. Often a 5% or 10% reduction in body weight has a major impact on these conditions. Cigarette smoking, another strong risk factor for heart and vascular disease as well as cancer, actually has a small impact on reducing weight.

A number of approaches have been suggested to address the epidemic of obesity in the United States. An increasing number of drugs are being developed and approved to treat obesity. A surgical approach called gastric bypass surgery or more generally bariatric or weight loss surgery have been demonstrated to have efficacy using randomized controlled trials, including long-term weight loss and reduction in complications especially among those with a BMI greater than 40.

Newer dietary approaches, such as low-carbohydrate diets, have been shown in randomized controlled trials to increase weight loss over the short run, but like other diets, the low-carb diet has less impressive results over longer periods of time. A variety of sugar substitutes have been investigated and introduced in recent years. It is controversial whether these sugar substitutes have had a substantial impact on obesity.

Other approaches attempt to get at the cultural influences on obesity, including the fact that the average portion size in restaurants has increased over the last few decades. Efforts to limit the size of high-calorie soft drinks are one example of this approach. Focusing on children and adolescents by restricting the availability of food with high sugar and carbohydrates in school lunches and offering healthier alternatives is also being tried. Taxing high-calorie, low-nutrition food is another option being debated. Increasing requirements for physical activity in schools is yet another policy change being advocated.

The answers to the weighty question of obesity in the United States remain a great challenge. What do you think we should do about it?

## Discussion Questions

1.  Identify the contributions of social determinants of health, including cultural factors, to the increased rate of obesity in the United States. Explain.
2.  Discuss the relationship between obesity and other health conditions that lead to cardiovascular disease, including the interactions that occur.
3.  Which of the interventions discussed in this case would you endorse? Explain why, including considering the positive and negative aspects of each intervention.
4.  How would you combine the interventions that you selected in question number 3 to effectively address the national epidemic of obesity?

## ▶ Changing Behavior—Cigarette Smoking

It was not going to be easy for Steve to stop smoking. He had been at it for 30 years—ever since he took it up on a dare at age 16 and found that it was a good way to socialize. In his 20s, it seemed to make dealing with the work pressure easier, and in those days, you could smoke in your office and did not even need to shut the door—much less deal with those dirty looks he was getting now.

Steve was always confident that he could take cigarettes or leave them. He would quit when he was good and ready, and a few cigarettes could not hurt. But then he talked to some friends who had quit a decade or more ago and said they would go back in a minute if they thought cigarettes were safe. *Maybe for some people, those cravings just never go away*, he worried to himself. However, there was that bout of walking pneumonia, and then the cough that just did not seem to go away. The cough was so bad that he had trouble smoking more than a few cigarettes a day. The physician assistant let him know that these symptoms were early warning signs of things to come; however, Steve just was not ready to stop. So the physician assistant gave him a fact sheet and let Steve know there was help available when he was ready.

It might have been his fears about his 10-year-old son that finally tipped the scales. "Daddy, those cigarettes are bad for you," he said. Or maybe it was when he found cigarette butts in the backyard after his 16-year-old daughter's birthday party. Steve knew enough to believe that a father who smokes has a child who smokes. So this time, he would do it right.

Steve's physician assistant recognized that Steve was finally ready to quit. He let him know in no uncertain terms that it was important to quit totally, completely, and forever. He also informed Steve that he could rely on help—that he was not alone. With the encouragement of his physician assistant, Steve joined a support group, set a quit date, and announced the date to his friends and family. The new medication he was prescribed seemed to relieve the worst cravings and the feeling he called "crawling the walls."

His wife, Dorothy, was supportive. She cleared the cigarette butts and ashtrays out of the house and dealt with the smell by having all the drapes cleaned. She also helped by getting him up after dinner and taking a walk, which kept him from his old habit of having a cigarette with dessert and coffee. It also helped keep him from gaining too much weight, which she confided was her greatest fear. Dorothy's quiet encouragement and subtle reinforcement without nagging worked wonders.

Saving a five to ten of dollars a day did not hurt. Steve collected those dollars and put them in a special hiding place. On his first year anniversary of quitting, he wrapped up the dollar bills in a box and gave them to Dorothy as a present. The note inside said: "A trip for us for as long as the money lasts." Dorothy was delighted, but feared the worst when Steve began to open up his present to himself. As he unwrapped a box of cigars, he smiled a big smile and said, "I am congratulating myself on quitting smoking."

## Discussion Questions

1. How are each of the phases in the stages of change model illustrated in Steve's case?
2. What other theories or models can be applied to the public health issue described in this case? Explain.
3. What effective individual and group approaches are illustrated in this case? Explain.
4. Which effective public health (or population) approaches are illustrated in this case? Explain.
5. What is the impact of combining individual clinical approaches with public health (or population) approaches?

# ▶ The New Era of E-Cigarettes

Randy had smoked for three decades since his teens and he was hooked. When he tried to quit, the withdrawal was more than he could take. He found himself smoking in the morning along with his two cups of coffee in order to get his day started. His doctor told him that was a sure sign of addiction. And addicted he was, try as he might to quit, nothing seemed to work. Nicotine patches and nicotine gum helped a little but that deep puff on a cigarette couldn't be beat.

Then to Randy's amazement along came e-cigarettes. Like cigarettes he could breathe in nicotine to his heart's content. Also, instead of being shut out from places he wanted to go or be given stares which screamed "don't you know any better" things changed. Now people looked at him as if to say, glad to see you are trying to quit. Well Randy wasn't really trying to quit, though he did gradually cut back. He became an advocate for e-cigarettes, speaking out for their safety and ability to help those like him who had smoked for years to finally take control of their lives.

One day Randy's 15-year-old son Noah picked up his father's e-cigarettes and gave them a try. Wow, he liked the feeling when he inhaled deeply. "I can see why my Dad likes them so much" Noah said to himself. Soon Noah was buying his own e-cigarettes which were easier to get than the old fashioned kind. Like his Dad, Noah soon found himself using e-cigarettes almost around the clock. "Must run in the family" he thought. E-cigarettes were all Noah needed, though a few of his friends starting smoking e-cigarettes but then moved on the "the real thing".

Randy and Noah both were hooked on e-cigarettes. They cost almost as much as tobacco cigarettes and they were certainly addictive, but at least e-cigarettes were safe they both agreed. Then they heard that the FDA was considering regulating e-cigarettes. What, they asked, was the FDA trying to achieve? Would they put age restrictions on who could buy e-cigarettes? Would they restrict how much nicotine they could contain? Would they put them "behind the counter" or otherwise restrict how they could be sold? Randy and Noah agreed they didn't like what they saw coming as they had a father-son talk, puffing away on their e-cigarettes.

1. What are the positive aspects of e-cigarettes? Explain.
2. What are the negative aspects of e-cigarettes? Explain.
3. Do e-cigarettes pose special danger for children? Should the FDA focus on banning sales to children and prohibiting flavors which might appeal to children? Justify your answer.
4. What actions do you think should or should not be taken when regulating e-cigarettes such as prohibiting advertising, restricting indoor public use as with cigarettes, or taxing them the same as cigarette etc.? Justify your answer.

## ▶ The Elderly Driver

It was late in the afternoon on a sunny April day. Maybe it was the sun in her eyes, but 82-year-old Janet found herself in her car in a ditch at the side of the road, unsure of how she got there. Once at the hospital, her son and daughter joined her and heard the good news that Janet had escaped with just a broken arm. The police report strongly suggested that she had swerved off the road, but it was not clear why.

This was not Janet's first driving "episode"; in fact, her driving had been a constant worry to her daughter for over 2 years. Her daughter often offered to take her Mom shopping and insisted that she do the driving when they were together. "Don't you trust me?" was the only thanks the daughter received. When alone, Janet continued to drive herself, staying off the freeway and increasingly driving only during the day. She knew it was not as easy as it used to be, but it was her lifeline to independence.

Then, a few months after the April incident, the form for Janet's license renewal arrived. A vision test and a physical exam were required, along with a doctor's certification that Janet was in good health and capable of driving; however, no road test was required. So Janet made a doctor's appointment, and at the end of it, she left the forms with a note for the doctor saying, "To the best doctor I have ever had. Thanks for filling this out. You know how much driving means to me."

On Janet's way home from the doctor's office, it happened. She was driving down the road when suddenly she was crossing that yellow line and heading toward an oncoming car. The teenage driver might have been going a little fast, but Janet was in the wrong lane and the head-on collision killed the 16-year-old passenger in the front seat who was not wearing a seat belt. The 18-year-old driver walked away from the collision unharmed, thanks to a seat belt and an inflated airbag.

Janet was never the same emotionally. And despite escaping the collision with just a few bruises, the loss of her driver's license symbolized the end for her. Those lost weekly shopping trips and the strangers in the assisted living center were not the same as living in her own home. The young man in the collision screaming for help woke her up almost every night. It was only a year after the collision when Janet died, and it was just like she had said: "Take my license away and it will kill me."

### Discussion Questions

1. How does this case reflect the important issue of balancing the legal rights of the individual and the rights of society as a whole?
2. What role do you believe healthcare providers should play in implementing driving laws and regulations?
3. Identify any changes you would make to prevent the types of outcomes that occurred in this case study.
4. How would you communicate the lessons learned in this case to new and inexperienced drivers?

# SECTION III
# Preventing Disease, Morbidity, and Mortality

There are currently over 2.5 million deaths per year in the United States. The Centers for Disease Control and Prevention (CDC) reports that the top 10 causes of death that appear on death certificates account for approximately two-thirds of these deaths as indicated in **TABLE S03.1**.[1]

To better understand the causes of death in the United States the CDC has developed the concept of **actual causes** which provides additional insights into the underlying causes of death. It provides a way of organizing what we know about the prevention of disease and disability into categories that we can measure. Thus, it allows us to ask a key question: How many deaths result from preventable disease?[2]

Actual causes of disease can then be linked to three basic categories: noncommunicable diseases, communicable diseases, and environmental diseases and injuries. **FIGURE S03.1** illustrates the framework

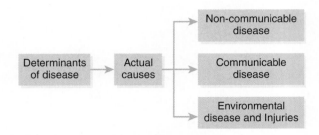

**FIGURE S03.1** Public Health Framework for Diseases and Injuries

we will use in this section to connect determinants of disease, actual causes, and categories of disease and injury.

The concept of actual causes of disease is a relatively new idea that has been successfully applied to the causes of death, though not to disability. **TABLE S03.2** provides the most recent data on the actual causes of death. It indicates that nearly half of all deaths in the United States are related to nine potentially preventable actual causes.

The concept of actual causes of disease provides us with a framework for thinking about the underlying problems that lead to death. As indicated in the table, nearly half of all deaths can be ascribed to one of these actual causes. Actual causes can help guide us in prioritizing where we should put our attention and spend our money to prevent disease.

A substantial portion of the actual causes of death are related to the development of noncommunicable diseases, including tobacco, diet and physical inactivity, alcohol consumption, and illicit drug use. Communicable disease remains an important category related not only to microbial agents, but also to sexual behavior. Finally, a broad range of environmental diseases and injuries are related to toxic agents, motor vehicle–related injuries, and firearm-related injuries. The recently recognized contribution played by small particle air pollution in producing coronary artery disease has increased our understanding of the importance of environmental factors.

Let us also take a look at the major causes of morbidity in the United States. Leading causes of morbidity in the United States are displayed in **TABLE S03.3** in the order of their impact. The data comes from the Burden of Disease study which has produced important information on the impact of morbidity and mortality throughout the world.[3]

Notice that the major causes of mortality and morbidity are very different. Musculoskeletal disorders including arthritis and mental health disorders

| **TABLE S03.1** Ten Leading Causes of Mortality in the United States | |
|---|---|
| **Cause of death on death certificates** | **Approximate number of deaths 2015** |
| Heart disease | 633,000 |
| Cancer | 595,000 |
| Chronic lower respiratory diseases | 155,000 |
| Unintentional injuries (including overdoses) | 146,000 |
| Stroke | 140,000 |
| Alzheimer's disease | 110,000 |
| Diabetes | 79,000 |
| Influenza and pneumonia | 57,000 |
| Kidney disease | 49,000 |
| Intentional self-harm (suicide) | 44,000 |

Reproduced from Centers for Disease Control and Prevention. Leading causes of death. https://www.cdc.gov/nchs/fastats/leading-causes-of-death.htm. Accessed July 21, 2017.

**TABLE S03.2** Actual Causes of Death in the United States[a]

| Actual cause | Number of deaths |
|---|---|
| Tobacco | 435,000 |
| Diet and physical inactivity | 365,000 |
| Alcohol consumption | 85,000 |
| Microbial agents (infections) | 75,000 |
| Toxic agents | 55,000 |
| Motor vehicles | 43,000 |
| Firearms | 29,000 |
| Sexual behavior | 20,000 |
| Illicit drug use | 17,000 |
| Total | 1,124,000 (total deaths 2,403,351) |

[a] This is the most recently available data but does not fully reflect the current actual causes of death in the United States. In recent years there has been a large increase in drug related deaths from both illicit drug use and prescription drug use. Deaths from antibiotic resistant bacterial infections have increased in recent years raising the number of deaths from microbial agents (infections). Deaths due to diet and physical activity are increasing and those due to tobacco are beginning to fall resulting in roughly equal numbers for these two actual causes.

Data from Mokdad AM, Marks JS, Stroup DF, Gerberding JL. Actual causes of death in the United States 2000. *JAMA*. 2004;291:1238–1245.

are the leading causes of morbidity. Dental disease, especially gum disease or periodontitis, may be under-represented in this list since it occurs in approximately 50% of adults and is the leading cause of tooth loss. Major causes of mortality including diabetes, chronic obstructive lung disease, Alzheimer's, ischemic heart disease, stroke, and chronic kidney disease make up only about 15% of the overall impact of morbidity among these 30 conditions.

The data from the Burden of Disease study suggests that the impact of morbidity on healthy years lived is almost as great as the impact imposed by premature deaths. The total impact from these 30 conditions on the number of healthy years lived by the average American is approximately 10% of the potential healthy years of life. That is, approximately 10% of the average American's healthy life is lost due to disability.

When looking at the impacts of conditions on health it is important to look not only at premature death but also at the impact that a condition has on reducing the quality of life; that is, on disability or morbidity.

In Chapters 6, 7, and 8, we will address non-communicable and communicable diseases, review environmental health and injury, and examine the public health strategies that have been used to address each of them. We will aim to better understand the burden of disease, both premature mortality and morbidity, and strategies for addressing them. Let us begin with the largest category of disease in the United States today—noncommunicable diseases.

**TABLE S03.3** The 30 Leading Causes of Morbidity in the United States

| Cause of morbidity—in order of impact | Number of years lived with disability (YLD) in thousands* |
|---|---|
| Low back pain | 3180 |
| Major depressive disorder | 3048 |
| Other musculoskeletal disorders | 2602 |
| Neck pain | 2134 |
| Anxiety disorders | 1866 |
| Chronic obstructive pulmonary disease | 1745 |
| Drug use disorders | 1295 |
| Diabetes | 1164 |

*(continues)*

| TABLE S03.3 The 30 Leading Causes of Morbidity in the United States | *(continued)* |
|---|---|
| Osteoarthritis | 994 |
| Asthma | 932 |
| Falls | 864 |
| Alcohol use disorders | 835 |
| Alzheimer's disease | 829 |
| Schizophrenia | 825 |
| Migraine | 805 |
| Ischemic heart disease | 685 |
| Stroke | 628 |
| Bipolar disorder | 578 |
| Hearing loss | 559 |
| Dysthymia—persistent depressive disorder | 545 |
| Sickle cell disorder | 472 |
| Chronic kidney disease | 410 |
| Rheumatoid arthritis | 403 |
| Benign prostate hypertrophy | 396 |
| Eczema | 390 |
| Vision loss | 375 |
| Road injuries | 373 |
| Edentulism-loss of teeth | 314 |
| Diarrheal diseases | 283 |
| Epilepsy | 260 |

*YLD is measured as the prevalence of the condition multiplied by the weight that reflects the health loss associated with the condition on the basis of surveys of the general population. Thus the YLD reflect the relative impacts of the condition.

Data from US Burden of Disease Collaborators. The state of US Health, 1990–2010: Burden of diseases, injuries, and risk factors. *JAMA, 310(6):591–608, 2013.*

## Key Words

Actual causes

## References

1. Centers for Disease Control and Prevention. Leading causes of death. https://www.cdc.gov/nchs/fastats/leading-causes-of-death.htm. Accessed October 14, 2017.
2. Mokdad AM, Marks JS, Stroup DF, Gerberding JL. Actual causes of death in the United States 2000. *JAMA.* 2004;291:1238–1245.
3. US Burden of Disease Collaborators. The state of US health, 1990–2010: burden of diseases, injuries, and risk factors. *JAMA.* 2013;310(6):591–608.

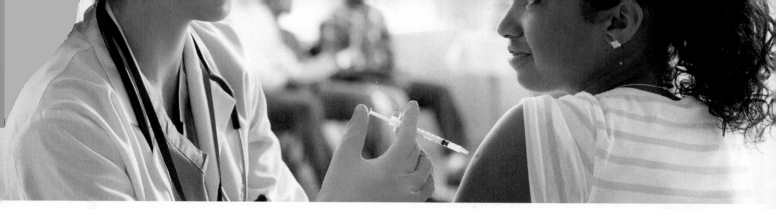

# CHAPTER 6

# Noncommunicable Diseases

## LEARNING OBJECTIVES

By the end of this chapter, the student will be able to:

- describe the burden of noncommunicable diseases on mortality and morbidity in the United States.
- describe the ideal criteria for a screening program.
- explain why two or more tests are nearly always required to screen for asymptomatic disease.
- explain the multiple risk factor intervention approach to control a noncommunicable disease.
- describe the meaning of "cost-effectiveness."
- describe several ways that genetic interventions can affect the burden of noncommunicable diseases.
- describe approaches to reducing the adverse impacts of treatments including overdoses of prescription drugs.
- describe ways that population interventions can be combined with individual interventions to more effectively reduce the burden of noncommunicable diseases.

Sasha did not want to think about the possibility of breast cancer, but as she turned 50, she agreed to have a mammogram which, as she feared, was positive or "suspicious," as her doctor put it. Waiting for the results of the follow-up biopsy was the worst part, but the relief she felt when the results were negative brought tears of joy to her and her family. Then she wondered: Is it common to have a positive mammogram when no cancer is present?

The first sign of Michael's coronary heart disease was his heart attack. Looking back, he had been at high risk for many years because he smoked and had high blood pressure and high bad cholesterol. His lack of exercise and obesity only made the situation worse. Michael asked: What are the risk factors for coronary heart disease,

and what can be done to identify and address these factors for me and my family?

John's knee injury from skiing continued to produce swelling and pain, greatly limiting his activities. His physician informed him that the standard procedure today is to look inside with a flexible scope and do any surgery that is needed through the scope. It is simpler and cheaper, and does not even require hospitalization. "We call it 'cost-effective,'" his doctor said. John wondered: What does "cost-effective" really mean?

Looking back, JoAnn realized she had been living with depression all her life. As a teenager it affected her ability to form friendships and later an intimate personal relationship. After the birth of her child, depression robbed her of much of the joy of motherhood. As a maturing adult she realized how much more she could be enjoying life. Thank God, I got help, she said to herself, or suicide could have been in my future.

Jennifer and her husband, George, were tested for the cystic fibrosis gene, and both were found to have it. Cystic fibrosis can lead to chronic lung infections and greatly shortens the length of life. They now ask: What does this mean for our chances of having a child with cystic fibrosis? Can we find out whether our child has cystic fibrosis early in pregnancy?

Fred's condition deteriorated slowly, but persistently. He just could not remember anything and repeated himself endlessly. The medications helped for a short time, but before long, he did not recognize his family and could not take care of himself. The diagnosis was Alzheimer's, and he was not alone. Almost everyone in the nursing home seemed to be affected. No one seems to understand the cause of Alzheimer's disease. The family asked: What else can be done, not only for Fred, but also for those who come after Fred?

Alcohol use is widespread on your campus. You do not see it as a problem as long as you walk home or have a designated driver. Your mind changes one day after you hear about a classmate who nearly died from alcohol poisoning as a result of binge drinking. You ask yourself: What should be done on my campus to address binge drinking?

Each of these scenarios represents one of the approaches to noncommunicable diseases that we will examine in this chapter.

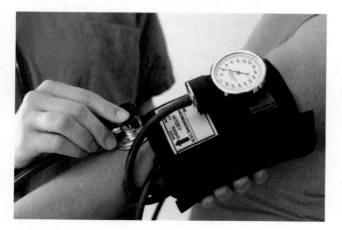

## ▶ What Is the Burden of Noncommunicable Disease?

Noncommunicable disease represents a wide range of diseases, from cardiovascular disease, cancers, and depression, to Alzheimer's and chronic arthritis. Together, they represent the majority of causes of death and disability in most developed countries. Today, cardiovascular diseases and cancer alone each represent nearly 25% of the causes of death as reflected on death certificates in the United States.

The impact of noncommunicable diseases on death only reflects part of the influence of these diseases on people's lives. Chronic disabilities, largely due to noncommunicable diseases, are now the most rapidly growing component of morbidity in most developing as well as developed countries. As populations age, noncommunicable diseases increase in frequency. The presence of two or more chronic diseases makes progressive disability particularly likely. The consequences of the rapidly growing pattern of disability due to noncommunicable diseases have enormous economic implications. The great increase in direct costs for health care is in part due to the increased burden of noncommunicable diseases. The impact extends beyond healthcare costs, as it affects the quality of life and may limit the ability of those who wish to work to continue to do so.

Until recently mental health conditions have not been treated as a major public health issue and accurate data were not available. As we have seen, evidence now suggests that mental health conditions are at or near the top of the reasons for disability and morbidity in the United States. At the top of the list of mental health conditions producing disability and morbidity as well as mortality is major depression. **BOX 6.1** looks at depression and its impacts throughout the life span.[1,2]

Noncommunicable diseases have not always dominated the types of diseases that impact a society. **BOX 6.2** discusses the **epidemiological transition**[4] and provides a perspective on where we stand today.

There are a wide range of preventive, curative, and rehabilitative approaches to noncommunicable diseases. However, there are a limited number of basic strategies being used that are part of the population health approach, including:

- Screening for early detection and treatment of disease
- Multiple risk factor interventions
- Identification of cost-effective treatments
- Genetics counseling and intervention
- Research

**BOX 6.1** Depression Throughout the Life Span

Major depression affects one in six persons during their lifetime. It can include mood producing sadness or loss of interest in previously enjoyable activities severe enough to interrupt daily activities over a period of at least 2 weeks. Depression may produce changes in sleep, appetite, energy, ability to concentrate, or self-esteem. Major depression may be associated with thoughts of suicide.

Depression may occur in episodes over an entire life span, but it may express itself differently in children, adolescents, and adults. Depression can be diagnosed among children as young as 3 and is most common between those aged 14–24. Over 10% of women experience post-partum depression, and the incidence greatly increases for those with previous post-partum depression, pregnancy loss, as well as those with low level of emotional support.

Depression has been referred to as the "under disease" since it is often under-diagnosed, under-discussed, and under-treated. Adult women are believed to experience depression more than twice as frequently as men, and far fewer men seek help.

Randomized controlled trials have established the efficacy of a wide range of medications, cognitive behavioral therapy and other talk treatments, and even electrical stimulation of the brain. Treatment can reduce the severity of depression, the length of the depression, and the chances of suicide. It is important, however, to recognize that new generations of increasingly effective antidepressants are associated with a small increase in suicidal thoughts among those aged 18–29.

Early diagnosis of depression may result in more successful treatment and may prevent suicide. The United States Preventive Services Task Force recommends screening for depression as part of primary care practice, including during pregnancy and post-partum. A system of follow-up care is an important part of a successful screening program.[3]

New research is producing a better understanding of the biology of depression and may lead to better methods of prevention, diagnosis, and treatment in the not-too-distant future.

We will take a look at each of these approaches. Finally, we will see how many of these approaches can be combined using the population health approach. Let us begin with what we call **screening** for disease.

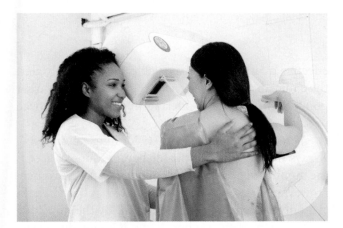

© Tyler Olson/Shutterstock

## ▶ How Can Screening for Disease Address the Burden of Noncommunicable Diseases?

Screening for disease implies the use of tests on individuals who do not have symptoms of a specific disease. These individuals are **asymptomatic**. This implies that they do not have symptoms related to the disease being investigated. They may have symptoms of other diseases. Screening for disease can result in detection of disease at an early stage under the assumption that early detection will allow for treatment that will improve outcome. Screening has been successful for a range of noncommunicable diseases, including breast cancer and colon cancer, as well as childhood conditions, including vision and hearing impairments. In all of these conditions, screening has resulted in reduced disability and/or deaths. Not all noncommunicable diseases, however, are good candidates for screening, and in some cases, screening programs have yet to be devised and studied for some noncommunicable diseases for which early detection could be useful.

Four criteria need to be fulfilled for an ideal screening program.[5] While few, if any, health conditions completely fulfill all four requirements, these criteria provide a standard against which to judge the potential of a screening program. These criteria are:

1. The disease produces substantial death and/or disability.
2. Early detection is possible and improves outcome.
3. There is a feasible testing strategy for screening.
4. Screening is acceptable in terms of harms, costs, and patient acceptance.

---

**BOX 6.2** The Epidemiological Transition and Noncommunicable Diseases

Disease patterns have not always been the same, and they will continue to evolve. To gain a big picture understanding of this process of change, it is useful to understand the concept known as the epidemiological or public health transition.

The epidemiological transition describes the changing pattern of disease that has been seen in many countries as they have experienced social and economic development. Its central message is that prior to social and economic development, communicable diseases—or microbial agents, using the term from actual causes—represent the dominant cause of disease and disability. In countries in early stages of development, infections are a key cause of mortality, either directly or indirectly. For instance, in undeveloped countries, maternal and perinatal conditions, as well as nutritional disorders, are often identified as the causes of death. Microbial agents play a key role in maternal and perinatal deaths, as well as deaths ascribed to nutrition. Most maternal deaths are due to infection not necessarily transmitted from others, but related to exposure to microbial agents at the time of birth and in the early postpartum period.

Similarly, most deaths among young children in undeveloped countries are related directly or indirectly to infection. Inadequate nutrition predisposes children to infection and interferes with their ability to fight off infection when it does occur. Many of the deaths among children with malnutrition are related to acute infections, especially acute infectious diarrhea and acute respiratory infections.

As social and economic development progresses, noncommunicable diseases—including cardiovascular diseases, diabetes, cancers, chronic respiratory ailments, and neuropsychiatric diseases, such as depression and Alzheimer's—predominate as the causes of disability and death. Depression is rapidly becoming one of the major causes of disability, and the World Health Organization (WHO) estimates that it will produce more disability than any other single condition in coming years. In addition, illicit drug use has become a major cause of death among the young and includes not only illegal use of drugs, but increasingly the use of addictive prescription drugs.

In much of the developing world, the same basic patterns are occurring in the developing regions within these countries. Often, earlier distributions of disease dominated by communicable diseases coexist with patterns of noncommunicable diseases typical of developed countries. Thus, it is not unusual to find that malnutrition and obesity are often present side-by-side in the same developing country.

The epidemiologic transition does not imply that once countries reach the stage where noncommunicable diseases dominate that this pattern will persist indefinitely. Newly emerging diseases, such as HIV/AIDS, pandemic flu, and drug-resistant bacterial infections, raise the possibility that communicable diseases will once again dominate the pattern of disease and death in developed countries.

---

The first criterion is perhaps the easiest to evaluate. Conditions such as breast and colon cancer result in substantial death and disability rates. Breast cancer is the second most common cancer in terms of causes of death and is the most common cancer-related cause of death among women in their 50s. Colon cancer is among the most common causes of cancer death in both men and women. Childhood conditions, such as hearing loss and visual impairment, are not always obvious; however, they cause considerable disability.

Determining whether early detection is possible and will improve outcomes is not as easy as it may appear. Screening may result in early detection, but if effective treatment is not available, it may merely alert the clinician and the patient to the disease at an earlier point in time without offering hope of an improved outcome.

Screening cigarette smokers for lung cancer using X-rays would seem reasonable because lung cancer is the number one cancer killer of both men and women. However, X-ray screening of smokers has been beneficial only in terms of early detection. By the time lung cancer can be seen via chest X-ray, it is already too late to cure. This early detection without improved outcome is called **lead-time bias**.[a]

As indicated in the third criterion, in order to implement a successful screening program, there

---

a  The concept of lead time implies that screening produces an earlier diagnosis that may be effectively used to intervene prior to diagnosis without screening. If there is little that can be done to improve outcomes, the extra lead time may result in lead-time bias. It should be noted that a newer screening test for lung cancer called spiral computerized tomography (CT) does meet most of these criteria. Unfortunately it is a very expensive and has only a small impact on the outcome of lung cancer. Therefore use of spiral CT has become a controversial issue.

must be a feasible testing strategy.[b] This usually requires identification of a high-risk population. It also requires a strategy for using two or more tests to distinguish what are called **false positives** and **false negatives** from those who truly have and do not have the disease. False positives are individuals who have positive results on a screening test but do not turn out to have the disease. Similarly, false negatives are those who have negative results on the screening test but turn out to have the disease.

Screening for asymptomatic disease usually identifies more false positives than **true positives**. True positives are individuals who have a positive test and also have the disease. This is true for most screening tests, as discussed in **BOX 6.3** on **Bayes' theorem**.

How can we develop feasible testing strategies?[6] To understand the need for and use of feasible testing strategies, it is important to recognize that screening for diseases is usually conducted on groups that are at an increased risk for the condition. For instance, screening men and women for colon cancer and women for breast cancer is often conducted on people aged 50 years and older. This type of group is considered high risk, usually with a chance or risk of having the disease of 1% or more. Use of high-risk groups like these allows tests that are less than perfect to serve as initial screening tests.

As we have seen, screening for diseases such as breast cancer almost always requires two or more tests. These tests need to be combined using a testing strategy. The most commonly used testing strategy is called **sequential testing**, or consecutive testing. This approach implies that an initial screening test is followed by one or more definitive or diagnostic tests. Sequential testing is used in breast cancer, hearing, and vision testing, and most other forms of screening for noncommunicable diseases. It is generally the

© Radu Bercan/Shutterstock

most cost-effective form of screening because only one negative test is needed to rule out the disease.

Sequential testing by definition misses those who have false negative results because when a negative test occurs, the testing process is over, at least for the immediate future. Thus, a testing strategy needs to consider how to detect those missed by screening. We need to ask: Is there a need for repeat screening, and if so, when should it occur?[c]

---

b  A prerequisite to the use of tests in screening and other situations is establishing the cutoff line that differentiates a positive test and a negative test. Often this is done by using what is called a reference interval. The range of the reference interval is often established by utilizing populations that are believed to be free of a disease. The central 95% of the range of values (or the mean plus or minus 2 standard deviations) for this population is then used as the reference interval, or range of normal. This approach has a number of limitations, including equating existing levels on a test with desirable levels. When data is available on the desirable levels, it is preferable to utilize these levels to establish a reference interval and to define a positive and negative test result. Establishing the desirable level for a test result requires long-term follow-up. For such measurements as blood pressure, cholesterol, and fasting blood sugar, desirable levels are now available.

c  A sequential testing strategy also requires a decision on the order of administering the tests. Issues of cost and safety are often the overriding considerations in determining which test to use first and which to use to confirm an initial positive test. At times, a testing strategy known as **simultaneous testing**, or **parallel testing**, is used. In this scenario, two tests are used initially if one test can be expected to detect one type of disease and the other test can be expected to detect a different type of disease. Traditionally, flexible sigmoidoscopy, which examines the lower approximately 35 cm of the colon, has been used along with tests for occult blood in the stool. Tests for occult blood attempt to screen for cancer in the large section of colon proximal to the sigmoid region. Using both of these tests has been shown to be more accurate for screening than use of either test alone because each attempts to find cancer in different anatomical sites. Stool testing for DNA is currently being increasingly used as the initial screening test rather than utilizing simultaneous testing with two tests.

## BOX 6.3 Bayes' Theorem

**Bayes' theorem** is a mathematical formula that has very practical applications to interpreting the meaning of diagnostic and screening tests. Bayes' theorem provides the connection between the probability of disease before a test is conducted, or the **pretest probability of disease**, and the probability of disease after knowing whether the test result is positive or negative, or the **posttest probability of disease**. To understand Bayes' theorem, we need to appreciate its three elements:

- The meaning of the pretest probability of the disease
- The measures used to summarize the information provided by the results of a test
- The meaning of the posttest probability of the disease when the test is positive and when the test is negative

*Pretest probability of disease:* The pretest probability of a disease is an estimate based on combining information about the prevalence of the disease and risk factors for the disease.[a]

*Measure to summarize information provided by the test:* The measures used to summarize the information provided by a test are called **sensitivity** and **specificity**. Sensitivity is the probability that the test will be positive in the presence of the disease (positive-in-disease). Specificity is the probability that the test will be negative in the absence of the disease (negative-in-health). Ideally, tests have 100% sensitivity and 100% specificity, in which case the test results are always correct. Unfortunately, most tests have a lower sensitivity and specificity, more in the range of 90%, as is the situation with use of mammography for screening for breast cancer.

*Posttest probability of disease:* The posttest probability of disease is the probability of disease after taking into account the pretest probability of disease as well as the sensitivity and specificity of the test. If a test is positive, the posttest probability of disease is called the **predictive value of a positive**. If the test result is negative, the posttest probability that the disease is absent is called the **predictive value of a negative**.

Let us look at how this process works using the example of screening for breast cancer using mammography among women 50 years of age and older. We will assume that the pretest probability of breast cancer among women 50 years of age and older is 1%.

We begin by creating what we call a 2 × 2 box. In the 2 × 2 box, the mammography results positive (+) or negative (−) appear on the left, while the actual presence or absence of breast cancer, as established by a definitive or gold standard test, appears across the top. For illustration purposes, we are assuming that there are 1000 women 50 years and older in this population. Because we are assuming that the pretest probability of disease is 1%, we can conclude that 10 of the 1000 women actually have breast cancer, and 990 do not have breast cancer, as is indicated along the bottom row.

|  | Breast cancer present | Breast cancer absent |  |
|---|---|---|---|
| Mammography (+) |  |  |  |
| Mammography (−) |  |  |  |
|  | 10 | 990 | 1000 |

Now let us include the information provided by the test. We are assuming that mammography has a 90% sensitivity and a 90% specificity. The following boxes illustrate what happens when we apply a test with 90% sensitivity and 90% specificity to a group with a 1% pretest probability of a disease.

|  | Breast cancer present | Breast cancer absent |  |
|---|---|---|---|
| Mammography (+) | 9 | 99 | 108 |
| Mammography (−) | 1 | 891 | 892 |
|  | 10 | 990 | 1000 |

---

a When signs or symptoms of a disease are present, the pretest probability of disease also takes these into account. When screening a population or group of people, we include only individuals who are asymptomatic; that is, they do not have any signs or symptoms of the disease for which screening is being conducted. Often when screening for disease, the pretest probability is low—that is, 1% or even less. For instance, the recommendations for screening women over 50 years of age for breast cancer and screening men and women over 50 for colon cancer are based on data showing that the prevalence of the disease in these risk groups is in the range of 1%.

Because the sensitivity of mammography is assumed to be 90%, among the 10 women with breast cancer, 9 will be detected by the test, allowing us to fill in the 9 and 1 in the left-hand column. Similarly, because we are assuming that the specificity of mammography is also 90%, there are 891 women without breast cancer (0.9 × 990) who will have a negative mammography. That leaves 99 women without breast cancer who will have a positive mammography.

This 2 × 2 box form of Bayes' theorem lets us calculate the probability of breast cancer if the mammography is positive. Note that there are 108 positive mammography tests out of 1000 tests, but only 9 reflect breast cancer. The positive mammographies that reflect breast cancer are called true positives. The positive mammographies that do not reflect breast cancer are called false positives. Therefore, only 9 out of 108, or less than 9% of the positive tests, are true positives.

This implies that if a mammography is positive, the chance, or probability, of breast cancer is still less than 10%.

As we have seen in this illustration, the pretest probability of breast cancer was 1%, while the posttest probability of breast cancer after obtaining a positive mammography was less than 10%. The bottom line of this illustration is that the pretest probability of the disease is a major factor in determining the posttest probability of the disease unless the test is nearly perfect—that is, unless its sensitivity and specificity are nearly 100%.

One key implication of Bayes' theorem for screening for disease is that most screening tests cannot do the job on their own. Follow-up testing, which provides more definitive evidence of disease, is almost always needed. For instance, with breast cancer, a biopsy is often done to make the diagnosis. Most of the time, the biopsy will be negative after a positive mammography, so it is important not to jump to conclusions based on a screening test.

Finally, an ideal screening test should be acceptable in terms of harms, costs, and patient acceptance. Harms must be judged by looking at the entire testing strategy—not just the initial test. Physical examination, blood tests, and urine tests often are used as initial screening tests. These tests are virtually harmless. The real question is: What needs to be done if the initial test is positive? If a large number of invasive tests, such as catheterization or surgery, are required, the overall testing strategy may present substantial potential harms.

Screenings and diagnostic tests themselves can be quite costly. In addition, costs are related to the length of time between testing. Testing every year will be far more costly than testing every 5 or 10 years. The frequency of testing depends on the speed at which the disease develops and progresses, as well as the number of people who can be expected to be missed on the initial test. Mammographic screening is traditionally conducted every year because breast cancer can develop and spread rapidly. In the case of colon cancer, however, longer periods between testing are acceptable because the disease is much slower to develop. Thus, cost considerations may be taken into account when choosing between

technologies and when setting the interval between screenings.[d]

Finally, patient acceptance is key to successful screening. Many screening strategies present little problem with patient acceptance. However, colon cancer screening has had its challenges with patience acceptance because many consider sigmoidoscopy and colonoscopy to be invasive and uncomfortable procedures. Fewer than half the people who qualify for screening based upon current recommendations currently pursue and receive colon cancer screening. This contrasts dramatically with mammography, where a substantial majority of women over 50 now receive the recommended screening.

Screening tests that completely fulfill these ideal criteria are few, and many more screening tests are used despite not fulfilling all these criteria. Screening may still be useful as long as we are aware of its limitations and prepared to accept its inherent problems. **TABLE 6.1** illustrates how commonly used screening tests for risk factors for cardiovascular disease and common cancers perform based upon the four criteria we have outlined.

These criteria also help identify types of screening that should not be done. In general, we do not screen

---

d  Today, there is a wide range of methods for screening for colon cancer, including colonoscopy, which examines the entire colon, and virtual colonoscopy, which does not require an internal examination. These newer tests are much more costly than sigmoidoscopy and occult stool testing. Which is the most accurate and cost-effective test remains controversial. However, the need for and benefits of screening for colon cancer are widely accepted.

**TABLE 6.1** Examples of Screening Tests for Heart Disease and Cancer and Ideal Criteria

| | Substantial mortality and/or morbidity | Early detection is possible and alters outcome | Screening is feasible (can identify a high-risk population and a testing strategy) | Screening is acceptable in terms of harms, costs, and patient acceptance |
|---|---|---|---|---|
| Hypertension | Contributory cause of strokes, myocardial infarctions, kidney disease | High blood pressure precedes bad outcomes often by decades and effective treatment is available | Test everyone—desirable range has been established | Screening itself is free of harms, low cost, and acceptable to patients Treatments, however, may be complicated and have harms, costs, and side effects |
| Low-density lipoprotein (LDL) cholesterol | Contributory cause of strokes, myocardial infarctions, and other vascular diseases | Precedes the development of disease by decades and treatment is effective in altering outcome | Test everyone—desirable range has been established | Screening itself is free of harm, low cost, and acceptable to patients Treatment has rare side effects, which can be detected by symptoms and low-cost blood tests |
| Breast cancer | 2nd most common fatal cancer among women and most common for women under 70 | Early detection improves outcome | For those 50 and over, combination of mammography and follow-up biopsy shown to be feasible | Harm may occur due to false positives, low risk of harm from radiation, patient acceptance good, but test can be somewhat painful Screening younger women increases costs and false positives |
| Cervical cancer | If undetected and untreated—may be fatal | Early treatment dramatically reduces the risk of death | Pap smear and follow-up testing have been extremely successful | Pap results in substantial number of false positives New DNA, or deoxyribonucleic acid, testing may be used to separate true and false positives |
| Colon cancer | Second most common fatal cancer in men and third in women | Early detection of polyps reduces development of cancer, and early detection of cancer improves chances of survival | Men and women 50 and older, plus those with high-risk types of colon disease Options for screening include: fecal occult blood testing, plus flexible sigmoidoscopy, colonoscopy, and virtual colonoscopy. Newer DNA stool test may become initial screening test. | Patient acceptance for use of sigmoidoscopy and colonoscopy has been major barrier, small probability of harm from procedure, substantial cost for colonoscopy and virtual colonoscopy |

for disease when early detection does not improve outcome. We do not screen for rare diseases, such as many types of cancers, especially when the available tests are only moderately accurate. Finally, we do not screen for disease when the testing strategy produces substantial harms. Screening for disease is not the only population health approach that can be used to address the burden of noncommunicable disease. Multiple risk factor reduction is a second strategy that we will examine.

## ▶ How Can Identification and Treatment of Multiple Risk Factors Be Used to Address the Burden of Noncommunicable Disease?

As we have seen, the concept of risk factors is fundamental to the work of public health. Risk factors ranging from high levels of blood pressure and LDL cholesterol to multiple sexual partners and anal intercourse help us identify groups that are most likely to develop a disease. Evidence-based recommendations often focus on addressing risk factors, and implementation efforts often address the best way(s) to target high-risk groups. Thus, identifying and reducing risk factors is an inherent part of the population health approach to noncommunicable diseases.

A special form of intervention aimed at risk factors is called **multiple risk factor reduction**. As the name implies, this strategy intervenes simultaneously in a series of risk factors, all of which contribute to a particular outcome, such as cardiovascular disease or lung cancer. Multiple risk factor reduction is most effective when there are constellations, or groups of risk factors that cluster together in definable groups of people. It may also be useful when the presence of two or more risk factors increases the risk more than would be expected by adding together the impact of each risk factor.

The success in the last half century in addressing coronary artery disease exemplifies multiple risk factor reduction. **BOX 6.4** discusses the impact of this strategy on coronary artery disease. Multiple risk factor reduction strategies are being attempted for a range of diseases, from asthma to diabetes.

Multiple risk factor reduction is most successful when a number of risk factors are at work in the same individual. As we have seen with asthma, factors like indoor and outdoor air pollution, cockroaches and other allergens, and a lack of adherence to medications tend to occur together and may be most effectively addressed together. Similarly, obesity and lack of exercise tend to reinforce each other, often requiring a comprehensive multiple risk factor reduction approach.[e]

Screening for disease and multiple risk factor reduction are key approaches to using testing as part of secondary intervention.[f] The enormous burden of noncommunicable disease cannot be totally prevented, even by maximizing the use of these strategies. It is important to couple them with cost-effective treatment. Thus, a third population health strategy for addressing the burden of noncommunicable disease is to develop cost-effective interventions to treat common diseases.

## ▶ How Can Cost-Effective Interventions Help Us Address the Burden of Noncommunicable Diseases?

Clinicians today have a wide range of interventions to treat disease. Many of these interventions have some impact on the course of a disease. The proliferation of interventions means that it is especially important to identify which provide the greatest benefits at the

---

e   In some situations, the existence of multiple risk factors does more than add together to produce disease. At times, the existence of two or more factors multiplies the risk. In these situations, addressing even one of the factors can have a major impact on disease. For instance, it is now well established that asbestos exposure and cigarette smoking multiply the risks of lung cancer. Thus, if the relative risk for cigarettes is 10 and the relative risk for asbestos exposure is 5, then the relative risk if both factors are present is approximately 50. If an individual who has previously been exposed to both risk factors stops smoking cigarettes and the effects of cigarette smoking are immediately and completely reversible, we can expect the relative risk of lung cancer to decline from approximately a fifty-fold increase to a five-fold increase. This type of interaction is increasingly central to addressing complex public health issues.

f   The principles of testing discussed here are not limited to screening for disease and identification of risk factors. They are also useful as part of a cost-effective approach to diagnosis of symptomatic diseases. In addition, testing is often used for a range of applications in medicine and public health, including monitoring response to treatment, identifying side effects, identifying genetic predictors of disease, and establishing baseline levels for future testing. Public health applications include the use of environmental testing and testing for disease prevalence.

## BOX 6.4 Coronary Artery Disease and Multiple Risk Factor Reduction

An epidemic of coronary artery disease and subsequent heart attacks spread widely through the United States in the mid-1900s. Sudden death, especially among men in their 50s and even younger, became commonplace in nearly every neighborhood in the suburban United States. To better understand this epidemic, which caused nearly half of all deaths in Americans in the 1940s and 1950s, the National Institutes of Health began the Framingham Heart Study in the late 1940s.[7]

In those days, there were only suggestions that cholesterol and hypertension contributed to heart disease, and little, if any, recognition that cigarettes played a role. The Framingham Heart Study enrolled a cohort of over 7000 individuals in Framingham, Massachusetts, questioning, examining, and taking blood samples from them every other year to explore a large number of conceivable connections with coronary artery disease—the cause of heart attacks. Now well into its second half century, after thousands of publications and hundreds of thousands of examinations, the Framingham Heart Study continues to follow the children and grandchildren of the original Framingham cohort.

The study has provided us with extensive long-term data on a cohort of individuals. These form the basis for many of the numbers we use to estimate the strength of risk factors for coronary artery disease. It has helped demonstrate not only the risk factors for the disease, but also the protective, or resilience, factors. The use of aspirin, regular exercise, and modest alcohol consumption has been suggested as protective factors despite the fact that no one ever thought of them in the 1940s.[a]

The Framingham Heart Study demonstrated that high blood pressure precedes strokes and heart attacks by years and often decades. It took the Veterans Administration's randomized controlled trials of the early 1970s to convince the medical and public health communities that high blood pressure needs and benefits from aggressive detection and treatment. Through a truly joint effort by public health and medicine, high blood pressure detection and treatment came to public and professional recognition as a major priority in the 1970s.

The impact of elevated levels of LDL, the bad cholesterol, was likewise suggested by the Framingham Heart Study, but it was not until the development of a new class of medications called statins in the mid-1980s that treatment of high levels of LDL cholesterol took off. These drugs have been able to achieve remarkable reductions in LDL and equally remarkable reductions in coronary artery disease with only rare side effects. These drugs have been so successful that some countries have made them available over the counter. Clinicians are using them more and more aggressively to achieve levels of LDL cholesterol that are less than half those sought a generation ago.[b]

Although diabetes has been treated with insulin since the 1920s and with oral treatments beginning after World War II, the treatment of diabetes to prevent its consequences—including coronary artery disease—was not definitely established as effective until the 1990s. Our current understanding of diabetes has come from a series of randomized controlled trials and long-term follow-ups that demonstrate the key role that poorly controlled diabetes can play in diseases of the heart and blood vessels and the impressive role that aggressive treatment can play in reducing the risks of these diseases.

Efforts aimed at early detection and treatment of heart attacks and prevention of second heart attacks through the use of medications has become routine parts of medical practice. Medical procedures, including angioplasty and surgical bypass of diseased coronary arteries, have also been widely used. Widespread availability of defibrillators in public areas is one of the most recent efforts to prevent the fatal consequences of coronary artery disease.

Between the 1950s and the early years of the 2000s, the death rate from coronary artery disease has declined by over 50%. The impact is even greater among those in their 50s and 60s. Sudden death from coronary artery disease among men in their 50s is now a relatively rare event.

For years, medicine and public health professionals debated whether public health and clinical preventive interventions or medical and surgical interventions deserved the lion's share of the credit for these achievements. The evidence suggests that both prevention and treatment have had important impacts.[9] When medicine and public health work together, the public's health is the winner.

---

a  The data developed for the surgeon general's reports on smoking and health in the 1960s and beyond strongly pointed to substantial effects of cigarettes not only on lung disease, but on coronary artery disease as well. In fact, given the large number of deaths from coronary artery disease compared to lung disease, it became evident that in terms of number of deaths, the biggest impact of cigarette smoking is on heart disease, not lung disease.

b  Recent data even suggests that for individuals with levels of LDL cholesterol within the currently accepted range of normal, statins may be beneficial in the presence of evidence of inflammation as measured by a test called C-reactive protein.[8]

lowest cost. In order to understand how cost-effective interventions can help address the burden of noncommunicable disease, we need to understand what we mean by "cost-effective."

**Cost-effectiveness** is a concept that combines issues of benefits and harms with issues of financial costs. It starts by considering the benefits and harms of an intervention to determine its **net-effectiveness** or net benefit. Net-effectiveness implies that the benefits are substantially greater than the harms, even after the value (or utility), as well as the timing of the harms and benefits, are taken into account. Only after establishing net-effectiveness do we take into account the financial costs.

Cost-effectiveness compares a new intervention to the current or standard intervention. It usually asks: Is the additional net-effectiveness of an intervention worth the additional cost? At times, it may also require us to ask: Is a small loss of net-effectiveness worth the considerable savings in cost? **FIGURE 6.1** is a tool for categorizing interventions in order to analyze their costs and net-effectiveness. **BOX 6.5** provides more details on the use of cost-effectiveness analysis.[10]

Preventive interventions often undergo cost-effectiveness analysis. Many interventions, ranging from mammography to most childhood vaccinations to cigarette cessation programs, get high or at least passing grades on cost-effectiveness. However, many widely used treatment interventions do not or would not meet the current standards of cost-effectiveness. The application of cost-effectiveness criteria to common clinical interventions is considered a population health intervention aimed at getting maximum value for the dollars spent.

The results of cost-effectiveness analysis have already had an impact on a number of common clinical procedures. For instance, cost-effective treatments include the use of minimally invasive orthopedic surgery, such as knee surgery; the reduced length of

intensive care and hospitalization for coronary artery disease; and the use of home health care for intravenous administration of antibiotics and other medications. These efforts to increase the cost-effectiveness of routine healthcare procedures are becoming key to maximizing the benefits obtained from the vast amount of money spent on health care in the United States.

In addition to screening, multiple risk factor reduction, and cost-effective interventions using **prediction rules**, the revolution in genetics has opened up other possible strategies for addressing the burden of noncommunicable diseases.

## ▶ Can Genetic Testing Help Predict Disease and Disease Outcomes and Allow More Personalized Medicine?

Interventions for diseases with a genetic component have been part of medical and public health practice since at least the 1960s, when it was recognized that abnormalities of single genes for such conditions as Tay-Sachs disease (found among Ashkenazi Jews) and sickle-cell anemia (found among African Americans) could be detected by testing potential parents who could then be counseled on the risks associated with childbearing.

It was also recognized that chromosomal abnormalities that produce Down syndrome, the most commonly recognized cause of mental retardation, could be detected at an early stage in pregnancy. In addition, certain genetic defects, such as phenylketonuria (PKU), can be recognized at birth, and in the case of PKU, relatively simple dietary interventions can prevent the severe retardation of mental development that would otherwise occur.

The early years of the 21st century have seen rapid growth in our understanding of human genetics and the ability to economically test for genetic information. This new capability has led to great enthusiasm for the possibility of using genetic information to predict the development of disease and the outcome of disease including individual responses to specific drugs.

Potential uses of genetic testing has been categorized as follows:[11]

*Predicting the risk of a disease*—Predictive genetic testing identifies gene variants that increase an individual's risk of developing a disease. For example, if a woman who has breast cancer is found to have

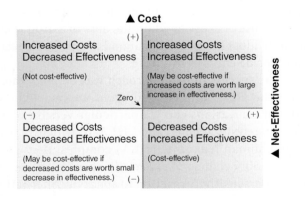

**FIGURE 6.1** The Four Quadrants of Cost- and Net-Effectiveness

## BOX 6.5 Cost-Effectiveness and Its Calculations

Cost-effectiveness is often judged by comparing the costs of a new intervention to the cost of the current, standard, or state-of-the-art intervention. A measure known as the **incremental cost-effectiveness** ratio is then obtained. This ratio represents the additional cost relative to the additional net-effectiveness.

Net-effectiveness may measure a diagnosis made, a death prevented, a disability prevented, etc. Operationalizing the concept of net-effectiveness requires us to define, measure, and combine the probabilities and utilities of benefits with the probabilities and utilities of harm and take into account the timing of the benefits and the harms. Thus, the process of calculating net-effectiveness can be quite complex.

Similarly, calculating costs can be challenging. Most economists argue that the costs are not limited to the costs of providing the intervention and the current and future medical care, but should also include the cost of transportation, loss of income, and other expenses associated with obtaining health care and being disabled. Thus, calculating a cost-effectiveness ratio has become a complex undertaking.

The criteria for establishing cost-effectiveness have changed over time. Most experts in cost-effectiveness prefer the use of a measurement called quality-adjusted life years, or QALYs. QALYs ask about the number of life-years, rather than the number of lives, saved by an intervention. Thus, one QALY may be thought of as 1 year of life at full health compared to immediate death.

In cost-effectiveness analysis, a financial value is usually placed on a QALY, reflecting what a society can afford to pay for the average QALY as measured by its per capita gross domestic product (GDP). In the United States, where the GDP is approximately $50,000, there is a general consensus that a QALY currently should be valued at $50,000. Thus, when you hear that a formal cost-effectiveness analysis has shown that an intervention is cost-effective, it generally implies that the additional cost is less than $50,000 per QALY.[a]

The ideal intervention is one in which the cost goes down and the effectiveness goes up. Cost-saving, quality-increasing interventions have a negative incremental cost-effectiveness ratio. That is, QALYs go up while the costs go down. These cost-reducing, QALY-increasing interventions, while highly desirable, are very rare. Usually, we need to spend more to get additional QALYs. One example of an intervention that reduces costs and at the same time produces additional QALYs is treatment of hypertension in high-risk individuals, such as those with diabetes.[b]

---

a  It is important to note that an increase of one QALY may be the result of obtaining small improvements in utility from a large number of people. For instance, if ten people increase their utility from 0.1 to 0.2, the result is an increase of one QALY. Setting the value of a QALY at $50,000 reflects how much we can afford to pay rather than strictly reflecting how much we think a QALY is worth.

b  Another example is the use of the influenza vaccine among the elderly and those with chronic disease predisposing them to the complications of influenza. It is important to distinguish these types of interventions from those that reduce the costs, but also reduce the QALYs, because at times, both are referred to as cost-saving measures.

---

a breast cancer gene variant (*BRCA1*), a hereditary breast–ovarian cancer syndrome, her relatives can be offered the option of being tested to determine whether they carry the variant. Women who carry the gene have an 80% lifetime risk of developing breast cancer.

The ability to use predictive testing has been limited. For many diseases having a gene associated with disease may only slightly increase the chance of developing the disease. This is known as **incomplete penetrance.** Prediction of outcomes for individuals is a very difficult assignment and has limited the ability so far to use genetic information to predict disease.

*Pharmacogenetic testing* provides information about how individuals will respond to drugs. Pharmacogenetics has the potential to help identify the best drug(s) to use for a condition such as cancer and to prevent use of drugs or adjust the dose of a drug when an individual has a high likelihood of an allergic reaction or side effect from a drug.

The success of this approach was demonstrated with the HIV antiretroviral agent abacavir. Up to 10% of Caucasians carry a particular version of an immune-system gene called HLA-B, which is part of the human leukocyte (HLA) complex, that gives them a 50% chance of experiencing a life-threatening hypersensitivity reaction to abacavir. Alternative drugs exist which can be used when HLA-B is present.[12]

*Reproductive Genetic Testing* aims to identify people who are at increased risk for having a child who has a genetic disease. **Carrier tests** are used to identify people who are at increased risk for having a child who has a genetic disease. Carrier tests usually aim to identify people who are heterozygous for or "carry" one variant copy and one normal copy of a gene for a disease that requires both copies of the gene to clinically express the disease. Carriers generally do not show signs of the disease, but they have the ability to pass on the variant gene to their children.

For example the gene for cystic fibrosis, the most common genetic disorder among whites in the United States, has been identified, and screening of large numbers of couples is now possible. Even among whites without a history of cystic fibrosis, the chance of carrying the gene is about 3%. If both the mother and the father carry the gene, the chance of having a child with cystic fibrosis is 25% with each pregnancy. The severity of cystic fibrosis, however, may vary from mild to severe.

Current guidelines recommend that all pregnant women be offered maternal serum screening tests to identify pregnancies that are at increased risk for a trisomy disorder such as Down syndrome or for a neural-tube defect such as spina bifida.

The use of genetic testing is likely to increase in the coming years, but evidence that it improves patient outcomes will be needed. In addition there are ethical, legal, and social implications of genetic testing which raise questions such as:

- Should we identify diseases when little can be done to prevent or treat them?
- Should genetic risk information be shared among family members?
- How can we prevent stigma or discrimination based on genetic information?
- How do we ensure that the benefits of genetic testing will not be restricted to those with expensive health insurance plans?

High tech solutions to health problems such as genetic testing are very attractive. However, it is important to remember that our interventions can also produce undesirable side effects. The next approach to noncommunicable disease relates to how we can prevent mortality and morbidity from our treatments.

# ▶ What Can Be Done to Prevent Long-Term Mortality and Morbidity from Our Treatments?

We are seeing a rapid increase in the number and types of interventions available to potentially improve health outcomes. Some of these produce short-term benefits but longer-term problems. Our growing ability to successfully suppress the immune system using drug treatments has been successful in the short-term treatment of such hard to control conditions as rheumatoid arthritis, psoriasis, and inflammatory bowel disease.

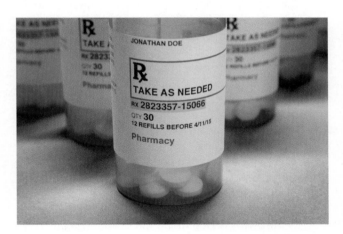

© Burlingham/Shutterstock

Advertisement for drugs to treat these diseases, often for young people, hold out great short-term promise which is associated with greatly increased risks of serious infections and life-threatening cancers. It is key that potential users understand both the benefits and the harms.

The introduction of new types of prescription opioid drugs in the 1990s and beyond has become perhaps the most striking example of the potential for long-term harm from prescription medication. Death from drug overdoses in the United States increased by over 500% since 1990 and now total over 50,000 more than automobile crashes and homicides put together. These deaths are usually due in whole or in part from prescription drug overdoses, most often including opioid drugs, and have become the fastest growing cause of death in many part of the United States. **BOX 6.6** describes the history and impact of the opioid epidemic.[13]

---

**BOX 6.6** The Opioid Epidemic and the Role of Prescription Drugs

Opioids are a class of highly addictive narcotics that are derived from the poppy plant or its derivatives. The term narcotics generally refer to all psychoactive drugs which are either illegal or controlled or restricted by the Food and Drug Administration (FDA).

Opioid abuse in the United States can be traced to the Civil War and even before. Heroin was introduced as a wonder drug in the 1890s and soon was widely used for a range of ailments including cough suppression. Injection of heroin soon became a widespread form of addiction, but it took until the 1920s to outlaw heroin. Today heroin is an inexpensive illegal opioid that is often widely available to those who are already addicted to prescription opioids.

The role of prescription opioids in the current opioid epidemic began in the 1990s. Short-term studies in the 1990s suggested that opioids could be successfully used to treat chronic pain. A new type of immediately active prescription opioids were approved by the FDA in the mid-1990s including OxyContin. Fentanyl—an extremely strong opioid—was made available as a skin patch and in other easy to use forms which rapidly increased its use.

The use of immediately active prescription opioids grew very rapidly in the late 1990s and well into the 21st century. This use was often endorsed by medical experts and encouraged by a Joint Commission on Accreditation of Hospital's requirement that all hospitalized patients be assessed for pain.

By the 2010s the combination of widespread prescription of immediate acting opioids, the widespread availability of inexpensive heroin, and the passive or active endorsement of the medical profession and the FDA helped lead to the opioid epidemic.[14]

In recent years the opioid epidemic has been recognized as a major public health issue. The Director of the CDC wrote in the New England Journal in 2016 "We know of no other medication routinely used for a nonfatal condition that kills patients so frequently."[15] He cited evidence that showed that use of opioids for chronic pain may actually worsen pain and functioning, possibly by increasing pain perception. He indicated that opioid dependence may be as high as 26% for patients using opioids for chronic noncancer pain.[16]

Fatal overdoses usually involve the use of multiple drugs including opioids, alcohol, and antianxiety medications. Those addicted to opioids may not recognize the life threatening potential of these other drugs when added to their usual opioid dosages.

Overdoses of opioids can be rapidly reversed by drugs such as naloxone which are increasingly being carried by first responders. New approaches to pain management, greater education of prescribers of opioids, more available treatment for those addicted, and research into new approaches is bringing hope that the impact of the opioid epidemic can be reversed. However, it took nearly 20 years for the full scale epidemic to develop. and it will take time to reverse its impact on public health.

---

# ▶ What Can We Do When Highly Effective Interventions Do Not Exist?

Alzheimer's is among the most rapidly increasing conditions among those that we classify as noncommunicable diseases. The aging of the population has been and is expected to be associated with many more cases of Alzheimer's, which primarily affects the quality of life with its progressive damage to memory—especially short-term memory.[g]

Today, we have limited treatment options for those afflicted with Alzheimer's. Several drugs are available that have modest positive impacts on memory. Efforts to stimulate mental activity through keeping active mentally and physically have also been shown to have positive, yet modest, impacts. Public health efforts have encouraged the use of these existing interventions, especially when there is evidence that they allow individuals to function on their own or with limited assistance for longer periods of time.

The population health approach to Alzheimer's disease, however, also stresses the need for additional research. Epidemiological research has helped produce the modest advances in preventing progression and treating the symptoms of the disease. A population health approach, however, needs to acknowledge

---

g  Not all cases of memory loss or dementia are due to Alzheimer's. Additional causes include strokes and cerebral vascular disease, chronic alcoholism, thyroid disease, specific infectious diseases (such as syphilis and AIDS), as well as the effects of drugs and a long list of rare diseases. Today, however, Alzheimer's is the most common and the most important cause of memory loss and dementia. We tend to classify a disease as noncommunicable unless there is convincing evidence that it can be transmitted or that it is due in large part to environmental exposures or injuries. Despite the fact that we do not yet know the etiology of Alzheimer's disease, it is generally classified as noncommunicable.

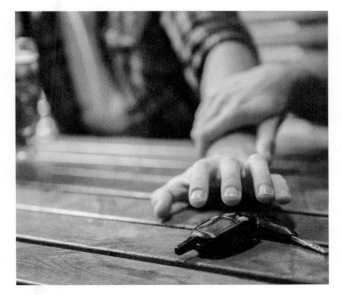

© George Rudy/Shutterstock

the need for a basic biological understanding of what causes Alzheimer's.

Biological, medical, and public health research is actively pursuing a better understanding of the cause or etiology of Alzheimer's as well as investigating new interventions.[17] Pathological studies have demonstrated increases in a protein called amyloid-B deposited in the brains of patients dying with Alzheimer's disease. Observational studies support a role for amyloid-B in the development of Alzheimer's. Unfortunately randomized controlled trials of drugs that reduce the deposition of amyloid-B have had little success in preventing or reversing the disease. New data and new theories including infectious disease and trauma are being advanced to address the still to be explained development of Alzheimer's. We will

hopefully see important progress in this increasingly important public health problem.

We have now explored the major population health strategies for addressing noncommunicable diseases. These include screening, multiple risk factor reduction, cost-effective treatments, genetic counseling, preventing long-term harms of treatment, and more research. A complex problem often requires us to combine many of these approaches.

## ▶ How Can We Combine Strategies to Address Complex Problems of Noncommunicable Diseases?

Multiple interventions combining health care, traditional public health approaches, and social interventions are often needed to address the complex problems presented by noncommunicable diseases. The combined and integrated use of multiple interventions is central to the population health approach. **BOX 6.7** looks at what we can learn about the population health approach to noncommunicable diseases from the long history of alcohol use and abuse, as well as the substantial recent success in addressing disease due to alcohol.[18]

We have now taken a look at strategies to control noncommunicable diseases, which are currently the most common reason for disability and death in most developed countries. Now, let us look at a second category that has been central to the history of public health and threatens to become central to its future: communicable disease.

---

**BOX 6.7**  Alcohol Abuse and the Population Health Approach

Alcohol has been a central feature of U.S. society and U.S. medicine and public health since the early days of the country. It was among the earliest painkillers and was used routinely to allow surgeons to perform amputations during the Civil War and earlier conflicts. The social experiment of alcohol prohibition during the 1920s and early 1930s ended in failure as perceived by a great majority of Americans.

Efforts to control the consequences of alcohol took a new direction after World War II. Americans began to focus on the consequences of alcohol, including liver disease, fetal alcohol syndrome, motor vehicle injuries, and intentional and unintentional violence.

Population health interventions became the focus of alcohol control efforts. For instance, taxation

of alcohol based upon 1950s legislation raised the price of alcohol. Restrictions on advertising and higher taxes on hard liquor, with its greater alcohol content, eventually contributed to greater use of beer and wine. Despite the continued growth in alcohol consumption, the number of cases of liver disease and other alcohol-related health problems have declined. In recent years, efforts to alert pregnant women to the health effects of drinking through product labeling and other health communications efforts have had an impact.

The highway safety impacts of alcohol use have led to population health efforts in cooperation with transportation and police departments. Greatly increased police efforts to catch drunk drivers and stripping of the licenses of repeat offenders have become routine and has contributed to impressive reductions in automotive accidents related to alcohol. Efforts such as the designated driver movement originated by Mothers Against Drunk Driving (MADD) have demonstrated the often-critical role that private citizens can play in implementing population health interventions.

Focusing on high-risk groups, as well as using what we have called "improving-the-average" strategies, has had an important impact. Alcoholics Anonymous (AA) and other peer support groups have focused on encouraging individuals to acknowledge their alcohol problems. These groups often provide important encouragement and support for long-term abstinence.

Medical efforts to control alcohol consumption have been aimed primarily at those with clear evidence of alcohol abuse—often those in need of alcohol withdrawal, or "drying out." Drugs are available that provide modest help in controlling an individual's

alcohol consumption. Screening for alcohol abuse has become a widespread part of health care. These interventions have been aimed at those with the highest levels of risk. The combination of individual, group, and population interventions has reduced the overall impact of alcohol use without requiring its prohibition. In fact, modest levels of consumption, up to one drink per day for women and two for men, may help protect against coronary artery disease.

The issue of alcohol and public health has not gone away. The focus today has returned to identifying high-risk groups and intervening to prevent bad outcomes. A key risk factor today is binge drinking, with its risk of acute alcohol poisoning, as well as unintentional and intentional violence. College students are among the highest risk group. One episode of binge drinking dramatically increases the probability of additional episodes, suggesting that intervention strategies are needed to reduce the risk. We've made a great deal of progress controlling the impacts of alcohol, but we clearly have more to do.

## Key Words

| | | |
|---|---|---|
| Asymptomatic | Incomplete penetrance | Posttest probability of disease |
| Bayes' theorem | Lead-time bias | Screening |
| Carrier test | Multiple risk factor reduction | Sensitivity |
| Cost-effectiveness | Net-effectiveness | Sequential testing |
| Epidemiological transition | Prediction rules | Simultaneous testing |
| False negatives | Predictive value of a negative | Specificity |
| False positives | Predictive value of a positive | True positives |
| Incremental cost-effectiveness | Pretest probability of disease | |

## Discussion Questions

Take a look at the questions posed in the following scenarios, which were presented at the beginning of this chapter. See now whether you can answer them.

1. Sasha did not want to think about the possibility of breast cancer, but as she turned 50, she agreed to have a mammogram, which, as she feared, was positive or "suspicious," as her doctor put it. Waiting for the results of the follow-up biopsy was the worst part, but the relief she felt when the results were negative brought tears of joy to her and her family. Then she wondered: Is it common to have a positive mammogram when no cancer is present?

2. The first sign of Michael's coronary heart disease was his heart attack. Looking back, he had been at high risk for many years because he smoked and had high blood pressure and high bad cholesterol. His lack of exercise and obesity only made the situation worse.

Michael asked: What are the risk factors for coronary heart disease, and what can be done to identify and address these factors for me and my family?

3. John's knee injury from skiing continued to produce swelling and pain, greatly limiting his activities. His physician informed him that the standard procedure today is to look inside with a flexible scope and do any surgery that is needed through the scope. It is simpler and cheaper, and does not even require hospitalization. "We call it cost-effective," his doctor said. John wondered: What does cost-effective really mean?

4. Looking back, JoAnn realized she had been living with depression all her life. As a teenager it affected her ability to form friendships and later an intimate personal relationship. After the birth of her child, depression robbed her of much of the joy of motherhood. As a maturing adult she realized how much more she could be

enjoying life. Thank God, I got help, she said to herself, or suicide could have been in my future.

5. Jennifer and her husband, George, were tested for the cystic fibrosis gene and both were found to have it. Cystic fibrosis can cause chronic lung infections and greatly shortens the length of life. They now ask: What does this mean for our chances of having a child with cystic fibrosis? Can we find out whether our child has cystic fibrosis early in pregnancy?

6. Fred's condition deteriorated slowly, but persistently. He just could not remember anything and repeated himself endlessly. The medications helped for a short time, but before long, he did not recognize his family and could not take care of himself. The diagnosis was Alzheimer's, and he was not alone. Almost everyone in the nursing home seemed to be affected. No one seems to understand the cause of Alzheimer's disease. The family asked: What else can be done, not only for Fred, but also for those who come after Fred?

7. Alcohol use is widespread on your campus. You do not see it as a problem as long as you walk home or have a designated driver. Your mind changes one day after you hear about a classmate who nearly died from alcohol poisoning as a result of binge drinking. You ask yourself: What should be done on my campus to address binge drinking?

## References

1. National Institute of Mental Health. Depression. https://www.nimh.nih.gov/health/topics/depression/index.shtml. Accessed July 21, 2017.

2. Centers for Disease Control and Prevention. Depression. https://www.cdc.gov/mentalhealth/basics/mental-illness/depression.htm. Accessed July 21, 2017.

3. Siu AL, the US Preventive Services Task Force (USPSTF). Screening for depression in adults: US Preventive Services Task Force Recommendation Statement. *JAMA*. 2016;315(4):380–387. doi:10.1001/jama.2015.18392.

4. Omran AR. The epidemiologic transition: a theory of the epidemiology of population change. *The Milbank Memorial Fund Quarterly*. 1971;49(4):509–538.

5. Riegelman RK. *Studying a Study and Testing a Test: Reading the Evidence-Based Health Research*. Philadelphia, PA: Lippincott, Williams & Wilkins; 2013.

6. Gordis L. *Epidemiology*. 4th ed. Philadelphia, PA: Elsevier Saunders; 20014.

7. Framingham Heart Study. History of the Framingham heart study. https://www.framinghamheartstudy.org/about-fhs/history.php. Accessed July 21, 2017.

8. Ridker PM, Danielson E, Foneseca FAH, et al. Rosuvastatin to prevent vascular events in men and women with elevated C-reactive protein. *New England Journal of Medicine*. 2008;259(21):2195–2207.

9. Critchley J, Capwell S, Unal B. Life-years gained from coronary heart disease mortality reduction in Scotland—prevention or treatment? *Journal of Clinical Epidemiology*. 2003;56(6):583–590.

10. Gold MR, Siegel JE, Russell LB, Weinstein MC. *Cost-Effectiveness in Health and Medicine*. New York, NY: Oxford University Press; 1996.

11. National Academies of Sciences, Engineering, and Medicine. *An Evidence Framework for Genetic Testing*. Washington, DC: The National Academies Press; 2017. doi:10.17226/24632.

12. Drew L. Pharmacogenetics: the right drug for you. *Nature*. September 2016;537:S60–62. doi:10.1038/537S60a12.

13. Centers for Disease Control and Prevention. CDC Wonder. https://wonder.cdc.gov/. Accessed July 21, 2017.

14. CNN. Opioid history: from 'wonder drug' to abuse epidemic. http://www.cnn.com/2016/05/12/health/opioid-addiction-history/. Accessed July 21, 2017.

15. Frieden TR, Houry D. Reducing the risks of relief—the CDC opioid-prescribing guideline. *New England Journal of Medicine*. 2016;374:1503. doi:10.1056/NEJMp1515917.

16. Frieden TR, Houry D. Reducing the risks of relief—the CDC opioid-prescribing guideline. *New England Journal of Medicine*. 2016;374:1501–1504. doi:10.1056/NEJMp1515917.

17. Alzheimer's Association. What we know today about Alzheimer's disease. http://www.alz.org/research/science/alzheimers_disease_causes.asp. Accessed July 21, 2017.

18. Room R, Babor T, Rehm J. Alcohol and public health. *Lancet*. 2005;365(9458):519–530.

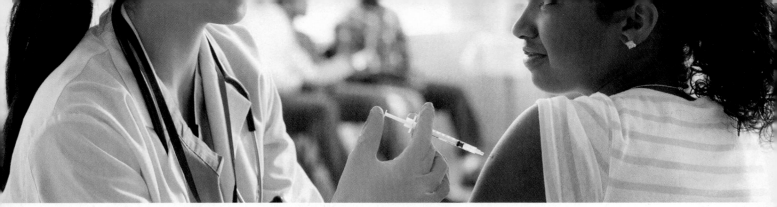

© KidStock/Blend Images/Getty

# Communicable Diseases

## LEARNING OBJECTIVES

By the end of this chapter, the student will be able to:

- describe the burden of disease caused by communicable diseases.
- describe the criteria that are used to establish that an organism is a contributory cause of a disease.
- identify factors that affect the transmissibility of a disease and the meaning of *R* naught.
- identify the roles that barrier protections play in preventing communicable diseases.
- identify the roles that vaccinations can play in preventing communicable diseases.
- identify the roles that screening, case finding, and contact treatment can play in preventing communicable diseases.
- identify the conditions that make eradication of a disease feasible.
- describe a range of options for controlling the HIV/AIDS epidemic.

Your college roommate went to bed not feeling well one night, and early the next morning, you had trouble arousing her. She was rushed to the hospital just in time to be effectively diagnosed and treated for meningococcal meningitis. The health department recommends immediate antibiotic treatment for everyone who was in close contact with your roommate. They set up a process to watch for additional cases to be sure an outbreak is not in progress. Fortunately, no more cases occur. You ask yourself: Should your college require that all freshmen have the meningococcal vaccine before they can register for classes?

As a health advisor to a worldwide HIV/AIDS foundation, you are asked to advise on ways to address the HIV and developing tuberculosis (TB) epidemics. You are asked to do some long-range thinking and to come up with a list of potential approaches to control the epidemics, or at least ways to reduce the development of TB. The first recommendation you make is to forget about eradicating HIV/AIDS. How did you come to that conclusion?

You are a principal at a local high school. One of your top athletes is in the hospital with a spreading bacterial infection due to staphylococcus bacteria resistant to all known antibiotics. The infection occurred after what appeared to be a minor injury during practice. As the principal, what do you decide to do?

Just before your exams begin you develop a fever, runny nose, sore throat, and a dry cough. In the past, antibiotics seemed to help. You know this infection is going to make it hard for you to get that A you need. You make an appointment to be seen at your school health center. After a long wait you hope at least you will be prescribed antibiotics to shorten the course of your infection and give you more time to study. You are discouraged and a bit angry when the nurse practitioner tells you that you have a viral infection and antibiotics won't help. You wonder why the doctor back home usually prescribed antibiotics.

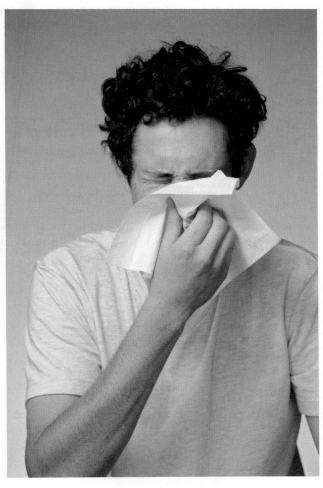

© Matt_Brown/E+/Getty Images

Diseases due to infection form a large part of the history of public health, and are again a central part of its present and its future. Infections of public health importance are primarily those that are communicable; that is, they can be transmitted from person to person or from animals or the physical environment to humans. **Communicable disease** may be caused by a wide variety of organisms, ranging from bacteria, to viruses, to a spectrum of parasites, including malaria and hookworm. Let us examine the burden of disease due to communicable diseases.[a]

## ▶ What Is the Burden of Disease Caused by Communicable Diseases?

For many centuries, communicable diseases were the leading cause of death and disability among all ages, but especially among the young and the old. Communicable diseases are not only the causes of widespread **epidemics** of disease, but they can also become **endemic** or be regularly present and become routine causes of death.[b] Communicable and noncommunicable infectious diseases play a key role in maternal deaths associated with childbirth, infant, and early childhood deaths, as well as deaths of malnourished infants and children.

The last half of the 20th century saw a brief respite from deaths and disabilities caused by communicable diseases and other infections. This was due in large part to medical efforts to treat infections with drugs and public health efforts to prevent infections (often with vaccines) and to eradicate or control other infections. Even as these great accomplishments were under way, warning signs of bacteria resistant to antibiotics began to appear. Staphylococcus organisms resistant to current antibiotics began to plague hospitals in the 1950s until new antibiotics were developed. Resistance of gonorrhea and pneumococcus to a range of antibiotics became widespread. World Health Organization (WHO) and U.S. government–sponsored programs, such as those to promote the eradication of malaria and TB, were not able to have sustained impacts, and the goals were trimmed back to control rather than eradicate.

Over a dozen previously unknown infections have emerged in recent decades in the United States. The presence of Lyme disease and the West Nile virus

---

a The term **infectious disease** is intended to include both communicable disease and disease caused by organisms that are not communicable. The central feature that distinguishes communicable disease from other diseases caused by organisms is its ability to be transmitted from person to person or from animals or the physical environment to humans. Other **infections** of public health interest are caused by organisms, such as the bacteria pneumococcus (*streptococcus pneumoniae*), which usually coexist with healthy individuals, but are capable of causing disease when relocated to areas of the body with increased susceptibility or when they are provided opportunities to multiply or invade new areas because of an individual's decreased resistance. It is important to note that the distinction between infectious diseases and communicable diseases is not always made, and at times they are considered synonyms.

b Epidemic implies that a disease has increased in frequency in a defined geographic area far above its usual rate. Endemic implies that a disease is present in a community at all times but at a relatively low frequency.

was unknown in the United States until the late 20th century, but have now spread to extensive areas of the country. Long-established mosquito-borne diseases, such as malaria and dengue fever, are extending their geographic range, and have the potential to return to the United States.

The early 21st century saw the return of infections that were previously under control, as well as an emergence of new diseases. TB, the great epidemic of the 1700s and 1800s, has returned in force, partially as a result of HIV/AIDS. **BOX 7.1** looks at the history of TB and the historical and current burden of disease caused by it.[1]

In addition to the large number of epidemic communicable diseases, a few diseases have the potential to produce a **pandemic**. A pandemic is an epidemic occurring worldwide, or over a very wide area, crossing international boundaries and affecting a large number of people. As we will discuss, pandemics of influenza have occurred multiple times in the past, and are likely to occur in the future as ongoing mutations produce new strains capable of person-to-person transmission.

History suggests that public health and medical interventions have and will continue to have major impacts on the burden of communicable diseases. In order to understand a potentially communicable disease, we need to demonstrate that a particular organism is in fact capable of being transmitted and producing the disease, which is the hallmark of a communicable disease. Let us take a look at what is needed to establish that an organism is a contributory cause of a communicable disease.

## ▶ How Do We Establish That an Organism Is a Contributory Cause of a Communicable Disease?

Establishing that an organism is a contributory cause of a disease traditionally relied on Koch's postulates.[2] Koch's postulates hold that in order to definitively establish a cause-and-effect relationship, all of the following four conditions must be met:

1. The organism must be shown to be present in every case of the disease by isolation of the organism.
2. The organism must not be found in cases of other disease.
3. Once isolated, the organism must be capable of replicating the disease in an experimental animal.

4. The organism must be recoverable from the animal.

Ironically, TB could not be shown to fulfill Koch's postulates. However, a very useful set of Modern Koch's postulates has been developed by the National Institute of Allergy and Infectious Disease. Modern Koch's postulates require:

1. Evidence of an epidemiological association between the presence of the organism and the presence of a disease in human beings
2. Isolation of the organism from most of those with the disease
3. Transmissions to definitively establish that an organism is a contributory cause of the disease[3]

These criteria may be referred to as association, isolation, and transmission. At times, researchers have been able to directly isolate and transmit diseases from person to person. For instance, fluid from chickenpox skin was collected and transferred to other individuals, resulting in active cases of chickenpox.

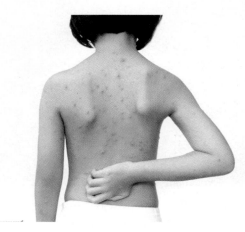

© frank60/Shutterstock

This type of direct evidence of transmission is unusual in humans. Nonetheless, outbreaks of disease can often provide the evidence needed to fulfill Modern Koch's postulates, as illustrated in the case of the bacteria *Neisseria meningitidis,* which has been established as the organism that causes meningococcal meningitis and sepsis.

Meningococcal meningitis, an important cause of meningitis and blood-borne infection, or sepsis, was first recognized during an epidemic in Geneva, Switzerland, in 1805, and occurred in epidemic form especially during military conflicts throughout the 1800s. The bacteria *N. meningitidis* was first cultured

## BOX 7.1  The Burden of TB

*If the importance of a disease for mankind is measured by the number of fatalities it causes, then tuberculosis must be considered much more important than those most feared infectious diseases, plague, cholera and the like. One in seven of all human beings die from tuberculosis. If one only considers the productive middle-age groups, tuberculosis carries away one-third, and often more.*[1]

—Robert Koch, March 24, 1882

The history of TB goes back to ancient times, but beginning in the 1700s, it took center stage in much of Europe and the United States. It has been estimated that in the two centuries from 1700 to 1900, TB was responsible for the deaths of approximately one billion human beings. The annual death rate from TB when Koch made his discovery was approximately seven million people.[1] Considering the current population that would be the equivalent of over 30 million people today.

Robert Koch's discovery of the association between the tuberculosis bacilli, its culture and isolation, and its transmission to a variety of animal species provided a clear demonstration that the bacilli are a contributory cause of the disease. While the tuberculosis bacilli are clearly a contributory cause of the disease TB, they are not sufficient alone to produce disease. A large percentage of the world's population harbors TB. Other factors are needed to produce active disease. These factors include reduced immunity and nutrition, as well as genetic factors.

The discovery of the tuberculosis bacilli actually followed the development of what was called the sanitarium movement, which began in Europe and the United States. Sanitariums isolated TB victims, while providing good nutrition and clean air. The sanitarium movement was coupled in the early 20th century with the use of the Bacillus Calmette-Guérin vaccine, purified protein derivative skin tests, and the recently invented chest X-ray. These three early and rather crude technologies are still in use today, and are designed to prevent and diagnose TB.

In addition, the understanding of the epidemiology of the TB bacteria led to a clear victory for public health. The near elimination of TB from the milk supply through pasteurization early in the 20th century largely eliminated bovine TB.

Even before the ability to actively treat TB, public health interventions were able to dramatically reduce the frequency of the disease, at least in Europe and the United States. A second round of efforts to control TB began in the 1940s with the discovery of streptomycin, the first anti-TB drug, followed over

the next decade by para-aminosalicylic acid and isoniazid (INH). Combination drug treatments proved highly effective. In addition, INH was found to be effective on its own to prevent skin-test-positive TB from progressing to active disease. Public health and medical efforts to conduct screening for positive skin tests and selectively treating with INH became widespread.

By the late 1950s and 1960s, TB was brought under control by the combination of medical and public health advances. The success of this effort resulted in the closing of TB sanitariums, gradual cutbacks in screening and treatment programs, and a general loss of interest in TB. Beginning in the mid-1960s, there was little interest in or research on TB. TB became a treatable disease usually handled as part of routine medical care. Most medical and public health practitioners regarded it as a disease ready for eradication.

Unfortunately, TB was prematurely pronounced dead. It had never come under control in many parts of the world, and approximately 33% of those living in developing countries today are estimated to harbor the TB bacillus. That is, they carry TB organisms that may multiply and spread in the future.

Soon after the beginning of the AIDS epidemic in the 1980s, active TB came back with a vengeance. AIDS patients with latent TB often developed active TB quite early in their battle with AIDS. They then became contagious to others. TB may be more difficult to diagnose and may progress faster in AIDS patients.

Coupled with the return of TB as a public health problem, resistance to TB drugs began to emerge. The problem was successfully combated in the 1990s by the simple public health intervention known as directly observed therapy (DOT). DOT helped ensure that patients received all the prescribed treatment, thus greatly increasing adherence to effective treatment.

Nonetheless, in the early years of the 21st century, resistance to multiple TB drugs increased all over the world. We were faced with a triple threat of limited recent research, leaving us without modern diagnostic aids or new drugs; a rapidly emerging threat from multiple-drug-resistant TB; and a spreading epidemic of HIV/AIDS, predisposing patients to active TB. Each of these can be addressed by coordinated public health and medical actions, which have been occurring in recent years. In the past, TB has been exceptionally responsive to a wide range of public health and medical efforts to control its spread. There is hope that with increased awareness and further research, this will happen again.[2]

from patients with acute meningitis in 1887. Efforts to fulfill **Koch's postulates** were not successful because transmission to animals was not possible, and a large number of humans were carriers without developing the disease.

The ability to culture or isolate the bacteria in sick individuals in the meninges and the blood, areas of the body that should be free of bacteria, was key evidence in establishing the causal role of *N. meningitidis* in the disease. Transmission from person to person has been documented in outbreaks of the disease, and has been used to confirm the final criteria of **Modern Koch's postulates**.

Understanding the mechanism of transmission is important for establishing etiology, but it is also important for appreciating the degree of communicability of a disease and in designing interventions to reduce its spread. Let us take a look at how we measure the potential impact of a communicable disease.

## How Do We Measure the Potential Impact of a Communicable Disease?

### $R_0$ (R naught)

$R_0$ (**R naught**) has gained wide visibility through movies and the media as an indication of the potential of a disease to cause an epidemic. $R_0$ is increasingly being used as a measure of the potential for transmission of a communicable disease.

$R_0$ is intended to measure the average number of infections produced by an infected individual exposed to an otherwise entirely susceptible population. $R_0$ has been used to estimate the degree of communicability of a disease and the potential of the disease to lead to an epidemic.[4]

When $R_0$ is greater than 1, it implies that each infected individual will on average infect more than one previously uninfected individual. Therefore, an $R_0$ of greater than 1 implies that the number of infections will increase over time and produce an epidemic.

**TABLE 7.1** provides examples of the $R_0$ that have been calculated for different diseases.

Influenza usually has an $R_0$ of less than 1.5, but the $R_0$ of the 1918 pandemic strain has been retrospectively estimated as 2–3.

**BOX 7.2** provides additional information on the uses and limitations of $R_0$.

**TABLE 7.1** Examples of $R_0$ for Communicable Diseases

| Disease | Estimated $R_0$ |
| --- | --- |
| Measles | 18 |
| Mumps | 10 |
| HIV | 4 |
| Severe acute respiratory syndrome (SARS) | 4 |
| Ebola | 2 |
| Hepatitis C | 2 |

Data from Ramirez VB. What Is $R_0$?: Gauging Contagious Infections. Healthline. https://www.healthline.com/health/r-nought-reproduction-number.

The following factors have a major impact on $R_0$:

- Transmission probability—probability of infection being transmitted during contact. The **route of transmission** greatly affects transmission probability with airborne infections—especially those transmitted by sneezing—having the highest rate of transmission.
- Period of communicability—the period during which the infection can be transmitted, including frequency and duration. The more contact made while the disease can be transmitted the greater the $R_0$. The longer the period of communicability, the greater the $R_0$, especially if the disease is transmissible in the absence of symptoms.

These factors suggest ways to evaluate the potential impacts of interventions to prevent epidemics. For example:

- Quarantine may reduce the number of contacts.
- Effective treatment may reduce the period of communicability.
- Barriers such as masks or condoms may reduce the probability of transmission.
- Vaccination can reduce the probability of transmission after contact.

Let us take a closer look at the route of transmission and period of communicability.

### Route of Transmission

A wide range of possible routes of transmission have been demonstrated for communicable disease.

**BOX 7.2** Uses and Limitations of $R_0$ [5,6]

$R_0$ can also be used to estimate the proportion of the population which needs to be protected by vaccination to prevent the development of an epidemic. Protection requires effective immunizations so it is important to estimate both the effectiveness of the vaccine and the proportion of the population who are vaccinated. The proportion of the population who need to be effectively vaccinated is calculated as

$$1 - 1/R_0$$

This formula predicts the following:

- When the $R_0$ is 1.2 an epidemic may be prevented by effective immunization of approximately 17% of the population
- When the $R_0$ is 1.5 an epidemic may be prevented by effective immunization of approximately 33% of the population
- When the $R_0$ is 2.0 prevention of an epidemic may require effective immunization of approximately 50% of the population
- When the $R_0$ is 4.0 prevention of an epidemic may require effective immunization of approximately 75% of the population
- When the $R_0$ is 10 or greater prevention of an epidemic requires effective immunization of 90% or more of the population.

This suggests that control of diseases with a large $R_0$ such as measles and mumps requires very high levels of effective immunization which are very difficult to obtain and maintain.

$R_0$ does not allow us to predict how long it will take for an epidemic to develop, but it can be used alone to predict the proportion or percentage of the population which will eventually be infected if no effective intervention(s) are implemented.

Despite the usefulness of $R_0$, it is important to recognize its inherent limitations and cautions in its application. Standard estimates of $R_0$ assume not only that everyone is susceptible to the disease, but that all individuals have an equal probability of exposure. In diseases such as HIV and hepatitis B the probability of infections is largely limited to high-risk groups.

$R_0$ also assumes that there is an average transmission probability. In some diseases such as SARS "super spreaders" have been recognized who may infect large number of individuals and play a disproportionate role in producing an epidemic. In addition, transmission probability may vary throughout the course of a disease. For instance HIV often has a very high initial probability of transmission followed by much lower levels of transmission once the acute infection is controlled.

$R_0$ has become an important measurement in the investigation and control of communicable disease. However, it is important to understand its meaning, uses, and limitations.

Communicable diseases may be transmitted from person to person or from animal species or from the physical environment to humans. **TABLE 7.2** outlines the major methods of transmission of human disease, and provides examples of each of the methods.[7]

## Period of Communicability

Diseases with the potential to create human epidemics are often diseases that can be transmitted from person to person while the individual is free of symptoms. Classic examples include influenza, chickenpox, measles, and mumps. Transmission often occurs in the days or weeks prior to the development of symptoms, but it can also occur from individuals who never develop signs or symptoms of the disease.

In addition to those who transmit the disease as part of their initial exposure to it, other individuals may transmit the disease after they have recovered from the clinical disease or after they are infected with it but do not develop symptoms. Those individuals without symptoms but with the ability to chronically transmit the disease are called **chronic carriers**. Examples of disease that often lead to chronic carriers are HIV and hepatitis B and C.

Now let us turn our attention to the tools that are available to public health to deal with communicable diseases.

## What Public Health Tools Are Available to Address the Burden of Communicable Diseases?

A range of public health tools are available to address the burden of communicable diseases. Some of these are useful in addressing noncommunicable diseases as well, but they have special applications when directed toward infections. These include:

- Barrier protections, including isolation and quarantine

**TABLE 7.2** Methods of Transmission of Human Disease

| Method of transmission | Examples |
| --- | --- |
| Insects | Malaria, Lyme disease, West Nile virus, dengue fever, Zika, and yellow fever |
| Other animals | Rabies, avian flu, anthrax, and plague |
| Airborne—person-to-person | Influenza, SARS, measles, chickenpox, TB, and the common cold |
| Sexual transmission/open sores | Gonorrhea, syphilis, herpes genitalis, chlamydia, hepatitis B, and HIV |
| Water/food | Hepatitis A and cholera |
| Fecal/oral | Polio and salmonella |
| Transfusions/blood/contaminated needles | HIV and hepatitis B, C, D, and E |
| Transplacental | Rubella and HIV |
| Breastfeeding | HIV |
| Contaminated articles ("fomites") | Chickenpox, common cold, and influenza |

Data from Timmreck TC. *An Introduction to Epidemiology*. 3rd ed. Sudbury, MA: Jones and Bartlett Publishers; 2002:34.

■ Immunizations designed to protect individuals as well as populations
■ Screening and case finding
■ Treatment and contact treatment
■ Efforts to maximize the effectiveness of treatments by preventing resistance

Let us look at each of these tools.

## How Can Barriers Against Disease Be Used to Address the Burden of Communicable Diseases?

Examples of barriers to the spread of infections are as old as handwashing and as new as insecticide-impregnated bed nets, which have had a major impact on the rate of malaria transmission. Barrier protection, such as condoms, is believed by many to be the most successful intervention to prevent sexually transmitted diseases. The use of masks may be effective in reducing the spread of disease in health-care institutions, such as hospitals. The same measures may be preventative in the community at large and are a routine part of winter weather habits in much of Asia.

A special form of barrier protection consists of separating individuals with disease or potential disease from the healthy population to prevent

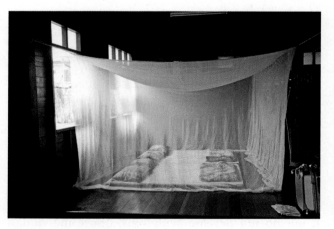

© Anirut Thailand/Shutterstock

exposure. Isolation occurs when individuals with symptoms of a disease are separated from those who do not have symptoms. Quarantine occurs when those suspected of having a disease but without current symptoms are separated from others. As we discussed previously, isolation in sanitariums had a major impact in reducing outbreaks of TB in the 1800s and the first half of the 20th century. The 2014–2016 outbreak of Ebola brought attention to the continuing limited use of quarantine to observe those exposed to a disease during its **incubation period** or the expected time between contact and development of symptoms.

A second traditional public health approach to communicable and noncommunicable infections is the use of immunizations. Let us take a look at a range of ways that immunizations can be used to address the burden of communicable disease.

## How Can Immunizations Be Used to Address the Burden of Communicable Disease?

**Immunization** refers to the strengthening of the immune system to prevent or control disease. Injections of antibodies may be administered to achieve **passive immunity**, which may provide effective short-term protection. **Inactivated vaccine** (dead) and **live vaccines** (attenuated live) can often stimulate the body's own **antibody** production. Live vaccines utilize living but weakened organisms that also stimulate **cell-mediated immunity,** and produce long-term protection that more closely resembles the body's own response to infection.

Vaccines are now available for a wide range of bacterial and viral diseases, and are being developed and increasingly used to prevent infections as varied as malaria and hookworm.[8] Unfortunately, it has been difficult to produce effective vaccines for some diseases, such as HIV/AIDS. Vaccines, like medications, are rarely 100% effective and may produce side effects, including allergic reactions that can be life threatening. Live vaccines have the potential to cause injury to a fetus and can themselves produce disease, particularly in those with reduced immunity. Some vaccines are not effective for the very young and the elderly. Therefore, the use of vaccines requires extensive investigations to define their effectiveness and safety as well as to identify high-risk groups for whom they should be recommended.[c]

For instance, college students and military recruits who tend to live in close quarters represent two high-risk groups for meningococcal disease. This bacterial infection can be rapidly life threatening, and when present, it requires testing and antibiotic treatment of close contacts. Effective vaccination is now a key tool for controlling this disease.

Ideally, vaccination occurs before exposure. However, when an outbreak occurs, vaccination of large numbers of potentially exposed individuals living in the surrounding area may be key to effective control. Thus, public health uses of vaccines need to include consideration of who should receive the vaccine, when it should be administered, and how it should be administered.

Vaccine administration has traditionally been limited to injections as shots or ingestion as pills. New methods of administration, including nasal sprays, are now being developed. In addition, it is often possible to combine vaccines, increasing the ease of administration. Inactivated vaccines may not produce long-term immunity and may require follow-up vaccines or boosters. Thus, the use of vaccinations requires the development of a population health strategy that gives careful attention to "who," "when," and "how."

Some infections, especially those viruses that are highly contagious, can be controlled by vaccinating a substantial proportion of the population, often in the range of 70%–90%. In this situation, those who are susceptible rarely, if ever, encounter an individual with the disease. This is known as **herd immunity or population immunity**. When a population has been vaccinated at these types of levels for diseases—such as chickenpox, measles, and polio—those who have not been vaccinated are often protected. For some vaccines, such as live polio vaccine, herd immunity is facilitated by the fact that the virus in the vaccine can itself be spread from person to person, providing protection for the unvaccinated. Thus, public health authorities are interested in the levels of protection in

---

c   The potential for vaccinations to produce autism, especially the commonly used measles, mumps and rubella (MMR) was given widespread visibility after research was published suggesting a relationship. The data was later found to be falsified and the results were withdrawn by the publishing journal. No relationship has been found despite extensive research.[9] None-the-less a large percentage of the U.S. population continue to believe there is a relationship.

the community—that is, the level of protection of the unvaccinated as well as the vaccinated.

In addition to tools for preventing disease in individuals and populations, public health efforts are often directed at screening for disease and conducting what is called case finding.

## How Can Screening and Case Finding Be Used to Address the Burden of Communicable Disease?

Ideally, screening for communicable diseases fulfills the same criteria for noncommunicable diseases. Screening for communicable diseases has played a role in controlling the spread of a number of infections. For example, screening for TB and syphilis has been an effective part of the control of these infections even before they could be cured with antibiotics. Today, screening for sexually transmitted diseases, including gonorrhea and chlamydia, are a routine part of clinical care. HIV screening has long been recommended for high-risk individuals and for populations with an estimated prevalence above 1%.

Screening for communicable diseases has often been linked with the public health practice known as **case finding**. Case finding implies confidential interviewing of those diagnosed with a disease and asking for their recent close physical or sexual contacts. Case finding techniques have been key to the control of syphilis and to a large extent TB both before and after the availability of effective treatment. The advent of effective treatment meant that case finding was of benefit both to those diagnosed with the disease and those located through case finding.

Successful case finding aims to maintain confidentiality. However, when following up with sexual contacts, confidentiality is difficult to maintain. The potential for public recognition and the attendant social stigma has inhibited the use of case finding in HIV/AIDS in many parts of the world. The reluctance to utilize case finding may change in coming years, as early diagnosis and perhaps early treatment become more effective in controlling the epidemic.

In addition to the use of barrier protections, vaccination of individuals and populations, as well as the use of screening and case finding, public health tools also encompass treatment of those with disease and their contacts.

## How Can Treatment of Those Diagnosed and Their Contacts Help to Address the Burden of Communicable Disease?

Treatment of symptomatic disease may in and of itself reduce the risk of transmission. Successful treatment of HIV has been shown to reduce the viral load and thereby reduce the ease of transmission. Similarly, treatment of active TB reduces its **infectivity** or ease of transmission.

In addition to direct treatment, a public health tool known as **epidemiological treatment**, or treatment of contacts with the disease, has been effective in controlling a number of communicable diseases. Sexual partners of those with gonorrhea and chlamydia are routinely treated, even when their infections cannot be detected. This approach presumably works because early and low-level infections caused by these organisms may be difficult to detect. As we saw in the meningococcal scenario, epidemiological treatment may be the most effective way to halt the rapid spread of a disease.

Contact treatment of HIV/AIDS may become a routine part of controlling the disease. It is already recommended and widely used for treatment of needlestick injuries in healthcare settings.

Despite the progress that has been made against a wide array of infectious diseases, in recent years we are increasingly recognizing that we live with and benefit from an enormous ecosystem of bacteria and other microbes which is being called the **human microbiome**. Let us take a look at some implications of this new recognition and the dangers of disrupting these relationships.

## What Is the Human Microbiome and Why Is It Important?

We share many of our organ systems, including the pulmonary, skin, and especially the gastrointestinal system, with the human microbiome made up of billions of bacteria, viruses, and other microorganisms. According to Morens and Fauci of the National Institute of Allergy and Infectious Diseases:

Specifically, our gut flora represents a complex "external" organ system...that have evolved with us over millennia and appear to affect our health, including by preventing and modifying infection....Infants who start life with or develop "reduced" flora (e.g., via pre- or postnatal antibiotics) may be at increased risk of IDs (infectious diseases) and EIDs (emerging infectious diseases). Variations in the microbiome may also affect the occurrence of certain chronic diseases, allergies, and malnutrition.[10]

Humans have had a dramatic impact on our microbiome in recent years through extensive use of antibiotics and the development of antibiotic resistance. Today, the Centers for Disease Control and Prevention estimates that there are over 2 million infections per year with antibiotic resistant bacteria and over 20,000 deaths per year.[11]

Misuse of antibiotics in human medicine has been common. In many developing countries antibiotics are available over the counter. In addition to the use of antibiotics to treat specific human bacterial infection, it became common clinical practice to try antibiotics as a first line approach when the cause of the problem was not clear or was most likely due to a virus. Widespread use of low-dose antibiotics in farm animals for prevention of disease and increased growth has also contributed to the development of antibiotic resistance.

This is now rapidly changing. Today, routine feeding of medically important antibiotics for growth promotion is banned or will soon be banned in much of the developed world including the United States.

Considerable attention is now being focused on what can be done to reduce antibiotic resistance. Judicious use of therapeutic antimicrobials is an integral part of human and veterinary medical practice. It is key to maximizing therapeutic effectiveness and minimizing selection of resistant microorganisms. New drugs, greater use of vaccines, increased use of handwashing, more judicious use of antibiotics in humans, and reduced use of antibiotics in animals for growth and disease prevention are all being recommended as part of a concerted effort to address antibiotic resistance.[12] Hopefully we will look back in the not too distant future to the time when we turned the corner on misuse of antibiotics.

Let us now turn our attention to strategies that combine many of the specific public health tools designed to address the problems of communicable diseases. We will look at two basic strategies for combating complex infections: elimination and control.

## ▶ How Can Public Health Strategies Be Used to Eliminate Specific Communicable Diseases?

Smallpox was the first human disease to be eradicated. An international effort is hopefully nearing completion to eradicate polio. These two viral diseases are the only ones that have been successfully targeted for eradication. As we have discussed, programs to eradicate TB and malaria have never come close to meeting their goals. Talk of eradication of HIV/AIDS is even more unrealistic. Let us see what it takes to successfully eradicate a disease and why so few diseases are on the short list for potential eradication.[13]

The history of smallpox has a unique place in public health. The disease goes back thousands of years, and it played a prominent role in the colonial United States, where epidemics often killed a quarter or more of their victims, especially children, and left most others, including George Washington, with severe facial scars for life.

The concept of vaccination and the first successful vaccination were developed for smallpox. During the 1800s and early 1900s, smallpox was largely eliminated from most developed and developing countries through modest improvement on Jenner's basic approach to vaccination in which fluid from cowpox sores was placed under the skin to protect individuals against smallpox, despite the many side effects of this quite crude treatment.[d]

Despite the control of smallpox in most developed countries, there were still over 10 million cases annually of the disease in over 30 countries during the early 1960s. In 1967, the WHO began a campaign to eliminate smallpox. The success of the campaign over the next decade depended on extraordinary organizational management and cooperation, but the

---

d While the vaccine against smallpox is very effective, it has many side effects. The live virus contained in the vaccine can itself cause disease in those vaccinated, especially if they have widespread skin disease or have a compromised immune system. Today, these side effects may have prevented the widespread use of the smallpox vaccine because it could threaten the lives of the large number of HIV positive individuals, many of whom are unaware of their HIV infection. Allergic reactions to the vaccine are also quite common. Allergic reactions to the smallpox vaccine, including inflammation of the lining of the heart, prompted discontinuation of a campaign to vaccinate first responders and healthcare professionals soon after the 9/11 attack.

prerequisites for success were the unique epidemiological characteristics of smallpox that made it possible. Let us outline the characteristics of smallpox that made eradication possible:[14]

- *No animal reservoir*—Smallpox is an exclusively human disease. That is, there is no reservoir of the disease in animals. It does not affect other species that can then infect additional humans. This also means that if the disease is eliminated from humans, it has nowhere to hide and later reappear in human populations.

- *Short persistence in environment*—The smallpox virus requires human contact, and cannot persist for more than a brief time in the environment without a human host. Thus, droplets from sneezing or coughing need to find an immediate victim and are not easily transmitted except by human-to-human contact.

- *Absence of a long-term carrier state*—Once an individual recovers from smallpox, he or she no longer carries the virus and cannot transmit it to others. Smallpox contrasts with diseases such as HIV/AIDS and hepatitis B, which can maintain long-term carrier states and be infectious to others for years or decades.

- *The disease produces long-term immunity*—Once an individual recovers from smallpox, very effective immunity is established, preventing a second infection.

- *Vaccination also establishes long-term immunity*—As with the disease itself, the live smallpox vaccine produces very successful long-term immunity. Smallpox has not mutated to become more infectious despite the extensive use of vaccination.

- *Herd immunity protects those who are susceptible*—Long-term immunity from the disease or the vaccine makes it possible to protect large populations. At least 80% of the population needs to be vaccinated to interrupt the spread of the infection to the remaining susceptible people.

- *Easily identified disease*—The classic presentation of smallpox is relatively easy to identify by clinicians with experience observing the disease, as well as by the average person. This makes it possible to quickly diagnose the disease and protect others from being exposed.

- *Effective postexposure vaccination*—The smallpox vaccine is effective even after exposure to smallpox. This enables effective use of what is called **ring vaccination**. Ring vaccination for smallpox involves identification of a case of smallpox, vaccination of the individual's household and close contacts, followed by vaccination of all those within a mile radius of the smallpox case. In the past, households within 10 miles were typically searched for additional cases of smallpox. These public health surveillance and containment efforts were successful even in areas without high levels of vaccination.

The presence of all of these characteristics makes a disease ideal for eradication. While fulfilling all of them may not be necessary for eradication, the absence of a large number of them makes efforts at eradication less likely to succeed. **TABLE 7.3** outlines these characteristics of smallpox and compares them to polio—the current viral candidate for eradication—as well as to measles. Based upon the content of the table, you should not be surprised to learn that the polio campaign has been much more difficult and has taken much longer than that of smallpox. The potential for a successful measles eradication campaign is still being debated.[e]

Finally, take a look at **TABLE 7.4**, which applies these characteristics to HIV infection. It demonstrates why the eradication of HIV/AIDS is not on the horizon.

Unfortunately, eradication of most diseases is not a viable strategy. Thus, public health measures are usually focused on control of infections. In order to understand the range of strategies that are available and useful for controlling communicable diseases, we will take a look at three important and quite different diseases—HIV, influenza A, and rabies.

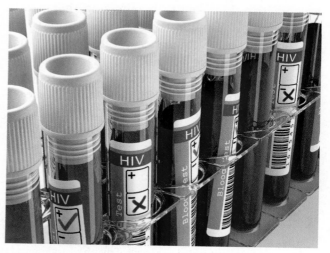

© ktsdesign/Shutterstock

---

e Efforts are under way for the eradication of Guinea worm, which exhibits a number of favorable characteristics for eradication.

**TABLE 7.3** Eradication of Human Diseases—What Makes It Possible?

| | Smallpox | Polio | Measles |
|---|---|---|---|
| Disease is limited to humans (i.e., no animal reservoir)? | Yes | Yes | Yes |
| Limited persistence in the environment? | Yes | Yes | Yes |
| Absence of long-term carrier state? | Yes | Yes—Absent, but may occur in immune-compromised individuals | Yes—Absent, but may occur in immune-compromised individuals |
| Long-term immunity results from infection? | Yes | Yes—But may not be sustained in immune-compromised individuals | Yes—But may not be sustained in immune-compromised individuals |
| Vaccination confers long-term immunity? | Yes | Yes—But may not be sustained in immune-compromised individuals Virus used for production of the live vaccine can produce polio-like illness and has potential to revert back to "wild type infection" | Yes—But may not be sustained in immune-compromised individuals |
| Herd immunity prevents perpetuation of an epidemic? | Yes | Yes | Yes |
| Easily diagnosed disease? | Yes | Yes/No—Disease relatively easy to identify, but large number of asymptomatic infections | No—Disease may be confused with other diseases by those unfamiliar with measles |
| Vaccination effective postexposure? | Yes | No | Partially effective if administered within 72 hours of exposure |

▶ # What Options Are Available for the Control of HIV/AIDS?

HIV/AIDS has been a uniquely difficult epidemic to control. An understanding of the biology of the HIV virus helps us understand many of the reasons for this. The HIV virus attacks the very cells designed to control it. The virus can avoid exposure to treatments by residing inside cells and temporarily not replicating. Many treatments work by interrupting the process of replication and thus are not effective when replication stops. The virus establishes a chronic carrier state, enabling long-term infectivity. High mutation rates reduce the effectiveness of drugs, as well as the effectiveness of the body's own immune system to fight the disease.

Despite these monumental challenges, considerable progress has been made by reducing the load of virus through drug treatment and preventing the transmission of the disease through a variety of public health interventions. To appreciate the efforts to control transmission of HIV/AIDS, it is important to understand the large number of ways that it can be transmitted.[13]

HIV is most infectious when transmitted directly by blood. Blood transfusions were an early source of the spread of the virus. The introduction of HIV virus testing in the mid-1980s led to a dramatic improvement in the safety of the blood supply. Nonetheless, the safest blood transfusions are those that come from an individual's

**TABLE 7.4** Potential for Eradication of HIV/AIDS

|  | HIV/AIDS |
|---|---|
| Disease is limited to humans (i.e., no animal reservoir)? | No—Animal reservoirs exist |
| Limited persistence in the environment? | No—May persist on contaminated needles long enough for transmission |
| Absence of long-term carrier state? | No—Carrier state is routine |
| Long-term immunity results from infection? | No—Effective long-term immunity does not usually occur |
| Vaccination confers long-term immunity? | No—None currently available and will be difficult to achieve |
| Herd immunity prevents perpetuation of an epidemic? | No—Large number of previously infected individuals increases the risk to the uninfected |
| Easily diagnosed disease? | No—Requires testing |
| Vaccination effective postexposure? | No—None currently available |

own blood. Thus, donation of one's own blood for later transfusion when needed has become a routine part of elective surgery preparation in many parts of the world.

The most dangerous forms of transfusions are those that come from blood or blood products pooled from large numbers of individuals. Hemophiliacs in many developed countries used pooled blood products to control their bleeding in the 1980s. They suffered perhaps the world's highest rate of HIV infection before this hazard was recognized and addressed. A more recent pooling of blood products occurred in China and contributed to a surge of the disease.

Unprotected anal intercourse is a highly infectious way to transmit HIV. This may help to explain the early spread of the disease among male homosexuals. Today, however, heterosexual transmission is the most common route of infection; additionally, there is a higher risk of transmission from male to female than from female to male. A series of public health interventions has now been shown to be effective: properly used latex condoms, male circumcision, and abstinence are being promoted in efforts to control the disease throughout the world. Additional interventions to provide protection before, during, and after intercourse are being investigated. Aggressive treatment of AIDS at an early stage reduces the viral load and the ease of transmission to others.[f]

Maternal-to-child transmission of HIV was a common, but not universal, event before the advent of effective drug treatment. The use of treatment during pregnancy and at the time of delivery has dramatically reduced the maternal-to-child transmission of the infection. Today, this route of transmission is close to being eliminated, which is an important public health achievement.

Breastfeeding represents an ongoing and more controversial route of transmission. Up to 25% of HIV-positive breastfeeding women may transmit HIV to their children. In countries where breastfeeding provides an essential defense against a wide range of infections, the issue of whether or not to breastfeed has been very controversial. Fortunately, drug treatment of HIV infections during breastfeeding has been shown to greatly reduce, but not eliminate, transmission.

Finally, HIV can be transmitted through contaminated needles. Thus, the risk of HIV transmission needs to be addressed in two very different populations—healthcare workers and those who abuse intravenous drugs and share needles. New needle technologies and better disposal methods have reduced the likelihood of needlestick injuries in healthcare settings. Postexposure treatment with drugs has been quite successful in reducing healthcare-related HIV infections.

---

f   It has been suggested that serial monogamy reduces the risk of HIV transmission in populations compared to having two or more concurrent partners. Serial monogamy contributes to only one chain of transmission at a time and thus may slow, if not halt, the speed or spread of the epidemic in a population.

Reductions in HIV transmission through intravenous drug use have also occurred in areas where public health efforts have focused attention on this method of transmission. Needle exchange programs have met resistance and remain controversial, but most likely contribute to transmission reductions when the programs are carefully designed and administered.

A range of existing interventions linked to the method of transmission of HIV have been moderately successful in controlling the disease. New methods of control are needed and are being investigated and increasingly applied. Unfortunately, vaccination is not yet a successful intervention. In fact, early randomized controlled trials demonstrated no substantial degree of protection from vaccinations and raised the concern that vaccination may actually increase the probability of acquiring HIV. More recent studies combining two or more types of vaccines have again provided hope for at least a partially effective vaccine in the years to come.

The recognition that highly effective vaccinations are not likely in the foreseeable future has brought forth a wide array of ideas on how to control the spread of infection. Antiviral creams, postcoital treatments, and early testing and case finding may become effective interventions. Antiviral creams may become both an adjunct to condom use and a substitute in those situations where condom use is not acceptable. The success of post needlestick interventions in the healthcare setting has raised the possibility that postexposure treatment may also be effective after high-risk sexual contact.

Finally, new diagnostic tests for HIV that allow for detection of the disease in the most contagious early weeks of the infection are being investigated for widespread use. To be effective, testing for early disease would need to be coupled with rapid case finding to identify and ideally treat contacts.

It is encouraging to know that existing and emerging interventions for HIV hold out the possibility of effective control. Public health and medical interventions complement each other and are both needed if we are to effectively address the most widespread epidemic of the 21st century.

## ▶ What Options Are Available for the Control of Influenza?

Pandemic influenza is not a new problem. The influenza epidemic of 1918 is estimated to have killed 50 million people in a world populated with 2 billion people. Today, that would translate to over 150 million deaths. The history of the 1918 influenza pandemic is briefly summarized in **BOX 7.3**. The 1958 pandemic of Asian flu caused a similar, if less deadly, pandemic. A number of less deadly influenza pandemics have occurred, the most recent in 2009–2010. Thus, we should not be surprised if pandemic flu returns in the coming years.

---

**BOX 7.3**  The Influenza Pandemic of 1918

The history of the influenza pandemic of 1918 is summarized by the United States National Archives and Records Administration as follows:[15]

*World War I claimed an estimated 16 million lives. The influenza epidemic that swept the world in 1918 killed an estimated 50 million people. One fifth of the world's population was attacked by this deadly virus. Within months, it had killed more people than any other illness in recorded history.*

The plague emerged in two phases. In late spring of 1918, the first phase, known as the "three-day fever," appeared without warning. Few deaths were reported. Victims recovered after a few days. When the disease surfaced again that fall, it was far more severe. Scientists, doctors, and health officials could not identify this disease which was striking so fast and so viciously, eluding treatment, and defying control. Some victims died within hours of their first symptoms. Others succumbed after a few days; their lungs filled with fluid, and they suffocated to death.

The plague did not discriminate. It was rampant in urban and rural areas, from the densely populated East coast to the remotest parts of Alaska. Young adults, usually unaffected by these types of infectious diseases, were among the hardest hit groups along with the elderly and young children. The flu afflicted over 25% of the U.S. population. In 1 year, the average life expectancy in the United States dropped by 12 years.

---

Influenza A is a viral infection that has long been capable of pandemic or worldwide spread.[g] Its ability to be rapidly transmitted through the air from person to person and its short incubation period have made it an ongoing public health problem. It often kills the

---

g  Influenza B can also cause epidemics of influenza; however, it is not thought to pose the same hazard of pandemic disease that is possible with influenza A.

very young, the very old, and those with chronic illnesses, particularly those with respiratory diseases and suppressed immune systems. In addition, the disease continues to mutate, creating new types against which previous infections and previous vaccinations have little or no impact. Thus, new vaccines are required every flu season. Seasonal influenza deaths vary widely from year to year. Influenza has killed approximately 3,000–49,000 people in the United States alone in recent years though these numbers can be expected to be reduced by the increasingly widespread use of vaccinations.[16]

A variety of public health and medical interventions have been and continue to be used to address the current and potential threat posed by influenza. They may well all be needed to address future threats. Let us take a look at a number of these interventions.

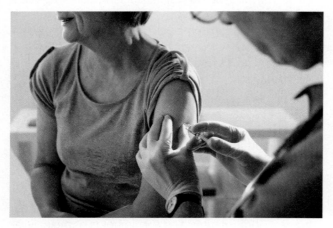

© Image Point Fr/Shutterstock

Inactivated or dead vaccines have been the mainstay of immunization against influenza. Unfortunately, current technology requires approximately 6 months lead time to produce large quantities of the vaccine. Thus, influenza experts need to make educated guesses about next year's dominant strains of influenza. In some years, they have been wrong and the deaths and disability from seasonal influenza have increased. New technologies for vaccine production are now available and should be able to help with this issue in the future.

In recent years, live vaccines administered through nasal spray have been developed and increasingly used. These vaccines are more acceptable than shots to most patients and are now considered safe for a wide range of age groups. Unfortunately recent data indicates that nasal spray vaccines have not been highly effective, and they are not currently being recommended by CDC.[16]

Medications to treat influenza and modestly shorten the course of the disease have also been developed. Influenza experts view these drugs as most useful to temporarily slow the spread of new strains, providing additional time for the development of vaccines to specifically target the new strain. Widespread use of influenza drugs has already resulted in resistance, raising concerns that these drugs will not be effective when we need them the most. Efforts are under way to develop new drugs and reserve their use solely for potential pandemic conditions.

Despite our best efforts, influenza is expected to continue its annual seasonal epidemic and to pose a risk of pandemic spread. The use of barrier protection such as masks, isolation methods, and even quarantine has been considered part of a comprehensive effort to control influenza. It is clear that we have a variety of public health methods to help control the impact of the disease. It is likely that we will need all of these efforts and new ones if we are going to control the potential deaths and disabilities due to influenza in coming years.[17]

Now, let us look at our last example of the development of public health strategies to control communicable diseases—that of rabies.

## ▶ What Options Are Available for the Control of Rabies?

Rabies is an ancient disease that has plagued human beings for over 4000 years. It is caused by a ribonucleic acid (RNA) virus that is transmitted through saliva of infected animals and slowly replicates. It spreads to nerve cells and gradually invades the central nervous system over a 20- to 60-day incubation period. Once the central nervous system is involved, the disease progresses almost inevitably to death within 1–2 weeks. Any warm-blooded animal can be infected with rabies, but some species are particularly susceptible—most commonly raccoons, skunks, and bats. Cats and dogs can also be infected and transmit the virus.

A multicomponent vaccination strategy has been very successful in preventing the development of rabies in humans. In most recent years, there have been between one and five fatal cases of rabies per year in the United States despite the persistence and periodic increase in rabies among wildlife populations. Let us take a look at how this quite remarkable control effort has occurred.

The ability to successfully vaccinate humans against rabies after the occurrence of a rabies-prone bite has long been a component of the success of rabies reduction among humans. The use of postexposure vaccination was first demonstrated by Louis Pasteur in 1887 and was used to dramatically save the life of a young victim. Early live vaccines had frequent and severe side effects. They were sequentially replaced by inactivated vaccines grown in animal nerve tissue. These replacement vaccines still led to occasional acute neurological complications and gave the treatment a reputation of being dangerous. The development of a vaccine grown in human cell cultures in the 1970s led to a safety record comparable to those of other commonly used vaccines. Today, over 30,000 rabies vaccination series are administered annually in the United States.

The success of rabies control is a result of a series of coordinated efforts to utilize vaccinations in different settings. Vaccines are administered to individuals who are bitten by suspicious species of wild animals, including raccoons, bats, skunks, foxes, and coyotes. Victims of suspected rabies bites by dogs and cats may await the results of quarantine of the animal and observation over a 10-day period. When substantial doubt still exists after this time period, vaccination is recommended. Laws requiring rabies vaccination of dogs and cats have been enforced in the United States for decades and have greatly reduced the number of reported infections in these animals. Today, only 10% or less of suspect rabies-prone bites comes from dogs and cats.

Wildlife remains the greatest source of rabies—wildlife epidemics occur with regularity. Rabies-prone bites still occur, especially from raccoons, which regularly feed from garbage cans in rural, suburban, and occasionally urban parts of the United States. The recent development of effective oral vaccinations that can be administered to wildlife through baits has been credited with reducing the number of infected animals, especially those residing in close proximity to humans.

Rabies illustrates the variety of ways that a key intervention—vaccination—can be used to address a disease. As with many complex diseases of public health importance, a carefully designed and coordinated strategy is required to maximize the benefit of available technology. In addition, ongoing research is needed to continue to develop new and improved approaches to the control of communicable diseases.[18]

HIV/AIDS, influenza A, and rabies represent three very different communicable diseases. However, they all require the use of multiple interventions, close collaboration between the public health and healthcare systems, and continuing efforts to find new and more effective methods for their control.

Efforts to control communicable diseases have increased in recent years along with the increase in emerging and reemerging infectious diseases and bacterial resistance to antibiotics. Technological advances have provided encouragement for the future, but at times have raised concerns about the safety of our interventions. New technology, new strategies for applying technology, and new ways to effectively organize our efforts are needed to ensure the effectiveness and safety of our efforts to prevent, eradicate, and control communicable diseases.

Whether you live in a dorm, are a public health professional, a clinician, a politician, or a high school principal, or are involved in almost any profession, communicable diseases are part of your present and your future.

Now let us turn our attention to our third category of disease: that of environmental diseases and injuries.

## Key Words

| | | |
|---|---|---|
| Antibody | Herd immunity or population | Immunization |
| Case finding | immunity | Koch's postulates |
| Cell-mediated immunity | Human microbiome | Live vaccines |
| Chronic carriers | Inactivated vaccine | Modern Koch's postulates |
| Communicable disease | Incubation period | Pandemic |
| Epidemic | Infections | Passive immunity |
| Epidemiological treatment | Infectious disease | Ring vaccination |
| Endemic | Infectivity | $R$ naught ($R_0$) |
| | | Route of transmission |

## Discussion Questions

Take a look at the questions posed in the following scenarios, which were presented at the beginning of this chapter. See now whether you can answer them.

1.  Your college roommate went to bed not feeling well one night, and early the next morning, you had trouble rousing her. She was rushed to the hospital just in time to be effectively diagnosed and treated for meningococcal meningitis. The health department recommends immediate antibiotic treatment for everyone who was in close contact with your roommate. They set up a process to watch for additional cases to be sure an

outbreak is not in progress. Fortunately, no more cases occur. You ask yourself: Should your college require that all freshmen have the meningococcal vaccine before they can register for classes?

2. As a health advisor to a worldwide HIV/AIDS foundation, you are asked to advise on ways to address the HIV and developing tuberculosis (TB) epidemics. You are asked to do some long-range thinking and to come up with a list of potential approaches to control the epidemics, or at least ways to reduce the development of TB. The first recommendation you make is to forget about eradicating HIV/AIDS. How did you come to that conclusion?

3. You are a principal at a local high school. One of your top athletes is in the hospital with a spreading bacterial infection due to staphylococcus bacteria resistant to all known antibiotics. The infection occurred after what appeared to be a minor injury during practice. As the principal, what do you decide to do?

4. Just before your exams begin you develop a fever, runny nose, sore throat, and a dry cough. In the past antibiotics seemed to help. You know this infection is going to make it hard for you to get that A you need. You make an appointment to be seen at your school health center. After a long wait you hope at least you will be prescribed antibiotics to shorten the course of your infection and give you more time to study. You are discouraged and a bit angry when the nurse practitioner tells you that you have a viral infection, and antibiotics won't help. You wonder why the doctor back home usually prescribed antibiotics.

## References

1. Nobelprize.org. Robert Koch and tuberculosis. http://www.nobelprize.org/educational/medicine/tuberculosis/readmore.html. Accessed July 21, 2017.
2. MedicineNet.com. Medical definition of Koch's postulates. http://www.medicinenet.com/script/main/art.asp?articlekey=7105. Accessed July 21, 2017.
3. National Institute of Allergy and Infectious Diseases. The evidence that HIV causes AIDS. http://www.niaid.nih.gov/topics/hivaids/understanding/howhivcausesaids/pages/hivcausesaids.aspx. Accessed July 21, 2017.
4. Ramirez, VB. What is $R_0$?: Gauging contagious infections. Healthline. http://www.healthline.com/health/r-nought-reproduction-number#R0values2. Accessed July 21, 2017.
5. Lamb E. Understand the Measles Outbreak with this One Weird Number: The basic reproduction number and why it matters. *Scientific American*. January 31, 2015. http://blogs.scientificamerican.com/roots-of-unity/understand-the-measles-outbreak-with-this-one-weird-number/. Accessed July 21, 2017.
6. Diekmann O, Heesterbeek JAP, Metz JAJ. On the definition and the computation of the basic reproduction ratio $R_0$ in models for infectious diseases in heterogeneous populations. *Journal of Mathematical Biology*. 1990;28:365–382.
7. Timmreck TC. *An Introduction to Epidemiology*. 3rd ed. Sudbury, MA: Jones and Bartlett Publishers; 2002:34.
8. Centers for Disease Control and Prevention. Vaccines. https://www.cdc.gov/vaccines/index.html. Accessed July 21, 2017.
9. Centers for Disease Control and Prevention. Measles, Mumps, and Rubella (MMR) Vaccine Safety. https://www.cdc.gov/vaccinesafety/vaccines/mmr-vaccine.html. Accessed July 21, 2017.
10. Morens DM, Fauci AS. Emerging infectious diseases in 2012: 20 years after the Institute of Medicine report. *mBio*. 2012;3(6):e00494-12. doi:10.1128/mBio.00494-12. http://mbio.asm.org/content/3/6/e00494-12.full. Accessed July 21, 2017.
11. Centers for Disease Control and Prevention. About Antimicrobial Resistance. http://www.cdc.gov/drugresistance/about.html. Accessed July 21, 2017.
12. Centers for Disease Control and Prevention. National Strategy to Combat Antibiotic Resistant Bacteria. http://www.cdc.gov/drugresistance/federal-engagement-in-ar/national-strategy/index.html. Accessed July 21, 2017.
13. Centers for Disease Control and Prevention. History and epidemiology of global smallpox eradication. https://www.cdc.gov/smallpox/history/history.html. Accessed July 21, 2017.
14. Sompayrac L. *How Pathogenic Viruses Work*. Sudbury, MA: Jones and Bartlett Publishers; 2002.
15. National Archives and Records Administration. The deadly vines: The influenza epidemic of 1918. http://www.archives.gov/exhibits/influenza-epidemic. Accessed July 21, 2017.
16. Centers for Disease Control and Prevention. Influenza (Flu). https://www.cdc.gov/flu/. Accessed July 21, 2017.
17. World Health Organization. Global agenda for influenza surveillance and control. http://archives.who.int/prioritymeds/report/append/62GlobAgenda.pdf. Accessed July 21, 2017.
18. Centers for Disease Control and Prevention. Rabies home. http://www.cdc.gov/rabies Accessed July 21, 2017.

# CHAPTER 8

# Environmental Health and Safety

## LEARNING OBJECTIVES

By the end of this chapter, the student will be able to:

- define the scope of morbidity and mortality caused by the physical environment including the unaltered environment, the altered environment, and the built environment.
- identify the components of environmental risk assessment, and apply them to an environmental hazard, such as lead.
- distinguish between a risk assessment, a public health assessment, and an ecological assessment.
- discuss the meaning of interactions and how they may impact the size of risks.
- describe how intentional and unintentional injuries can be addressed to prevent their occurrence and diminish their consequences.
- identify successes of outbreak investigations.

Joe grew up in an industrial district of town. His family lived in an old apartment building, and he played in a playground near a major intersection. By the age of 6, Joe was found to have high lead levels in his blood and was not doing well in school. Where could all that lead come from? his mother wondered.

Jill is pregnant and loves fish, which she has eaten almost daily for years as part of her effort to stay healthy. She hears that fish should not be eaten regularly during pregnancy. Why, she wonders, should I cut down on eating something as healthy as fish?

Ralph and Sonya, a prosperous professional couple, and their two children live in an older suburban home. They feel secure that their environment is safe. They were surprised to find

when they wanted to put their house up for sale that it did not pass the safety tests for radon. Where did the radon come from, they wondered, and what can be done about it?

Sandra worked for an international agency that had successfully addressed the danger of radiation due to the hole in the ozone layer. She was shocked when she was told that she had a life-threatening skin cancer called melanoma. She asked: What could cause melanoma? Could years of sun exposure have played a role?

You set out on your commute to work, and as you approach the subway station, you see police cars, ambulances, and dozens of emergency responders in hazmat suits. You are told the entire subway system will be shut down indefinitely, as

**163**

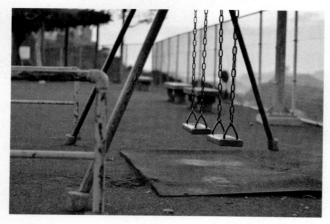

© TOMO/Shutterstock

there has been a suspected case of bioterrorism. You wonder how authorities were alerted to this situation, and what precautions are being taken to protect the health of those living in the city.

Alex suffered a traumatic brain injury when he was thrown from his motorcycle after colliding with a car in which the driver had an elevated blood alcohol concentration. Alex was not wearing a helmet. His family members wonder what is being done to prevent this from happening to others.

All of these situations are part of what we mean by the burden of environmental disease and injury. In order to understand the impact of the environment on health, we need to define what we mean by "environment" and appreciate the many ways that we interact with it.

## ▶ What Is Meant by "Environment"?

"Environment" is an ambiguous term. It is sometimes used to imply all influences other than genetic influences, including social, economic, and cultural influences. We will define the environment as the physical environment. The physical environment can be thought of in three categories: unaltered ("natural"), altered, and the built environment.[a] **FIGURE 8.1** diagrams the scope of environmental diseases and injuries.

The health of human beings was affected by the physical environment long before we had the capacity to substantially alter the environment. Floods, earthquakes, and volcanoes have always been a part of the physical environment. In addition to these intermittent and often isolated impacts, daily exposures to communicable diseases in water and food have always been a part of the unaltered environment.

In recent years, we have recognized more subtle impacts of the **unaltered environment**. Radon, a common naturally occurring breakdown product of uranium, increases the risk of lung cancer. Exposure to naturally occurring sunlight increases the chances of skin cancer, including melanoma—a potentially lethal skin cancer—especially among light-skinned individuals. Human activity has altered nearly every aspect of our physical environment. Some alterations to our environment may improve human health—from water treatment, to waste management, to mosquito and flood control. Nonetheless, we need to consider the overall impacts that these changes have on the physical environment.

The sheer growth in the number of human beings—the planet's population now exceeds 7.5 billion—is likely to magnify our impact on all aspects of our physical environment in the future. This population growth and increasing human activity are believed to be contributing to a range of environmental issues, from deforestation to global warming.

The impact on the physical environment of so many humans takes two major forms:

- Consumption of resources such as land, food, water, air, fossil fuels, and minerals
- Waste products as a result of consumption such as air and water pollutants, toxic materials, and greenhouse gases[1]

We often think of the **altered environment** as reflecting the impact of chemicals, radiation, and biological products that we introduce into the

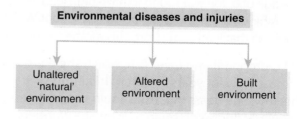

**FIGURE 8.1** Scope of Environmental Diseases and Injuries

---

a The term "natural" is used in quotations because it can be a misleading term. We often think that the term "natural disasters" implies that human actions had nothing to do with the events. Increasingly, human actions precipitate, worsen, and even cause "natural disasters." Construction on vulnerable lands increases the damage from storms, fires, earthquakes, and even volcanoes. Global warming caused by human activities is also beginning to have its impacts. Our planet has been altered in so many ways that the unaltered environment is becoming difficult to find.

environment. The list of intentional or unintentional introductions is in fact very long. It ranges from industrial chemicals, such as pesticides, benzene, and chlorofluorocarbons (CFCs), to elements mined from the earth, such as mercury and lead. It also includes radiation from nuclear energy and medical wastes. Biological impacts encompass the introduction of invasive species and the management of biological wastes.

The concept of the **built environment** is relatively new and includes all the impacts of the physical environment as a result of human construction. The impacts of human construction include injuries and exposures in the home, the transportation system, and where we work and play. They also include factors ranging from the way we build and heat our buildings and cook our food, to the way we travel from place to place. The built environment influences our safety through its impact on injuries and hazardous exposures. It also influences our activity levels and our social interactions, which impact our health.[2]

As we will see, we are coming to understand that the built environment may also affect our mood, social interactions, and social attitudes in ways that affects our health for the better or for the worse. The impact of the built environment is present throughout the world, but differs greatly by geography and stage of social and economic development.

Indoor air pollution from cooking is the most prominent source of air pollution in much of the developing world. Motor vehicle injuries are the most deadly consequences of the built environment in most developed countries. The built environment has subtle impacts as well. The way we build our cities affects the amount of exercise we get and the quantity of noise pollution we experience. Construction methods affect air systems in buildings and can increase our exposure to "sick buildings."

Now let us take a look at the burden of disease that results from the physical environment.

## ▶ What Is the Burden of Disease Due to the Physical Environment?

Measuring the impact of the physical environment on health is difficult because of the many types of impacts and the often subtle effects that occur. The impacts we experience today may pale in comparison to what we can expect in the future. Nonetheless, it is useful to appreciate the current estimates of the magnitude of the direct and indirect burden.

Motor vehicle injuries and exposure to toxic substances are two important actual causes of death that represent the largest known impact of the physical environment. Together, these incidents are estimated to cause nearly 100,000 deaths per year, representing about 20% of preventable deaths in the United States and approximately 10% of all deaths in the United States, according to the Centers for Disease Control and Prevention's (CDC) calculations.[3] Motor vehicle injuries and other unintentional injuries have especially heavy impacts on the young; in fact, they are the number one cause of death in the United States among those 1–24 years of age.[4] As a cause of disability, injuries also rank high especially considering their disproportionate impact on the young.

The impact of toxic substances on population health extends beyond acute symptoms such as skin and respiratory irritation to chronic conditions. The impact on death and disability is difficult to measure due to the length of time the substances may take to affect the body. It may be years after an exposure before an individual experiences negative health effects on their kidneys, liver, nerves, and other organs. **BOX 8.1** describes the impact of small particle air pollution on health, including the recent recognition of its long-term effects on the development of coronary artery disease. This link substantially increases the estimated impact the environment has on health outcomes.

In an effort to alert individuals to the air quality in their region, the Environmental Protection Agency (EPA) created an Air Quality Index (AQI).[6] The AQI is an index for reporting daily air quality. The AQI focuses on health effects that may be experienced within a few hours or days after breathing unhealthy air. The AQI is calculated for four major air pollutants regulated by the Clean Air Act: (1) ground level ozone, (2) particle pollution, (3) carbon monoxide, and (4) sulfur dioxide. **TABLE 8.1** displays the AQI and its health categories.

Many toxic exposures occur in occupational settings. In addition, approximately 5000 deaths due to

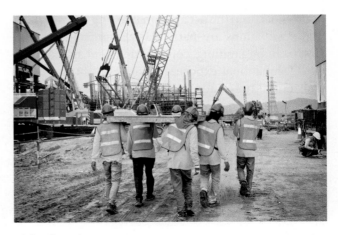

**BOX 8.1** Impact of Small Particle Air Pollution on Health[5]

Air pollution occurs when particulate matter, a mix of tiny solid and liquid particles, is suspended in the air. The particles can be comprised of a number of components, including acids, organic chemicals, metals, dust, and pollen and mold spores. The size of the particles makes a difference on their impact on health. Our body's natural defense mechanisms, such as coughing and sneezing, can dislodge larger particles. However, small particles, <10 μm in diameter, can be inhaled into the lungs and enter the bloodstream; therefore, they have potential to pose a great risk to health.

The smallest of these particles are referred to as fine particles. Fine particles measure <2.5 μm in diameter and, therefore, can only be seen with an electron microscope. When millions of these particles are suspended in the air, a haze forms, referred to as smog and often seen in cities largely due to exhaust from motor vehicles.

Everyone's health is at risk from small particle pollution; however, certain groups are at greater risk. Because children spend more active time outside, their lungs are still developing, and they are more likely to have asthma and acute respiratory disease, they face greater risk. Older adults also have an increased risk for health issues due to small particles because they are more likely to have heart or lung disease, which can be aggravated by inhalation of the particles. People of any age with heart or lung disease are also at increased risk for this reason.

Health effects from short-term exposure can include eye, nose, and throat irritation; shortness of breath; asthma attacks; and bronchitis. Long-term exposure to small particle pollution can contribute to reduced lung function, chronic bronchitis, and premature death.

A number of recent studies demonstrate a link between small particle air pollution and coronary artery disease. It is believed that exposure to fine particulate air pollution leads to thickening of the arteries, disrupting blood flow, which can lead to heart attacks and strokes. Attributing even a portion of deaths from coronary artery disease to air pollution substantially increases the estimates of the environmental burden of disease.

**TABLE 8.1** Air Quality Index for Particle Pollution

| Air Quality Index (AQI) Values | Levels of Health Concern | Colors |
|---|---|---|
| *When the AQI is in this range:* | *…air quality conditions are:* | *…as symbolized by this color:* |
| 0–50 | Good | Green |
| 51–100 | Moderate | Yellow |
| 101–150 | Unhealthy for sensitive groups | Orange |
| 151–200 | Unhealthy | Red |
| 201–300 | Very unhealthy | Purple |
| 301–500 | Hazardous | Maroon |

Reproduced from United States Environmental Protection Agency. Particulate Matter. Available at: https://www3.epa.gov/airnow/aqi_brochure_02_14.pdf. Accessed July 21, 2017.

injuries occur in the occupational setting per year. Certain occupations are particularly vulnerable to injuries, including mining, construction, and agriculture.

Occupational exposures that result in morbidity and mortality include lung diseases caused by exposures to hazardous dusts, hearing loss from loud noises, and back pain from excessive lifting, as well as a wide range of other mechanical problems, including carpal tunnel syndrome, which is often caused by repetitive motion of the hand and wrist.

Occupational injuries have been declining in recent years, but they remain an important cause of death and disability.[7] Cancer caused by occupational exposures has been of particular concern. As much as 5% of cancer deaths in males have been estimated to be due to occupational exposures. Cancers of the lung, bladder, and white blood cells (leukemia) are particularly likely to result from chronic exposures to chemicals, such as formaldehyde, benzene, and organic dyes. Reductions in occupational exposures in the last 30 years have resulted in a declining burden of disease from these exposures in the United States. The opposite is being seen in many newly industrializing countries, where current exposures are increasing and may result in more cases of cancer and other diseases in the not-too-distant future.[8]

Finally, we cannot evaluate the impact of toxic exposures solely by tracing them to human deaths and disabilities. The altered environment has impacts on entire ecosystems of plants and animals. The ecological impact of environmental factors can have long-term and largely irreversible consequences. Once chemicals, radiation, and biological products are released into the environment, the process cannot generally be easily reversed. Thus, we need to take a broad and long-term perspective when we address environmental health.

# How Do We Interact with Our Physical Environment?

To understand how the physical environment—be it the unaltered, altered, or built environment—affects health, we need to explore the myriad ways that we interact with it.[9] **BOX 8.2** discusses this concept.

---

**BOX 8.2** How We Interact with Our Environment

We are exposed to the physical environment every minute of our lives through multiple routes. For each of these routes of exposure, the body has mechanisms for protection. We are primarily exposed to the environment via the skin; the respiratory tract (from the nose to the lungs); the alimentary, or digestive, tract (from the mouth to the anus); and the genital-urinary tract.

Each bodily surface that is directly exposed to the physical environment has developed a form of barrier protection. The skin provides direct protection against radiation, organisms, and physical contact, as well as providing some protections against heat and cold. The respiratory tract is guarded by mucous production and by small hair like structures called cilia, whose motion in conjunction with coughing removes materials that we breathe into our lungs.

Cells called phagocytes literally consume organisms and large particles. Antibodies, along with cell-mediated immunity, also protect against access of harmful particles and organisms through the lungs. The alimentary, or digestive, tract is protected by saliva, mucous membranes, and antibodies, as well as strong acidity in the stomach. The genital-urinary tract is protected by mucous membrane barriers, antibody and cell-mediated immunity, and at times by an acid environment.[a]

Therefore, we need to recognize that the impacts of the environment on health are very complex.[7] We should expect to find that the following issues affect the risk:

- Route of exposure—The consequences of exposures to heavy metals including mercury, lead, and cadmium, for instance, depend on whether the exposure is via the skin or the respiratory or gastrointestinal tracts.
- Timing of exposure—Short-term high-dose impacts often will not be the same as long-term low-dose impacts, even if the total exposure and the routes of exposure are the same. For instance, a small number of severe episodes of sunburn during childhood have been found to greatly increase the risk of skin cancers far more than multiple milder adult sunburns. Chronic low-dose exposures may produce different and more subtle impacts.
- Stage of life—The impact on the very young and the very old is likely to be different than the impact on people at other stages of life. We need to be especially concerned about exposures during pregnancy, early childhood, and the later years of life.
- Other diseases—The presence of other diseases will affect how the body is impacted by an environmental exposure. We need to be especially concerned about environmental exposures for those with chronic lung diseases and those with suppressed immune systems, such as those living with AIDS.
- Special sensitivities—A few individuals will be hypersensitive to specific environmental exposures that have no measurable impact on the vast majority of individuals. We need to be concerned about how to identify and protect these individuals without depriving them of rights or opportunities.

---

a The effectiveness of our bodily defenses depends on a number of factors—for instance, genetic factors. Dark skin pigmentation reduces the penetration of radiation and reduces the risk of skin cancers, including melanoma, the most serious of skin cancers. Other diseases affect how well our defenses operate—for instance, chronic obstructive lung disease and cystic fibrosis can alter the ability of the cilia in the lungs to operate effectively. Age can affect the ability of our skin to serve as an effective barrier as well as the ability of the immune system to respond. The elderly are especially prone to the effects of heat and cold. They are also more susceptible to a range of infections and cancers. Our defense mechanisms can overreact to environmental stimuli and themselves produce ailments, including allergies and autoimmune disease. The impacts of certain environmental exposures may be limited to a small number of susceptible individuals whose immune systems react especially strongly to specific environmental exposures. For instance, allergies to peanuts or household or industrial chemicals can produce unusual, but severe, reactions in a small number of susceptible individuals.

Because of the complexity of the interactions between human beings and the physical environment, a range of approaches has been developed for addressing these issues. We will categorize and examine these approaches as follows:

- **Risk assessment**
- **Public health assessment**
- **Ecological assessment**
- **Interaction analysis**

We can think of these strategies as a progression of approaches of increasing complexity. We will organize our approach to environmental diseases and injuries starting with risk assessment and proceeding in order to examine each of these strategies.

## How Does Risk Assessment Address the Impacts of the Physical Environment?

Risk assessment is a formal process that aims to measure the potential impact of known **hazards**. A hazard indicates the inherent danger of an exposure, while a risk assessment aims to take into account not only the inherent danger, but also the quantity, route, and timing of the exposure.[7] The risk assessment approach to environmental hazards represents the mainstay of our current approach. The underlying principles have a long history in public health, often resulting from the investigation of specific occupational exposures.

One of the earliest occupational investigations occurred among chimney sweeps in England during the 1700s. Their high-dose exposure to carbon residues in smokestacks led to early and frequent testicular cancer. In the 1800s, industrializing countries also provided ample opportunities to study the impacts of work-related exposures. For instance, the dangers of radiation came to light after high levels of cancer were detected in workers who painted watches with radiation-containing paint for the purposes of nighttime illumination.

The dangers of asbestos became evident after high-dose exposures among ship workers during World War II resulted in cases of cancer many years later. The dangers of exposure to polyvinyl chloride, a common industrial compound, were recognized after five workers from the same manufacturing plant came down with a rare liver tumor in the 1970s.

Risk assessment today has become a complex technical effort requiring quantitative measures of the magnitude of the risk. The history of risk assessment in the United States is closely tied to the investigations and regulations surrounding benzene. **BOX 8.3** provides an overview of the history of the study and regulation of this chemical hazard.[10,11]

The formal process of risk assessment represents the current framework for assessing environmental hazards in the United States.[11,12] **FIGURE 8.2** illustrates the four-step risk assessment process as used by the U.S. EPA.

Risk assessment attempts to evaluate the impact of environmental exposures one at a time and to measure the types and magnitudes of the impacts. If a substantial risk is found to exist, the process then

---

**BOX 8.3** Benzene and Risk Assessment

Benzene is an organic chemical that is used as a solvent in the chemical and pharmaceutical industries. Because it readily becomes a gas at room temperature, airborne exposure is an important concern. Benzene is one of the most widely used organic chemicals. It is estimated that over 250,000 U.S. workers are exposed to benzene, particularly in the chemical, printing, paint, and petroleum industries.[a]

A range of toxic effects has been documented from benzene over the last 150 years. These include neurological effects of acute and chronic exposure, as well as life-threatening suppression of the production of red blood cells called aplastic anemia.

In the 1960s and 1970s, it was increasingly recognized that benzene causes cancer, particularly leukemia. Early

studies of benzene and leukemia were conducted by Muzaffer Aksoy, a Turkish physician, who observed leukemia among many shoemakers in Turkey where benzene was being used as a solvent in the manufacturing of leather products. His large cohort study helped establish the chemical as a presumed cause of leukemia.

Based on a series of studies that documented the risk of leukemia, in 1978 the federal government established a standard for exposure to benzene in the air of 1 part per million (1 ppm), as opposed to the former approach of limiting the exposure to 10 parts per million (10 ppm). One part per million is approximately the equivalent of 1 drop in 40 gallons of liquid. In 1980, the U.S. Supreme Court overturned the new standard based upon the

---

a  Benzene is also a component of gasoline; therefore, the entire population has some exposure to benzene. This discussion focuses on the hazard assessment of benzene in the occupational setting.

argument that the Occupational Safety and Health Administration (OSHA) had not documented the impact of the new 1 ppm standard in terms of the number of lives saved or compared it to the 10 ppm level.

The Supreme Court concluded that "safe" did not mean risk-free, giving the analogies of driving a car and breathing city air. The Supreme Court insisted that standards be set based upon the preponderance of evidence from a formal risk assessment. As a result of this Supreme Court decision, a risk-assessment approach was developed that grew into the current risk-assessment process. The 1 part per million standard was supported by quantitative measures of the impact: the federal government estimated that there would be 14–17 excess deaths per 1000 workers exposed to 10 ppm of benzene for a working lifetime, compared to being exposed to the new 1 ppm standard.

Thus, risk assessment today is a highly technical and quantitative activity designed to establish a maximum level of allowed exposure to one particular hazard. The goal is to protect workers and the public from the most important risks to health.

Data from Feitshans IL. Law and Regulation of Benzene. *Environ Health Perspect.* 1989; 82:299–307.

### The 4 Step Risk Assessment Process

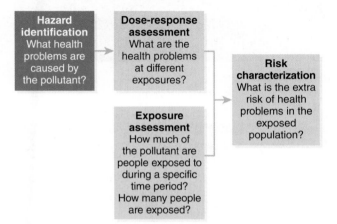

**FIGURE 8.2** The 4-Step Risk Assessment Process

Reproduced from United States Environmental Protection Agency. Risk Assessment Portal. Available at https://www.epa.gov/risk/conducting-human-health-risk-assessment#tab-2. Accessed July 21, 2017

reviews options to protect, detect, and react to the risk to minimize the burden of disease on humans.

The risk assessment process builds in a margin of error designed to provide extra protection for especially vulnerable individuals or populations. Thus, those exposed to levels above the recommended maximum levels of exposure will not necessarily experience adverse effects. **TABLE 8.2** outlines the four steps in the risk assessment process and uses a simplified example of how airborne exposure to benzene in occupational settings may be presented in this framework.

Other approaches to addressing risk should also be understood. Let us take a look at what we mean by public health assessment.

**TABLE 8.2** Four-Step Risk Assessment and Simplified Example—Benzene

| Components | Simplified example—benzene |
|---|---|
| **Hazard identification**<br>What health effects are caused by the pollutant? | Benzene causes leukemia<br>Strong evidence from cohort studies and supportive animal data exist |
| **Dose–response relationship**<br>What are the health problems at different exposures? | Strong dose–response relationship among occupational workers with level of 1 ppm over a working lifetime<br>The impact of exposure at 1 ppm is indistinguishable from unexposed, with rapid increase in rates of leukemia above that level |
| **Exposure assessment**<br>How much of the pollutant are people exposed to during a specific time period? How many people are exposed? | Industrial exposures above 1 ppm are common in a range of industries at the time the standard was set.<br>Over 250,000 workers exposed to benzene |
| **Risk characterization**<br>What is the extra risk of health problems in the exposed population? | 14–17 excess cases of leukemia per 1000 workers exposed to 10 ppm throughout a working lifetime |

Data from United States Environmental Protection Agency. Human health risk assessment. Available at http://www.epa.gov/risk_assessment/health-risk.htm. Accessed July 21, 2017.

# ▶ What Is a Public Health Assessment?

Risk assessment is distinguished from what is called a public health assessment. A public health assessment goes beyond a risk assessment by including data on actual exposure in a community.

Public health assessments have the potential for major impacts on large numbers of people because they address not just the risks in a specific location, such as in an occupational setting, but also the risks to large numbers of individuals and often to the population as a whole. These types of risk assessments have been very controversial and have taken years—often decades—to complete. A classic example of the importance and potential impacts of the public health assessment process and its ongoing challenges is discussed in **BOX 8.4**, which looks at the health risks due to lead.[13,14]

Risk assessments and public health assessments both focus exclusively on the health impacts on human beings. Let us take a look at an additional type of assessment conducted by the EPA that looks at the impact of an exposure on plants and animals.

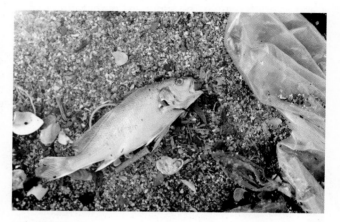

© NPDstock/Shutterstock

---

## BOX 8.4  Health Risks Due to Lead

Knowledge of the potential for lead poisoning goes back to ancient civilizations, when the metal was widely used—for example, it was a component of water pipes and part of the process of making wine. In Rome, lead was used as a method of abortion, and high-dose exposures led to a range of mental effects. It is said the Roman emperors were affected by the high levels of lead in Roman wine.

Benjamin Franklin listed every known profession for which lead posed a health hazard and predicted that many years would pass before the public health consequences of lead were addressed. Of course, Benjamin Franklin was right. Things were to get worse before they got better.

In the 1920s, lead was added to gasoline to make for smoother driving. It was highly effective in getting the "knocks" out of early versions of the piston engine, as well as elevating the level of lead in the air. Even today, the lead from gasoline lies in the soil of many playgrounds. High levels of lead also improved the performance of paints. Houses built before the 1970s, and especially before the 1950s, still pose a threat to children who often ingest peeling paint.

It was not until the 1970s that the effect of low-dose lead exposure on the development of intellectual function became clear. The studies of Dr. Herbert Needleman and subsequent investigators documented clear-cut negative effects on the intellectual development of young children even at low levels of

exposure. This prompted efforts to remove lead from gasoline, paints, and many other products. In recent years, new sources of lead, including toys, pottery, and water, have been given increased attention. In short, lead is a well-recognized hazard that is still with us.

Efforts to protect the environment have been coupled with efforts to detect and react to elevated lead levels. It is now standard practice in pediatrics and public health to monitor blood levels in high-risk children, investigate their home environments, and treat persistently elevated levels. Lead standards for playgrounds, lead abatement programs for homes, and lead monitoring of consumer products all aim to reduce or eliminate the hazards of lead. The system is by no means foolproof, and in recent years, elevated levels of the metal have been found from such divergent sources as toys manufactured in China and in glazes used in homemade pottery.

The most serious recent episode of lead exposure occurred in Flint, MI, when this poor, mostly African American community began using the Flint river as their water supply, and state officials failed to properly treat the water to prevent leakage of lead from old corroding pipes. Over 100,000 people were potentially exposed to extremely high levels of lead including a large number of children before the situation was addressed.

**TABLE 8.3** summarizes the potential exposures to lead, including their sources, and offers potential means of reducing or eliminating the hazard.

**TABLE 8.3** Where Does Lead in Our Bodies Come From and What Can Be Done About It?

| How lead enters our bodies | Where it comes from | Ways to reduce exposure |
|---|---|---|
| Inhalation | Workers in many lead-exposure industries, including mining, smelting, metal repair, or foundry work<br><br>Demolition and renovation activities that generate fumes and dust, including home renovations and hobby activities<br><br>Addition of lead to gasoline<br><br>Once inhaled deep into the lungs, it may remain for long periods and be absorbed into blood over time | Occupational controls<br><br>Phaseout of lead in gasoline in United States from 1976 to 1996 |
| Ingestion | Children—normal ingestion of dirt and dust by infants and young children, with up to 5% of children who ingest large quantities—a condition called "pica". Children absorb greater percentage of ingested lead than adults<br><br>Children's toys and objects that are placed in the mouth are especially important sources<br><br>Soil near old high traffic areas are often contaminated from previous lead in gasoline<br><br>Glazed pottery often includes lead that can leach into food | Removal of lead paint from older homes—lead levels in paint in the 1950s and earlier were as much as 50% lead<br><br>Enforce elimination of lead paint from children's toys<br><br>Monitoring and control of lead levels in soil in young children's play areas<br><br>Very high blood levels may require "chelation"—treatment to reduce lead levels in blood |
| Water | Pipes, especially in older water supplies and homes built before the mid-1980s, often contain lead<br><br>Lead used in pipes outside and within the home can leach into water—especially warm water—over time | Regulation of levels of lead in public water supply<br><br>Run home water before use—especially after away for extended period<br><br>Use cold water for cooking |
| In utero | Pregnant women absorb higher percentage of ingested lead compared to children, and lead can cross the placenta<br><br>Mother's previous lead exposure stored in her bones can be resorbed into her blood during pregnancy | Special effort to reduce exposure by pregnant women, including special care with home renovations during pregnancy, especially homes built before 1970 |

Data from Agency for Toxic Substance and Disease Registry. Case studies in environmental medicine-lead. Available at http://wonder.cdc.gov/wonder/prevguid/p0000017/p0000017.asp. Accessed July 21, 2017.

▶ # What Is an Ecological Risk Assessment?

Environmental health cannot be viewed solely on the basis of current impacts on human health. The impacts of environmental contamination or pollution on plants and animals and the ecosystems in which they exist often have important long-term consequences.

The modern environmental movement in the United States was ignited in large part by Rachel Carson's book, *Silent Spring*, which described how the widespread use of dichloro-diphenyl-trichloroethane (DDT) had threatened the American Eagle and other birds as it became deposited in and weakened their eggs.[15] Broader concern about the impacts of contaminants on ecological systems ranging from chemicals, to radiation, to genetically altered crops has made clear the importance of ecological risk assessments. Human health consequences remain an important, but not necessarily direct, consequence of the impacts of environmental contamination or pollution as described in **BOX 8.5**, which explores the impacts of mercury.[16,17]

Up to this point, we have addressed the impact of environmental exposures one at a time. Increasingly, we find that the interactions between exposures produce unexpectedly large impacts. Let us now look at a strategy that addresses more than one problem at a time and takes into consideration the interaction between multiple exposures. We will call it an interaction analysis.

---

### BOX 8.5 Health Risks of Mercury in the Environment

The impact of high-dose mercury on mental function has been recognized since the 1800s. More recently, it was established that much lower levels of mercury pose risks to the fetus. Neurological damage, including learning disabilities and hearing loss, have been documented at low levels of exposure. The human risks of mercury exposure need to be understood as part of the impact of mercury on an entire ecological system.

For much of the late 1800s and the 1900s, mercury was a common product of industry that heavily contaminated the Great Lakes of the United States. The impacts were not appreciated despite the high levels of contamination and the impacts on animal species. Mercury in bodies of water is filtered by fish species and can concentrate in their fat. Thus, certain fish species can and do accumulate high concentrations of mercury. These species may be eaten by fish-eating birds and pose a risk to a number of endangered avian species. There is no technologically feasible method for removing mercury from the Great Lakes or other bodies of water. Your children's children will most likely be living with mercury contamination.

Recommendations for limiting the consumption of fish, especially by pregnant women, have been the mainstay of efforts to address this problem. These efforts are complicated by the fact that the consumption of fish also carries health benefits. Today, the challenge is how to minimize the amount of mercury consumed by women without losing the benefits of fish consumption. Because some fish have much higher mercury levels than others, the March of Dimes recommends that pregnant women avoid shark, swordfish, king mackerel, and tilefish. They indicate that "it is ok" to eat a limited amount of fish that contain small amounts of mercury, including salmon, pollock, catfish, and canned light tuna.[18] The details of how much fish is safe for pregnant women to eat remains controversial. For today and many years to come, we will be living with the impacts of past environmental contamination on entire ecosystems.

---

## What Is an Interaction Analysis Approach to Environmental Diseases?

The term **interaction analysis** implies that to understand and control the impacts of environmental exposures, it is necessary to take into account the effect of two or more exposures. **BOX 8.6** describes the multiple interacting factors contributing to depletion of the ozone layer.

Risk assessment approaches make the assumption that each exposure stands on its own. Thus, if there is more than one type of exposure, we need to make the assumption that the total impact is the sum of the two impacts. For example, if one exposure has a relative risk of 4 and a second has a relative risk of 6, we assume that exposure to both results in a relative risk of 10. Many times, adding together the relative risks does provide an approximation of the risk of two or more exposures. However, in an increasing number of situations, we are recognizing that there are interactions between exposures themselves so that the presence of both exposures results in an overall impact much greater than expected. For instance, we may find that having both exposures results in a relative risk of a bad outcome of 4 times 6, or 24, instead of 10. This type of interaction is called **multiplicative interaction**. **BOX 8.7** examines the multiplicative interaction between radon and cigarette smoking.[19]

Not all risks for environmental disease require high-level or long-term exposure. In addition to causing lung cancer, asbestos has also been shown to cause a form of cancer called mesothelioma, which originates in the lining of the lung or pleura. Even small and short-term exposures to asbestos may cause mesothelioma, as evidenced by well-documented cases among household members who washed the clothing of those exposed. New technologies, such as nanotechnology, are raising concerns that the risks of low-level exposure need to be investigated as much as those of high-level exposure.

Low-dose environmental exposures to estrogen-like substances may pose threats to the reproductive health of animal species and could even affect the human rate of breast cancer. Addressing these types of issues requires us to focus on the interactions between multiple factors.

The process of risk assessment has been a slow and cumbersome process. In 2016 the U.S. Congress, with bipartisan support, passed legislation which

---

**BOX 8.6** Addressing the Problem of the Hole in the Ozone Layer[18]

It was first recognized in 1985 that the layer of ozone above Antarctica was being depleted at an alarming rate. Ozone in the upper atmosphere is known to protect against damaging radiation from the sun. Fears were raised that the hole in the ozone would expand progressively, encompass populated areas in the southern hemisphere, and involve the northern hemisphere as well.

It was quickly recognized that the problem was linked to multiple interacting human and naturally occurring systems. The use of CFCs in such products as refrigerators and air-conditioning equipment was quickly identified as a major contributor. In addition, commonly used aerosol sprays from deodorants and hair sprays contained CFCs. More concerning was the use of CFC in devices to deliver medications.

The timely accumulation of data, the rapid understanding of the multiple contributors to the problem, and a worldwide media campaign soon brought together a remarkably effective response to the problem. By 1987, an international agreement, known as the Montreal Protocol, was developed and quickly implemented by most nations. The agreement and subsequent revisions resulted in the rapid phaseout of most uses of CFC, with more gradual elimination of CFCs in medical devices.

The hole in the ozone layer continues to expand due to the extremely long half-life of CFCs. The projections, however, are for a turnaround in the near future and a resolution of the problem by 2050. The coordinated scientific, public health, health communications, and political responses have encouraged future efforts to recognize and jointly address multifactor environmental health problems.

Despite the great success seen with addressing the hole in the ozone, it has recently been recognized that the substitutes being used for CFC are themselves contributors to the greenhouse effect and climate change. Therefore, another round of interaction analysis is under way to identify and guide the use of chemicals that have minimum impact on the environment.

---

**BOX 8.7** Interaction Between Radon and Cigarettes

Radon is a naturally occurring radioactive gas. It is colorless and odorless. Radon is produced by the decay of uranium in soil, rock, and groundwater. It emits ionizing radiation during its radioactive decay. Radon is found all over the country, though there are areas of the country with substantially higher levels than other areas. Radon gets into the indoor air primarily by entering via the soil under homes and other buildings at the basement or lowest level.

Today, it is recognized that radon is the second most important cause of lung cancer after cigarettes and the most common cause of cancer among nonsmokers. The EPA estimates that radon accounts for over 20,000 cases of lung cancer, as compared with the over 100,000 cases attributed to cigarettes. The average indoor level in the United States is about 1.3pCi/L. The EPA has set a level of 2pCi/L as an attainable level and a level of 4pCi/L as the maximum recommended level. Approximately 15% of homes in the United States have basement radon levels above 4pCi/L.

Cigarette smoking and radon exposure are multiplicative; that is, when both are present, the hazard is multiplied. For instance, using the EPA's figures, the relative risk of lung cancer for the average smoker is approximately 9 times the risk compared to a nonsmoker. The relative risk from radon when the level is 10pCi/L compared to 2pCi/L is over 4.5. When both cigarette smoking and a level of radon exposure of 10pCi/L are present, the relative risk of lung cancer increases over 40 times.

The recognition that radon and also asbestos multiply the impacts of cigarette smoking has had a key impact on the approaches used to address these potential hazards. For smokers with exposure to these hazards, the risk can be greatly reduced by reductions in radon and asbestos, as well as by stopping smoking. Because both radon and asbestos are potentially controllable environmental exposures, there has been a great deal of attention and money given to the control of these hazards. Thus, the recognition of interactions that multiply or greatly increase the risk have become an important tool for setting priorities and developing approaches to risk reduction.

---

the President signed, to address many of the issues that have restricted the process of risk assessment in the United States. **BOX 8.8** summarizes the changes included in this law.

We have now taken a look at some of the impacts of the unaltered and altered environment. Let us now take a look at impacts on health of the built environment.

**BOX 8.8**   Toxic Substances Control Act and the Frank R. Lautenberg Chemical Safety for the 21st Century Act

In 1976 the Toxic Substances Control Act gave the U.S. EPA responsibility to regulate the over 60,000 chemical compounds then used in commerce other than food, drugs, and cosmetics regulated by the Food and Drug Administration (FDA). The EPA was expected to determine whether a chemical presented an "unreasonable risk" to health or the environment.

The EPA's authority to define, identify, and manage "unreasonable risks" was quite limited. These limitations included:

- The over 60,000 chemicals in use when the law was enacted were "grandfathered in" as safe, and the EPA had little authority to require testing for safety.
- To declare a new chemical as having "unreasonable risk" the EPA authority was limited by a need to balance the health risks with the economic consequences.
- No explicit protection of vulnerable populations such as children, pregnant woman, workers, and the elderly was provided.
- During the forty years after the passage of the 1976 law over 20,000 new chemicals were permitted to be manufactured and distributed with only a notification to the EPA.
- Only limited information on chemicals was available to the states and to health professionals if the manufacturer identified the information as "confidential business information."

For 40 years after the 1976 Toxic Substances Control Act was passed there were no changes in the legislation. In 2016, Congress, with bipartisan support, passed and the President signed the Frank R. Lautenberg Chemical Safety for the 21st Century Act (the Lautenberg Act). The Lautenberg Act retained

the basic approach to risk assessment which we have outlined but aimed to address each of the above limitations as follows:

- A process was put in place to prioritize the potential risk of the over 60,000 grandfathered in chemicals and conduct risk assessments on those determined by the EPA to be high priority.
- Unreasonable risk was separated into a determination of risk considering only human health and environmental impacts and a risk management decision which could consider costs and availability of alternatives.
- In considering the determination of unreasonable risk as well as the risk management decision the EPA was directed to consider vulnerable populations including but not limited to children, pregnant women, workers, and the elderly.
- New chemicals now require a determination of safety before they may be distributed.
- The use of the "confidential business information" category to limit distribution of information was greatly restricted.

The EPA was also given broad authority to require testing and the ability to charge fees to manufacturers to pay for a portion of the cost of the regulatory process. These and other provisions of the new law have the potential to allow a more comprehensive and transparent process to protect human health and the environment well into the 21st century.[20]

The Trump administration has begun implementation of this new EPA framework but critics have argued that the EPA "...intends to ignore more chemical uses and exposures at every stage of the regulatory process and label thousands of chemicals as safe in order to avoid review."[21]

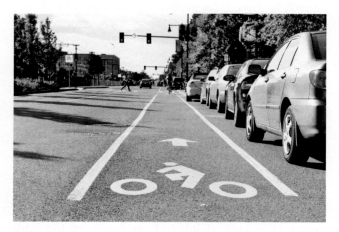

© Jorge Salcedo/Shutterstock

## ▶ What Are the Health Impacts of the Built Environment?

The impacts of the built environment are most evident in urban areas. The urban population of the United States continues to grow rapidly, with one in three Americans living in one of the 10 largest metropolitan areas and nearly all of the growth in population occurring in urban areas, with the most rapid growth now occurring in central cities. Over 85% of Americans now live in metropolitan areas of 50,000 or more.[22]

The impact of urban living has been widely recognized and has been a focus of public health since the 1800s. Crowded conditions were thought to contribute to tuberculosis, lack of clean water was a recognized cause of diarrheal diseases, uncollected garbage was thought to lead to an increase in rat borne disease, and noise was thought to contribute to mental illness. All of these conditions and other urban hazards were addressed as part of public health efforts in the late 1800s and early 1900s.

In recent years attention has been focused on the subtler impacts of the way cities are constructed. The dependence on the automobile for transportation has resulted in increased air pollution and reduced exercise. Efforts to provide greater public transportation have been the primary response to reliance on the automobile until recently. New efforts are now under way to increase bike lanes, walking paths, and construction of urban areas that allows many urban residents to walk to work or telecommute.

The impacts of the urban environment go even deeper than air pollution and lack of exercise. They also involve important social implications that are being recognized in a new movement called **Healthy Communities** or Healthy Cities. The Robert Wood Johnson Foundation (RWJ) has taken a lead role in defining an approach to Healthy Communities which they call "creating a culture of health." Creating a culture of health addresses a wide range of social issues from housing to employment, crime, social interactions, and recreational opportunities.

Underlying the culture of health concept is the concept of **health equity** which RWJ defines as follows: "… we cannot leave anyone behind. Everyone should have the opportunity to pursue the healthiest life possible, no matter where they live or work, the color of their skin, or the amount of money they have."[23, p10]

**BOX 8.9** looks at what is meant by creating a culture of health.

Now that we have examined health impacts of the unaltered, altered, and built environment, let us take a look at the safety component of environmental health and safety, starting with injuries.

## ▶ What Do We Mean by "Intentional and Unintentional Injuries"?

Injuries can occur in a wide array of settings and circumstances, including actions at work, home, and where we play. They can affect everyone, regardless of age, income, race, or ethnicity. It is estimated that, in the United States, one person dies every 3 minutes

due to violence or injury. Injuries are the leading cause of death among persons aged 1–44 years. Injuries do not always result in death and can result in long-term health effects, impacting quality of life. For instance recent evidence strongly suggests that athletic head injuries, previously considered of little health importance, can have lifelong impacts on mental and emotional function.[29]

In public health, we try to avoid the use of the term "accident" because "accident" implies that the reasons for the injury are beyond our control. Injuries can be categorized as intentional and unintentional. **Intentional injuries** are brought about on purpose, that is, by intention, whether the injury is self-inflicted or meant for others.

Intentional injuries can impact entire populations, such as bioterrorist actions that lead to fear and fatalities among a population, or can directly impact individuals, such as with suicide. Harms that occur not on purpose—that is, not by intention—are categorized as unintentional injuries. **Unintentional injuries** encompass injuries sustained in motor vehicle collisions, drownings, falls, fires, unintentional poisonings, and many other incidents.

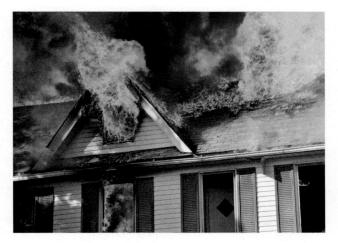

© Knumina Studios/Shutterstock

## ▶ What Is Being Done to Keep the Population Safe?

Safety is approached like many other public health issues: the problem is described; risk and protective factors are identified; and interventions and strategies are developed, implemented, evaluated, and disseminated. The formal steps of the evidence-based public health approach are often used to examine specific issues and interventions.

One of the most visible public health tools used to keep populations safe is outbreak investigations. These investigations conjure images of public health professionals serving as "disease detectives," tracking and responding to outbreaks of acute disease, and these investigations are often viewed as quintessential public health. **BOX 8.10** discusses some of the successes health departments and the CDC have had in outbreak investigations.

Public health's role in protecting the health of populations has evolved as new threats have emerged, including bioterrorism. **BOX 8.11** reviews the anthrax case that occurred shortly after the September 11, 2001 terrorist attack and describes its impact on public health.

In recent years, public health agencies have been increasingly integrated into a National Incident Management System (NIMS), which is part of the Department of Homeland Security (DHS). A central feature of the NIMS is an incident command system (ICS) widely used by police, fire, and emergency management agencies. The ICS attempts to establish uniform procedures and terminology, and an integrated communications system with established and practiced roles for each agency. The goal is to integrate these approaches into ongoing operations and not reserve them solely for emergency situations.[32]

The DHS has developed what is called an **all-hazards approach**. An all-hazards approach to public health preparedness uses the same approach to preparing for many types of disasters, including use of surveillance systems, communications systems, evacuations, and an organized healthcare response. The all-hazards approach has been widely endorsed by public health agencies and organizations in part at least because it recognizes the need for basic

---

**BOX 8.9**  Healthy Communities-Creating a Culture of Health

The RWJ has set out a wide ranging agenda to define and measure what is meant by a culture of health. The culture of health is a comprehensive approach to developing healthy communities which RWJ describes as follows:

> …the Robert Wood Johnson Foundation is working to eliminate barriers to healthy choices, and help communities create or expand upon the types of systems that many of the healthiest places have in common. For instance:

- Local policies that encourage healthy living, and make it easy to sustain a healthy lifestyle;
- Services that connect people to quality health care, transportation, housing, child care, after-school activities, and other critical supports;
- Access to educational and job opportunities that enable residents to support themselves and their families;
- Networks of individuals within and across communities who appreciate the many factors which shape health—and want to make a difference.[24]

The components of RWJ's framework are illustrated using their framework displayed in **TABLE 8.4**.

Each of the components of the RWJ culture of health framework includes measurements that can be used to assess where communities stand and what progress they are making. For instance, the first component "Making Health a Shared Value"[26] required a "sense of community" which RWJ describes as follows:

Research suggests that individuals who live in socially connected communities—with a sense of security, belonging, and trust—have better psychological, physical, and behavioral health, and are more likely to thrive. If people do not see their health as interdependent with others in their community, they are less inclined to engage in health-promoting behaviors or work together for positive health change.[27]

In addition, Making Health a Shared Value requires "civic engagement" which RWJ describes as follows:

Civic engagement creates healthier communities by developing the knowledge and skills to improve the quality of life for all. Voting is a key component of a healthy society, yet many Americans do not vote regularly. Activities such as volunteering, community organizing, and participating in community groups demonstrate that residents care about the outcomes of their community and want to cultivate positive change. Moreover, communities with strong civic engagement are better able to respond and recover during an emergency. These measures reflect whether Americans feel motivated and able to participate and make a difference.[28]

Making Health a Shared Value might be regarded as necessary to accomplish the other components of the framework since its premise is that we are all in it together.

The culture of health concept has helped put the impacts of the built environment on the national agenda and linked it with efforts to promote health equity. It will take many years to accomplish the goals of the culture of health, but RWJ has put forward a roadmap and scorecard to help us get there.

**TABLE 8.4** Culture of Health Action Framework[25]

# CULTURE OF HEALTH ACTION FRAMEWORK

| ACTION AREAS | DRIVERS | MEASURES |
|---|---|---|
| | MINDSET AND EXPECTATIONS | Value on health interdependence |
| | | Value on well-being |
| | | Public discussion on health promotion and well-being |
| | SENSE OF COMMUNITY | Sense of community |
| | | Social support |
| | CIVIC ENGAGEMENT | Voter turnout |
| | | Volunteer engagement |
| | ENUMERATION AND QUALITY OF PARTNERSHIPS | Local health department collaboration |
| | | Opportunities to improve health for youth at schools |
| | | Business support for workplace health promotion and Culture of Health |
| | INVESTMENT IN CROSS-SECTOR COLLABORATION | U.S. corporate giving |
| | | Federal allocations for health investments related to nutrition and indoor and outdoor physical activity |
| | POLICIES THAT SUPPORT COLLABORATION | Community relations and policing |
| | | Youth exposure to advertising for healthy and unhealthy food and beverage products |
| | | Climate resilience |
| | | Health in all policies |
| | BUILT ENVIRONMENT/PHYSICAL CONDITIONS | Housing affordability |
| | | Access to healthy foods |
| | | Youth safety |
| | SOCIAL AND ECONOMIC ENVIRONMENT | Residential segregation |
| | | Early childhood education |
| | | Public libraries |
| | POLICY AND GOVERNANCE | Complete Streets policies |
| | | Air quality |
| | ACCESS | Access to public health |
| | | Access to stable health insurance |
| | | Access to mental health services |
| | | Dental visit in past year |
| | CONSUMER EXPERIENCE AND QUALITY | Consumer experience |
| | | Population covered by an Accountable Care Organization |
| | BALANCE AND INTEGRATION | Electronic medical record linkages |
| | | Hospital partnerships |
| | | Practice laws for nurse practitioners |
| | | Social spending relative to health expenditure |

| OUTCOME | OUTCOME AREAS | MEASURES |
|---|---|---|
| | ENHANCED INDIVIDUAL AND COMMUNITY WELL-BEING | Well-being rating |
| | | Caregiving burden |
| | MANAGED CHRONIC DISEASE AND REDUCED TOXIC STRESS | Adverse child experiences |
| | | Disability associated with chronic conditions |
| | REDUCED HEALTH CARE COSTS | Family health care cost |
| | | Potentially preventable hospitalization rates |
| | | Annual end-of-life care expenditures |

Data from Robert Wood Johnson Foundation. Healthy communities. http://www.rwjf.org/en/our-focus-areas/focus-areas/healthy-communities.html. Accessed July 21, 2017.

## BOX 8.10 Outbreak Investigations

Outbreak investigations have been a key component of public health's effort to respond to epidemics and clusters of acute disease. These investigations are often successfully handled by local and state health agencies. The CDC, however, may be called in to assist with them. The CDC is involved in hundreds of outbreak investigations each year.

Famous investigations include the 1976 outbreak of what came to be called Legionnaires' disease. Hundreds of military veterans, called Legionnaires, gathering in Philadelphia in July to celebrate the nation's bicentennial, were infected, and many died from pneumonia. The CDC identified the cause as previously unrecognized bacteria—now called Legionella—that can grow in hot water and can be spread through the air.

In the early 1980s, an outbreak of life-threatening cardiovascular shock, known as toxic shock syndrome, was traced to a new type of absorbent tampon. It brought to light the need for surveillance of new products, even those not suspected of causing disease.

The most important outbreak of the late 20th century was investigated and brought to professional and public attention in 1981 by the CDC. It came to be called acquired immunodeficiency syndrome (AIDS).

Outbreak investigations are not limited to communicable diseases. In fact, the illnesses may originate, for example, from an environmental toxin, a food additive or supplement, or a drug reaction. For instance, eosinophilia-myalgia syndrome is an incurable and sometimes fatal neurological condition that often presents with vague flulike symptoms. It was traced by the CDC to poorly produced L-trytophan, an amino acid widely used as a food supplement. Reye's syndrome, an often fatal acute liver disease of children, was traced to the use of "baby aspirin" for healthy children during acute viral infections.

Thousands of outbreak investigations are conducted in the United States each year and are mostly handled by state and local health departments. These types of investigations can take months or even years to complete. Often the outbreak is over before the investigation can be completed. Outbreak investigations will remain an important part of public health. However, new technologies, new tracking systems, and better communications systems will hopefully make these critical investigations more rapid and efficient.[30]

## BOX 8.11 Bioterrorism and Anthrax[31]

Shortly after the terrorist attack on the United States on September 11, 2001, a second attack occurred that greatly altered the course of public health in the country. The attack occurred in the form of letters containing a powdered form of anthrax bacteria delivered through the U.S. mail to Congress and national news networks.

Anthrax is bacteria long known for its occasional spread from cattle to humans by close contact and its potential to cause a life-threatening pneumonia. It is considered a particularly deadly agent for bioterrorism, with the potential to kill tens of thousands of people. When prepared in the form of a weapon and delivered in quantity, it has the potential to widely disperse over an entire city or region. Early detection of the substance and treatment of its effects are key to controlling such an attack, including preventing the pneumonia through the early use of antibiotics.

The anthrax attack in 2001 made headlines for weeks, temporarily shutting down Congress and much of Washington, killing five people, and causing severe illness in 17 others. The episode also brought attention and funding to public health programs. It was soon recognized that even large health departments with extensive responsibilities and expertise were not prepared to address bioterrorism and ensure the availability of public health laboratories to diagnose anthrax-related illness and other potential agents of bioterrorism.

Preparation for bioterrorism also focuses on the unique characteristics of bioterrorism and the specific organisms that may be involved with it. The anthrax episode highlighted how terrorism, in general, and bioterrorism, in particular, differs from the types of emergencies and disasters that have become familiar.

First, they may involve the military, as well as law enforcement. Second, they require knowledge of agents that are often very rare. Little expertise exists in either the public health or medical communities about agents such as anthrax, botulism, smallpox, and plague. In addition, bioterrorism may not be easily detected, allowing the agent to spread widely before it is noticed and action can be taken. Finally, there is the potential for multiple simultaneous threats at multiple locations.

Thus, bioterrorism requires special preparation above and beyond the evolving preparedness system for emergencies and disasters. Public health agencies, including the CDC and local health departments, were on the front lines of the anthrax attack and will continue to be part of the first response to bioterrorism attacks if they occur in the future.

public health infrastructure to respond not only to the dramatic crisis or emergency, but to day-to-day needs as well.

New threats such as cyber-attacks have the potential to interfere with our basic infrastructure including our ability to communicate and generate electricity, as well as perform basic public health functions such as chlorination of the water and collection of garbage. Preparations and responses which connect public health with an all-hazards approach provides the best chance for preventing and responding to the expected and unexpected emergencies which are sure to come our way in the years ahead.

We have now looked at noncommunicable diseases, communicable diseases, and environmental health and safety as ways of organizing the major causes of disability and death. Now, let us turn our attention to the organized systems that have been developed for addressing these problems.

## Key Words

| | | |
|---|---|---|
| All-hazards approach | Hazard identification | Multiplicative interaction |
| Altered environment | Hazards | Public health assessment |
| Built environment | Health equity | Risk assessment |
| Dose–response relationship | Healthy communities | Risk characterization |
| Ecological assessment | Intentional injuries | Unaltered environment |
| Exposure assessment | Interaction analysis | Unintentional injuries |

## Discussion Questions

Take a look at the questions posed in the following scenarios, which were presented at the beginning of this chapter. See now whether you can answer them.

1. Joe grew up in an industrial district of town. His family lived in an old apartment building, and he played in a playground near a major intersection. By the age of 6, Joe was found to have high lead levels in his blood and was not doing well in school. Where could all that lead come from? his mother wondered.

2. Jill is pregnant and loves fish, which she has eaten almost daily for years as part of her effort to stay healthy. She hears that fish should not be eaten regularly during pregnancy. Why, she wonders, should I cut down on eating something as healthy as fish?

3. Ralph and Sonya, a prosperous professional couple, and their two children live in an older suburban home. They feel secure that their environment is safe. They were surprised to find when they wanted to put their house up for sale that it did not pass the safety tests for radon. Where did the radon come from, they wondered, and what can be done about it?

4. Sandra worked for an international agency that had successfully addressed the danger of radiation due to the hole in the ozone layer. She was shocked when she was told that she had a life-threatening skin cancer called melanoma. She asked: What could cause melanoma? Could years of sun exposure have played a role?

5. You set out on your commute to work, and as you approach the subway station, you see police cars, ambulances, and dozens of emergency responders in hazmat suits. You are told the entire subway system will be shut down indefinitely, as there has been a suspected case of bioterrorism. You wondered how authorities were alerted to this situation, and what precautions are being taken to protect the health of those living in the city?

6. Alex suffered a traumatic brain injury when he was thrown from his motorcycle after colliding with a car in which the driver had an elevated blood alcohol concentration. Alex was not wearing a helmet. His family members wonder what is being done to prevent this from happening to others.

## References

1. Nova. Population and the environment: A global challenge. http://www.nova.org.au/earth-environment/population-environment. Accessed July 21, 2017.
2. Robert Wood Johnson Foundation. Built environment and health. http://www.rwjf.org/en/our-focus-areas/topics/built-environment-and-health.html. Accessed July 21, 2017.2.
3. Mokdad AM, Marks JS, Stroup DF, Gerberding JL. Actual causes of death in the United States 2000. *JAMA*. 2004;291:1238–1245.
4. Centers for Disease Control and Prevention. Injury prevention and control. http://www.cdc.gov/injury/wisqars/LeadingCauses.html. Accessed July 21, 2017.

5.  U.S. Environmental Protection Agency. Particulate Matter (PM) Pollution. https://www.epa.gov/pm-pollution. Accessed July 21, 2017. (Note color table available on page 2)

6.  U.S. Environmental Protection Agency. Air quality index. https://www3.epa.gov/airnow/aqi_brochure_02_14 .pdf. Accessed July 21, 2017.

7.  Friis RH. *Essentials of Environmental Health*. 2nd ed. Burlington, MA: Jones & Bartlett Learning; 2012.

8.  Centers for Disease Control and Prevention. Occupational cancers. https://www.cdc.gov/niosh/topics/cancer/. Accessed April 7, 2017.

9.  Centers for Disease Control and Prevention. National Center for Environmental Health. http://www.cdc.gov/nceh /ehhe/about.htm. Accessed July 21, 2017.

10. Rom WN, Markowitz SB. *Environmental and Occupational Medicine*. Philadelphia: Lippincott, Williams & Wilkins; 2006.

11. Feitshans IL, Law and regulation of benzene. *Environmental Health Perspectives*. 1989;82:299–307.

12. U.S. Environmental Protection Agency. Human health risk assessment. http://www.epa.gov/risk_assessment/health-risk .htm. Accessed July 21, 2017.

13. Agency for Toxic Substance and Disease Registry. Toxic substance portal-lead. http://www.atsdr.cdc.gov/toxfaqs /tf.asp?id=93&tid=22. Accessed July 21, 2017.

14. Agency for Toxic Substance and Disease Registry. Case studies in environmental medicine-lead. http://wonder.cdc.gov /wonder/prevguid/p0000017/p0000017.asp. Accessed July 21, 2017.

15. National Defense Resource Council. The story of *Silent Spring*. http://www.nrdc.org/health/pesticides/hcarson.asp. Accessed July 21 2017.

16. U.S. Environmental Protection Agency. Mercury: Health effects. http://www.epa.gov/hg/effects.htm. Accessed July 21, 2017.

17. March of Dimes. Mercury and pregnancy. http://www .marchofdimes.org/pregnancy/mercury.aspx. Accessed July 21, 2017.

18. National Aeronautics and Space Administration. Ozone hole watch. http://ozonewatch.gsfc.nasa.gov/facts/hole.html#nav _bypass. Accessed July 21, 2017.

19. U.S. Environmental Protection Agency. Radon. http:// www.epa.gov/radon. Accessed July 21, 2017.

20. Environmental Defense Fund. A primer on the new Toxic Substances Control Act (TSCA) and what led to it. https://www.edf.org/sites/default/files/denison-primer-on -lautenberg-act.pdf. Accessed July 21, 2017.

21. U.S. News & World Report. EPA Sets Rules to Regulate Toxic Chemicals Under 2016 Law. https://www .usnews.com/news/politics/articles/2017-06-22 /epa-sets-rules-to-regulate-toxic-chemicals-under-2016 -law. Accessed October 15, 2017.

22. Washington Post. Metropolitan areas are now fueling virtually all of America's population growth. https:// www.washingtonpost.com/news/wonk/wp/2014/03/27 /metropolitan-areas-are-now-fueling-virtually-all-of -americas-population-growth/?utm_term=.9cc9768ba029. Accessed March 27, 2014.

23. Robert Wood Johnson Foundation. From vision to action: A framework and measures to mobility a culture of health, 2015, page 10. http://www.rwjf.org/content/dam/files /rwjf-web-files/Research/2015/From_Vision_to_Action _RWJF2015.pdf. Accessed July 21, 2017.

24. Robert Wood Johnson Foundation. Healthy communities. http://www.rwjf.org/en/our-focus-areas/focus-areas /healthy-communities.html. Accessed July 21, 2017.

25. Robert Wood Johnson Foundation. From vision to action: A framework and measures to mobility a culture of health, 2015, page 82. http://www.rwjf.org/content/dam/files/rwjf-web -files/Research/2015/From_Vision_to_Action_RWJF2015 .pdf. Accessed July 21, 2017.

26. Robert Wood Johnson Foundation. From vision to action: A framework and measures to mobility a culture of health, 2015, page 10. http://www.rwjf.org/content/dam/files/rwjf-web -files/Research/2015/From_Vision_to_Action_RWJF2015 .pdf. Accessed July 21, 2017.

27. Robert Wood Johnson Foundation. From vision to action: A framework and measures to mobility a culture of health, 2015, page 13. http://www.rwjf.org/content/dam/files /rwjf-web-files/Research/2015/From_Vision_to_Action _RWJF2015.pdf. Accessed October 16, 2017.

28. Robert Wood Johnson Foundation. From vision to action: A framework and measures to mobility a culture of health, 2015, page 13. http://www.rwjf.org/content/dam/files/rwjf-web -files/Research/2015/From_Vision_to_Action_RWJF2015 .pdf. Accessed October 16, 2017.

29. Centers for Disease Control and Prevention. Injury prevention and control. http://www.cdc.gov/injury/overview /index.html. Accessed July 21, 2017.

30. Centers for Disease Control and Prevention. Epidemiology intelligence service. https://www.cdc.gov/eis/history .html. Accessed July 21, 2017.

31. Hugh JM, Gerberding JL. Anthrax bioterrorism: Lessons learned and future directions. *Emerging Infectious Diseases*. 2002;8(10):1013–1014. doi:10.3201 /eid0810.020466.

32. Federal Emergency Management Administration. Emergency alert system. https://www.fema.gov/emergency-alert-system. Accessed July 21, 2017.

# SECTION III

# Cases and Discussion Questions

# ▶ High Blood Pressure: A Public Health and Healthcare Success

Elevated levels of blood pressure, or hypertension, have been observed since the development of blood pressure measurements in the 1800s. It was soon recognized that populations with a high frequency of elevated blood pressure were also populations with a high frequency of strokes, yet the dangers of high blood pressure often went unappreciated until recent years.

High blood pressure is a condition that historically has affected both the privileged and the underprivileged in our society. Presidents Woodrow Wilson and Franklin Delano Roosevelt both had high blood pressure and suffered strokes and heart disease. Today, the condition is disproportionately present among African Americans—15%–20% have some degree of elevated blood pressure.

For many years, high blood pressure was considered a consequence of disease rather than its cause. Clinicians seeing a patient with a stroke, for instance, often attributed their elevation in blood pressure to the stroke rather than the other way around. Long-term studies, such as the Framingham Heart Study, which followed a large number of individuals for many years, established that the high blood pressure actually preceded strokes and not the other way around.

High blood pressure as a contributory cause of strokes, as well as heart and kidney disease, was fully confirmed only after randomized controlled trials in the late 1960s and early 1970s established that lower blood pressure leads to reduced frequency of these diseases. Screening for high blood pressure became widespread in the same period in large part as a result of these investigations.

Elevated levels of blood pressure were initially defined as 140/100 or greater, the higher number indicating the systolic and the lower number indicating the diastolic blood pressure. This level was based upon a range of normal obtained by measuring the blood pressure on large numbers of adult Americans. What were once considered acceptable levels of blood pressure have been redefined as elevated levels in recent years.

Today, the desirable average level is considered 120/80 or lower. These changing levels are justified by follow-up data from a large number of individuals that demonstrates that even levels of blood pressure only slightly above 120/80 are associated with increased risk of stroke and heart disease. In addition, recent evidence suggests that even those with long standing elevation of the systolic blood pressure can benefit from reductions.

The fluctuating levels of blood pressure often make it difficult to establish an individual's average level. Electronic monitoring of blood pressure over a 24-hour period has become a feasible and acceptable gold standard for establishing an individual's average level. Early detection and successful treatments have been shown to effectively reduce the consequences of high blood pressure. Weight loss and salt restriction are often prescribed initially, with subsequent introduction of one or more drugs. Most, if not all, individuals with elevated blood pressure respond to drug treatment with tolerable or no side effects but need to continue treatment for many years—usually for the rest of their lives.

A national public health campaign began in the 1970s to encourage individuals to know their blood pressure and to urge clinicians to treat detected elevated levels. In recent decades, national surveys have indicated that a gradually increasing percentage of patients with elevated blood pressures are being successfully treated and that there has been a substantial reduction in strokes and deaths from strokes. Recent evidence showing that reducing the high salt levels in the U.S. diet can reduce the average level of blood pressure has prompted renewed public health efforts to change eating habits and the contents of commercial foods.

Today, treatment of high blood pressure is recognized as one of the most cost-effective interventions. Its cost per quality adjusted life-year saved is only a few thousand dollars a year for the average person. For high-risk groups, such as those with diabetes, it actually saves money to monitor and treat high blood pressure rather than allow it to cause or exacerbate other health problems requiring more expensive treatments.

## Discussion Questions

1. How does this history of high blood pressure demonstrate the problem description and etiology components of the P.E.R.I.E. process? What different types of studies were used to establish etiology or contributory cause?
2. How does this history of high blood pressure illustrate the evidence-based recommendations and implementation and evaluation components of the P.E.R.I.E. process?
3. Explain the justification for updating the definition of what is considered a "healthy" blood pressure level.

4.  How does this history of high blood pressure demonstrate the application of the four criteria for a successful screening program? Explain.

5.  Using the four quadrants of cost and effectiveness, how would you classify treatment of hypertension for the average person? For those with diabetes? Explain.

# ▶ Testing and Screening

Ken had just turned 40, and with a little encouragement from his wife, he decided that it was time to have a physical—it would be his first real visit to a doctor since he broke his arm as a kid. Seeing a doctor had not made sense to him before. He was in great shape, felt fine, and did not smoke.

Maybe it was his 65-year-old father's sudden death from a heart attack just a few weeks after his retirement that finally convinced Ken to find himself a doctor. He knew that his father had had high cholesterol, but he was told his own cholesterol level and electrocardiogram results were okay when he entered the military at age 18. Besides, Ken was not big on desserts and only ate a Big Mac when he took the kids out after their soccer games.

The examination was quite uneventful and Ken was reassured when the doctor could not find anything of concern. A few recommendations on nutrition and better ways to exercise were about all that came out of the visit. Then he got the call from the doctor's office—could he make a follow-up appointment to discuss his cholesterol?

His low-density lipoprotein (LDL, or "bad" cholesterol) was 165 and his high-density lipoprotein (HDL, or "good" cholesterol) was 40.

"We used to think these levels were okay because they are so common," his doctor began. "However, now we consider your LDL cholesterol too high because it increases your chances of developing heart and other blood vessel diseases. There is no evidence of heart disease at this point, but your cholesterol needs attention."

"What do you mean by 'attention'?" Ken replied. "I exercise, do not smoke, and generally keep my fats down."

Ken soon learned a lot more about cholesterol. He first tried his best at changing his diet—it helped a little, but just did not do the trick.

Ken's doctor told him: "For some people, there is a strong genetic component to high cholesterol levels, and while diet is still important, it just cannot always reduce LDL cholesterol enough by itself. Exercise helps, especially by increasing the good cholesterol, but it does not do much for the bad cholesterol. Medication may be needed, and there is now evidence that if taken regularly, it reduces the chances of having a heart attack or at least delays its occurrence."

Taking medication every day was not so easy for Ken, but he stuck with the plan. His doctor asked him to have his cholesterol levels checked every few months for the first year. Ken was amazed at how well the medicine worked. His LDL fell from 165 to less than 100 on only a modest dose. In addition to routine cholesterol checks, Ken had his blood tested for potential side effects from the medication, such as impacts to his liver, and he was told to report any long-lasting muscle aches and pains. The good news was that he could not tell he was taking the medication—he felt just fine.

Now that the cholesterol levels had dropped, he thought maybe he could go off the medication if he just watched his diet closely. His doctor let him try that for a month, but after the 30 days were up, his LDL level was back up to 160.

"Looks like you are hooked on medication for life," his doctor said with a wry smile, adding, "At least the extra cost is worth the extra benefit."

Ken and his wife were told the high cholesterol levels were a genetic condition. Not only did Ken need to take the medication on a permanent basis, but the pediatrician began testing his kids.

The doctors said, "We are beginning to understand the genetics behind this condition and would like to do some genetic testing on the children, including that new baby of yours."

Ken wondered if the information on his children's cholesterol levels would be part of their medical records for the rest of their lives. "You are not planning to put the results on the Internet, are you?" Ken joked nervously as they drew blood from his newborn son.

## Discussion Questions

1.  How are the range of normal and desirable-range approaches to establishing a reference interval and defining a positive and negative test illustrated in this case? Explain.

2.  What arguments are presented in this case that fulfills the criteria for screening for high LDL cholesterol? Explain.

3.  What definition of cost-effectiveness is being used to justify screening and treatment of elevated LDL cholesterol?

4.  What ethical issues need to be considered in screening for conditions such as elevated LDL cholesterol? Explain.

# ▶ *H. pylori* and Peptic Ulcers

Duodenal ulcers and benign stomach ulcers are frequently referred to as peptic ulcers. Peptic ulcers are among the digestive diseases with the highest incidence. Approximately 10% of the population experience a peptic ulcer at some point in their life, though a substantial proportion, perhaps a majority, are not medically diagnosed. Peptic ulcers generally heal even without prescribed treatment in 4–6 weeks. Approximately 1% of those with peptic ulcers experience complications, with potentially life-threatening perforation of the stomach or duodenum being the more serious complications. The disease often recurs, with a probability of recurrence in the range of 50%.

For many years, peptic ulcers were believed to be exclusively the result of excess acid production due to such factors as alcohol, aspirin, and other anti-inflammatory medications, spicy foods, and stress. The stomach and duodenum were known to be highly acidic, and it was believed that bacteria were unable to survive in this high-acid environment.

In the early 1980s, investigators observed a spiral-shaped bacterium, which they named *Helicobacter pylori*, or *H. pylori*, in a number of pathological specimens from patients with disease of the stomach and duodenum. Most scientists doubted the relationship to disease, often concluding that the organism must be a contaminant because of the belief that bacteria could not grow in highly acidic environments.

After many unsuccessful attempts, Australian researchers Barry J. Marshall, MD, and J. Robin Warren, MD, were able to culture the bacteria from the stomach and became convinced that the bacteria were actually the cause of peptic ulcers. They were frustrated in their attempts to demonstrate that *H. pylori* was the cause of the disease because of the absence of good animal models.

To attempt to establish causation, Marshall drank a flask of the cultured bacteria. He became ill and developed acute ulceration of the stomach. *H. pylori* was cultured from his ulcerations. This dramatic effort brought attention and extensive investigations to address whether *H. pylori* is a contributory cause of duodenal ulcers.

Subsequent studies in the United States and other countries established that *H. pylori* is a frequently occurring organism that increases with increasing age. Overall, over 20% of people in the United States have *H. pylori*; that is its prevalence is over 20% in the United States, with a higher prevalence beginning at an early age in many developing countries, as well as Japan. In case–control studies, *H. pylori* was found to have a strong association with duodenal ulcer, with over 70% of peptic ulcer patients having *H. pylori* at the time of their diagnosis.

Randomized controlled trials examined the recurrence rates of duodenal ulcers after treatment of the bacteria with antibiotics shown to eliminate *H. pylori*. In one study among those randomized to placebo, the recurrence rate was over 10 times as great as among those randomized to antibiotic treatment directed against *H. pylori*. This research led to a search for biological mechanisms. Extensive research established a greater understanding of the physiology of peptic ulcers, including identifying the production of an enzyme by *H. pylori* that reduces acidity and thus facilitates its growth in an acid environment.

New tests demonstrated that *H. pylori* is associated with the great majority of duodenal ulcers among outpatients. Randomized controlled trials and extensive clinical follow-up established the effectiveness and relative safety of antibiotic treatments of *H. pylori*. These investigations led to evidence-based recommendations for routine testing for *H. pylori* among outpatients diagnosed with peptic ulcers and treatment of *H. pylori* with antibiotics when it was detected.

## Discussion Questions

1. Describe the negative and positive roles that biological plausibility played in establishing causation.
2. Discuss what would be required to demonstrate that *H. pylori* is a cause of duodenal ulcers and stomach ulcers using Koch's modern postulates. Were these postulates established for *H. pylori*?
3. Discuss how the evidence linking *H. pylori* and peptic ulcers using randomized controlled trials fulfill the contributory cause criteria of association, prior association, and how altering the "cause" alters the "effect."
4. What grade (A, B, C, D, I) would you give the recommendation to treat *H. pylori* among those diagnosed with peptic ulcers and having a positive test for *H. pylori*? Explain based on the strength of the evidence and the magnitude of the impact.

# ▶ What to Do About Lyme Disease?

You have just moved into a new subdivision—your first home with your young family. The first week you are there, a neighbor tells you that her son has developed Lyme disease and now has chronic arthritis that requires extensive treatment.

Lyme disease is an increasingly common disease that can cause acute and chronic arthritis if not treated early and correctly. In rare instances, it can cause life-threatening heart disease and temporary paralysis often to one side of the face due to nerve damage. The disease is caused by an organism known as a spirochete, which is spread from deer ticks to humans via tick bites. Lyme disease is especially common in communities with large deer populations, which today includes much of the suburban United States as well as rural areas.

Ticks must remain in place on the human skin at least 12–24 hours in order to extract human blood and inject the spirochete organism at the site of the bite. Complete removal of the small but visible tick within 24 hours usually prevents the disease. Deer ticks are most abundant in the late spring and tend to live on tall grasses from which they can easily move to the bare legs of children and adults.

The disease frequently first appears as a circular red rash around the site of the bite. At this stage, early diagnosis and treatment with antibiotics is usually successful. Several weeks or months later, the onset of arthritis may occur and can be difficult to diagnose. A missed diagnosis may result in severe arthritis that is difficult to treat. A vaccine has been developed and briefly marketed to prevent the disease, but it was quite expensive and only partially successful.

In your new hometown, the local health department is charged with developing a plan for control or elimination of Lyme disease. As an informed and concerned citizen, you are invited to give input on the plan, identifying possible interventions.

## Discussion Questions

1. What primary interventions would you consider? Explain.
2. What secondary interventions would you consider? Explain.
3. What tertiary interventions would you consider? Explain.
4. What educational interventions do you recommend? Explain.
5. Can Lyme disease be eradicated? Can it be controlled? Explain.

## ▶ Sharma's Village

Sharma lives in a small farming village in south Asia, but she could just as well be living in Haiti, Ethiopia, Nigeria,

or several dozen other countries classified by the World Bank as low-income economies. Her home is a small hut, and she works daily with her mother to gather firewood for their small indoor fireplace, which acts as the kitchen stove. The smoke often makes her eyes water because there is no chimney or other ventilation.

At night, she sleeps with her extended family in a room where mosquitoes bite her regularly. Despite the fact that Sharma lives in a rural community, the villagers live in crowded quarters. The water the family drinks is carried by the women from a well several hundred yards from their home. The water sometimes tastes bad, but it is all they have to drink.

The family farms a small plot of land on the hillside, which had become eroded from years of cutting trees. The last big monsoon to hit the area created a landslide, which left the village underwater for several weeks, creating mold in nearly every home. Most of the adults have goiters from the lack of iodine in the soil. The addition of iodine to salt has prevented goiters in the children.

Pesticides are used widely to control mosquitoes and agricultural pests, but the farmers receive little education on their safe use. Recently, a new road was built, connecting her village with the neighboring towns. Despite the advantages of having the new road, cars and trucks now speed through her village, rarely stopping to let people cross the road.

In Sharma's village, the life expectancy is 49 years. Babies often die of diarrheal diseases in the first year of life, and mothers occasionally die in childbirth. Malaria is widespread and hookworm disease is present among those who farm the fields and in children, whose ability to learn is often affected. Malnutrition is also widespread despite the fact that farming is the major occupation in the village.

Chronic lung disease among adults and asthma among the young is surprisingly common, even though cigarette smoking is rare. Tuberculosis is widespread and a major cause of death, despite the fact that until recently, there have been few cases of HIV/AIDS in the area. Unexplained neurological diseases among farm workers occur regularly. The most common cause of death among teenagers is motor vehicle injuries along the new road, even though there is only one truck in the village.

## Discussion Questions

1. What environmental risk factors contributing to disease and other health conditions are illustrated in this case? Classify each as an unaltered, altered, or built environment factor.

2. Discuss at least two examples of how disease or other conditions found in the village can be explained by the environmental risk factors.

3. Identify at least two interventions that would make a large difference in the health of this village.

4. What changes do you expect to occur in this village as social and economic development take place?

# Type 2 Diabetes—An Epidemic Disease

Nearly everyone knows someone with type 2 diabetes. It may be your grandfather, mother, professor, or even the young person sitting next to you. Those with type 2 diabetes often do not talk about it and may not even realize they have it.

Type 2 diabetes mellitus is rapidly increasing in the United States in parallel with the increase in levels of obesity. Those with a family history are especially prone to developing the disease. Over 30 million people in the United States are living with type 2 diabetes and the medical care and social costs are estimated at over $300 billion dollars a year. It is predicted that by 2025 there will be over 50 million people with type 2 diabetes costing the country over $500 billion if current trends continue.

Type 2 diabetes is a progressive disease which affects blood vessels and nerves and thereby impacts nearly every organ in the body. The impact on the feet from neuropathy and diminished blood supply may lead to infections and amputations. The impact on the retina can lead to blindness while the impact on the kidneys is among the leading cause of renal failure requiring expensive hemodialysis or transplantation. The impact on the blood vessels also increases the probability of coronary artery disease and stroke. Most recently an increased risk of dementia has been recognized. Thus, type 2 diabetes ranks at the very top of the conditions classified as a 21st-century epidemic.

Testing for diabetes is increasingly being done as part of routine health care using the hemoglobin A1c blood test which measures average blood sugar control over a 2-month period. Many of the newly recognized diabetics have mild disease that would greatly benefit from weight loss.

Weight loss has been the approach to preventing and controlling type 2 diabetes for many years. Even loss of 5% of body weight can have a substantial impact on blood sugars. Approaches to weight loss include a variety of partially successful diets most of which can reduce weight in the short run, but all of which are difficult for individuals to maintain in the longer run. Gastric bypass surgery, despite its costs and potential side effects, has been shown to have an immediate effect on type 2 diabetes even before the impacts of weight loss occur. It is now often recommended for those with type 2 diabetes and a BMI of greater than 35.

Management of most patients with type 2 diabetes requires the efforts of several types of clinicians. A primary care clinician, and increasingly a nurse practitioner or physician assistant, is often key. Other health professionals who are needed for high quality preventive care may include nutritionists to work with patients on their eating habits, podiatrists to prevent and treat foot problems, as well as optometrists and ophthalmologists to identify and treat diabetic eye problems to prevent blindness.

Type 2 diabetes is often cited as a disease which requires shared decision-making and self-care. If insulin is required for management of the disease, adjustment to prevent high and low blood sugars often rests on the knowledge and engagement of patients and families.

Type 2 diabetes can be a very expensive disease to treat especially when hospitalization is required for very high blood sugar or for complications of the disease. Treatment of high blood pressure among type 2 diabetics has been shown to reduce costs as have annual influenza vaccinations. Early identification of damage to the retina from type 2 diabetes and laser treatment has been shown to be an effective and low cost approach to preventing blindness.

Studies of the underlying mechanism for the development and progression of diabetes may in the future lead to better methods for prevention and treatment. An increasing number of treatments for type 2 diabetes have been approved by the U.S. FDA. It is not yet clear which treatments work best and for whom they are most effective. Comparative effectiveness research is now under way to help clinicians tailor the available treatments to the individual patient.

## Discussion Questions

1. Identify interventions discussed in this case which can be classified as primary, secondary, and tertiary. Explain.

2. Identify ways that this case suggests that coordination of health care can improve the quality of care for type 2 diabetics. Explain.

3. Identify ways that this case suggests that the cost of care for type 2 diabetes can be reduced while increasing or maintaining quality. Explain.

4.  What role should society at large play in reducing the epidemic of obesity? How should it be accomplished?
5.  How would you suggest combining the approaches to type 2 diabetes discussed in this case to prevent and treat type 2 diabetes? Explain.

# ▶ Legal Drugs That Kill—Death from Prescription Drug Overdoses

Katie found herself flat on her back in pain after falling off her bicycle as she swerved to avoid a collision with a car. She was taken to the emergency department, where she was examined, X-rayed, and given a 5-day supply of a prescription pain-killer along with a note saying, "Make an appointment to see your doctor as soon as possible."

Though no one asked, Katie had a history of regular alcohol use and occasional binge drinking on weekends. Her father died of liver disease after many years of heavy drinking. Katie stayed away from most illegal drugs, though she tried marijuana a few times even though it was not legal in her state.

Katie had trouble filling her prescription after she left the emergency room late at night. Her nearest 24-hour pharmacy told her they do not carry narcotic pain medicine because they are a target for robberies. When she finally was able to fill her prescription, the pain was so bad that she took double the prescribed dose of medicine. She was running low before she could get an appointment with her doctor, but she found that if she took it with alcohol, it did the trick.

Her doctor agreed that her injuries were bad enough to require additional narcotic pain medications, which he prescribed for a month followed by a couple of refills. Katie quickly filled the prescription. On her way out of the pharmacy, she was stopped by a young man who offered to buy her medication for twice what she had paid. Katie turned the other way and rushed home to take her medication.

Katie could hardly get out of bed, the pain was so bad. After a few pills and a little alcohol, she was able to get going. Getting her work done was an ordeal, and she mostly looked forward to the weekends. Partying took on a new meaning now, as it was an escape from constant pain.

One Saturday night, several months after her injury, Katie's friends planned a party to celebrate her 30th birthday. Katie tried her best to get herself together to go to the party despite the pain. She thought a little extra medication and a few drinks were what she needed. She soon felt so tired that before getting ready for the party, she decided to lie down for a little nap. She never heard the knock on the door by her friends, who wanted to know why she did not show up at the party. By the time they had called the rescue squad and the responders had broken in the door, she was found lying in her bed without a heartbeat, a victim of an unintentional prescription overdose.

Katie's friends were astonished to hear that unintentional prescription overdoses now exceeds motor vehicle injuries, suicides, and firearms as causes of death among young people, far exceeding deaths from illegal drugs. Traditionally a cause of death among young males, deaths from unintentional drug overdoses are rapidly increasing among females. Drug overdoses often occur from a combination of prescription narcotic pain medicine and antianxiety medication with alcohol, which together form a common and deadly combination.

## Discussion Questions

1.  What underlying factors led to Katie's death?
2.  What educational interventions would you recommend to prevent unintentional overdoses? Explain.
3.  What motivational interventions directed toward prescribers or patients would you recommend to prevent unintentional overdoses? Explain.
4.  What obligation or legal interventions would you recommend to prevent unintentional overdoses? Explain.
5.  What changes in the rates of unintentional overdoses in the United States do you expect in the absence of the types of interventions that you identified in questions two, three, and four? Explain.

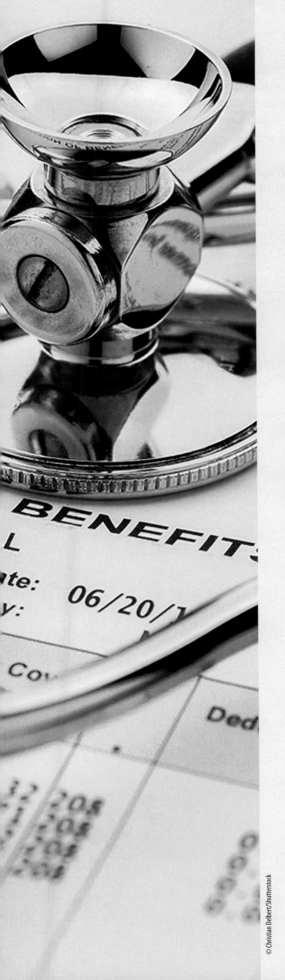

SECTION IV

# Health Professionals, Healthcare Institutions, and Healthcare Systems

In this section, we will take a look at healthcare systems, the people, institutions, and organizational structures that deliver health care to individuals. In the United States, the healthcare system consumes approximately $3 trillion in resources or over 18% of gross domestic product.

To understand how the U.S. healthcare system functions and is organized, we will start in Chapter 9 by taking a look at the people who provide health services. There are over 15 million people involved in the delivery of health services. We will focus on three of the largest groups: physicians, nurses, and public health professionals.

In Chapter 10, we will discuss the institutions involved in the delivery of healthcare services and how they interact or do not interact with each other. We will also examine methods for maximizing the quality of health care.

Finally, in Chapter 11, we will examine the health insurance system and the healthcare system as a whole. In this chapter, we will aim to understand how the U.S. system is financed and look at the issues of access to care, quality of care, and the costs of that care. As we do this, we will examine the issues that need to be addressed in reform of the U.S. health care and health insurance systems. To provide perspective, we will also examine the characteristics of some other healthcare systems in developed countries.

**FIGURE S04-1** displays the components of a healthcare system that will guide our discussion of this complex subject.

Let us begin in Chapter 9 by turning our attention to the types of clinical and public health professionals who are part of the health workforce.

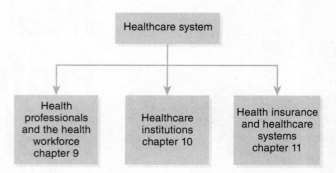

**FIGURE S04.1** An Approach to Examining Healthcare Systems

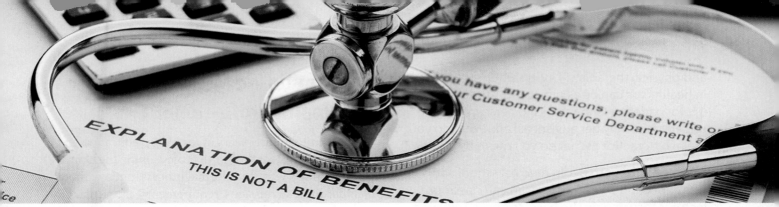

# CHAPTER 9

# Health Professionals and the Health Workforce

## LEARNING OBJECTIVES

By the end of this chapter, the student will be able to:

- describe roles that education and credentialing play in the development of health professions, such as medicine and nursing.
- describe the continuum of public health education and identify educational pathways for becoming a public health professional.
- identify recent changes in the education of physicians.
- describe the educational options in nursing and the growing role that nurses play in healthcare delivery.
- identify components of prevention and public health that are recommended for inclusion in clinical education.
- explain the concept of primary care and differentiate it from secondary and tertiary care.
- identify a range of mechanisms used to compensate clinical health professionals and explain their advantages and disadvantages.

Upon your arrival at the hospital, the nurse specialist examines you and consults with the radiologists, the gastroenterologist, and the general surgeon. Your medication is reviewed by the pharmacist and your meals by the clinical nutritionist. Throughout the hospitalization, you are followed by a hospitalist. Once you get back home, the home care team comes to see you regularly for the first 2 weeks, and the certified physician assistant (PA) and the doctor of nursing practice (DNP) see you in the office. You realize that health care is no longer just about doctors and nurses. You ask yourself: What roles do all of these health professionals play in the healthcare system?

Jenna decides that after college, she wants to become a doctor and see patients and practice medicine. "I thought there was only one kind of doctor who could diagnose disease and prescribe medicine," she mentions at a career counseling meeting. "Not so, anymore," says her advisor. "There are allopathic and osteopathic physicians. In addition, there are nurse practitioners (NPs) who are authorized to diagnose and prescribe medications, and there are PAs who do the same under a physician's supervision. The universe of 'doctors' now includes doctors of nursing practice, as well as other doctoral degree professionals, such as pharmacists, occupational therapists, and physical therapists." Understanding careers in health care can be as difficult for students as it is for patients, Jenna thinks to herself. Now she understands why her advisor asked: "What do you mean by 'practice'? What do you mean by 'doctor'?"

Sarah was about to begin medical school and was expecting 2 years of "preclinical" classroom lectures focusing on the basic sciences, followed by the study of clinical diseases. Then, as she had heard from her physician father, she expected 2 years of clinical hospital "rotations" and electives investigating specialties. She is surprised to find that medical school has changed. There are small-group, problem-based learning (PBL) sessions where she needs to be able to locate and read the research literature. There is contact with patients and their problems right from the beginning. There is increasingly a 4-year approach instead of a preclinical and clinical approach to medical education. She wonders: Are these changes for the better? What else needs to be done to improve medical education?

You are interested in clinical care, as well as public health. I need to make a choice, you think to yourself. "Not necessarily," your advisor says. "There are many ways to combine clinical care with public health." After a little investigation, you find out that undergraduate public health education is increasingly seen as preparation for clinical education, and clinical prevention and population health are increasingly becoming part of clinical care. In addition, many careers, from health administration, to health policy, to health education, to clinical research, combine the individual orientation of clinical care with the population perspective of public health. So what is the best pathway to a public health career for you?

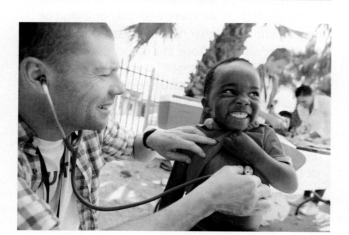

© laflor/E+/Getty Images

## ▶ What Do We Mean by a "Health Professional"?

Until the early years of the 1900s, education and practice for the health professions in the United States were an informal process, often without standardized admissions requirements, curricula, or even formal recognition of a profession. Throughout the 20th century and into the 21st century, there has been an ongoing movement to formalize and standardize the education process for health professionals.

These formal requirements have come to define what we mean by a "health professional" and include admission prerequisites, coursework requirements, examinations of competency, official recognition of educational achievements, and granting of permission to practice. Today, the list of formal health professions is very long. Clinical health professions include physicians, nurses, dentists, pharmacists, optometrists, clinical psychologists, podiatrists, and chiropractors. They also include NPs, PAs, health services administrators, and allied health practitioners.[1] "Allied health practitioner" is a broad and at times confusing category ranging from graduate degree–trained professionals, such as physical therapists, occupational therapists, and medical social workers, to technical specialists often with an associate's degree, such as dental assistants, sonographers, and laboratory technicians.

Education and training are central to the development and definition of most health professions. Education implies that a student is pursuing a degree or certificate from an accredited educational institution. Training is often organized and directed outside of educational institutions. Hospitals, health departments, and large group practices often have the responsibility of training new health professionals.

Before we take a look at specific health professions, let us step back and ask the more general question: How do education and training serve to define health professions?

## ▶ How Do Education and Training Serve to Define Health Professions?

Defining and enforcing educational requirements is central to creating and maintaining a profession. This can be accomplished using two basic approaches: **accreditation** and **credentialing**.

Accreditation implies a process of setting standards for educational and training institutions and enforcing these standards using a regularly scheduled institutional self-study and an outside review. Accreditation is used by most health professions to define and enforce educational expectations. At times, these expectations may be laid out in detail down to the level of square footage per student for laboratory space and the number of hours devoted to specific subjects. In other health professions, educational subject areas may be outlined and institutions left to judge how to best implement the curriculum.

Credentialing implies that the individual, rather than the institution, is evaluated. "Credentialing" is a generic term indicating a process of verifying that an individual has the desirable or required qualifications to practice a profession. Credentialing often takes the form of **certification**. Certification is generally a profession-led process in which applicants who have completed the required educational process take an examination. Successful completion of formal examinations leads to recognition in the form of certification.

Certification also has come to define specialties and even subspecialties within a profession. Successful completion of a specialty or subspecialty examination may entitle a health professional to call him- or herself "board-certified." Certification is often a prerequisite

for **licensure**, which is a state governmental function and usually requires more than certification. It may include local residency requirements, a criminal background check, continuing education requirements, etc. Licensure, when applicable, is usually required for practice of a health profession.

Thus, in order to understand what is meant by a particular health profession, it is important to understand the credentials that are expected or required. Let us take a look at the education required for public health, as well as for physicians and nurses.

## ▶ What Are the Educational Options Within Public Health?

Within public health, there is a growing array of health specialties. Some specialties require a minimum of a bachelor's degree, such as environmental health specialists and health educators. However, many public health roles require graduate degrees that focus on disciplines including epidemiology, biostatistics, environmental sciences, health administration and policy, and social and behavioral sciences. **BOX 9.1** discusses the development of what is being called the continuum of public health education.

---

**BOX 9.1** Development of the Continuum of Public Health Education[2]

The history of public health education as a formal academic activity in the United States dates back over 100 years to the 1915 Welch-Rose Report. Funded by the Rockefeller Foundation, this report set the stage for development of separate schools of public health focused on graduate education designed for those with previous professional education, particularly as physicians, nurses, and engineers.

The focus on graduate-level education of those with previous professional education remained the norm for half a century after the publication of the Welch-Rose Report. This began to change in the 1970s and 1980s with the growth of schools of public health as well as programs in public health, often located in medical schools. By the 1980s, a substantial portion of the students entering graduate training in public health had a bachelor's degree but no prior professional training.

In addition, graduate training in public health increasingly became specialized, with master of public health (MPH) degrees often focusing not only on a

generalist core but also on a specialty area, such as epidemiology, biostatistics, environmental health, health administration, health policy, health education, and health communications. This was accompanied by the growth of doctoral programs, including both academically oriented PhDs and practice-oriented doctor of public health (DrPH) degrees.

Undergraduate public health education began as specialty areas, such as health education, environmental health, and health services administration, during the last half of the 20th century. For instance, health education developed its own undergraduate degree programs, competencies, and certifying examination, the certified health education specialist.

A major change in public health education began in 2003 with the National Academy of Medicine's recommendation that "all undergraduates should have access to education in public health."[3,a] This recommendation launched what came to be known as the Educated Citizen and Public Health movement,

---

a  The National Academy of Medicine was previously known as the Institute of Medicine. The name change took effect on July 1, 2015 as part of a broader reorganization to integrate the work of the National Academies of Sciences, Engineering, and Medicine.

a collaborative effort of undergraduate education associations and public health education associations. The Educated Citizen and Public Health movement led to a series of recommendations by the Association of Schools and Programs of Public Health, including the Critical Component Elements of an Undergraduate Major in Public Health. These recommendations are now being used by the Council on Education for Public Health (CEPH) as part of the accreditation process for undergraduate majors in public health, including those that provide generalist education and specialty education, as well as those in institutions with and without graduate public health education.

As part of the 100th anniversary of the Welch-Rose Report, public health educators and practitioners joined with undergraduate educators and health profession leaders to form the Framing the Future Task Force: The Second Hundred Years of Education for Public Health. At the heart of the task force's deliberation was how to create a continuum of public health education. Key to the continuum was undergraduate public health education, including public health education as part of the curriculum of community colleges.

The task force produced the Community College and Public Health Report[4] with the League for Innovation in the Community College. The report includes prototype curriculum models that encourage articulation of community college associate degrees and bachelor's degrees in both specialty areas and generalist degrees.

In addition, community colleges are beginning to look at how to integrate public health into their own areas of strength and interest. Three "Health Foundations" courses: personal health with a population focus, health communication, and overview of public health are being recommended as part of nursing and allied health education as well as the education of first responders. Community colleges increasingly emphasize "guided learning pathways" which provide students with access to multiple programs in the same general area of study. The Health Foundation courses may become the entry curriculum for a guided learning pathway to health.

**Health navigation** education was also recommended by the Community Colleges and Public

Health Report as a certificate program or associate degree which provides skills and knowledge in prevention and community health, health systems, and health insurance as well as obtaining and using health information.

Health navigation education in community colleges is preparing those with an Associate's degree to help individuals navigate the complex public health, health care, and health insurance systems. These individuals may have a range of job titles including community health worker, patient navigator, and health insurance navigator. They may serve underserved populations but are also needed by the elderly, those with complex medical conditions, and an increasing number of individuals who need help navigating the complex U.S. health system. Nurses, medical social workers, and other health professionals may also take on these increasingly needed roles. This may require an additional certification program or integration of the necessary knowledge into a basic degree.

Thus, today, formal public health education includes degree programs at community colleges and 4-year colleges as well as at the master's and doctoral levels. The process of articulating these degrees and ensuring the development of career ladders is well underway. The continuum of public health education has been established as a goal and is rapidly becoming a reality.

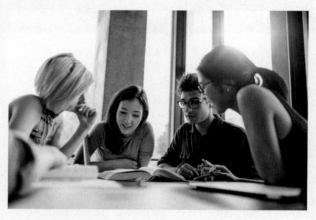

© Jacob Lund/Shutterstock

In addition to the educational options that lead to becoming a public health professional, a large and growing number of options are available to combine public health education with other professions. Combined or joint degrees with medicine, nursing, and PAs are widely offered. Combinations with law, social work, international affairs, and a range of other fields are also being offered. Combined or joint degrees often allow students to reduce the total number of credit hours required to satisfy the requirement for the two degrees.

Public health professionals today include those who specialize in a wide range of disciplines and work in a variety of settings, from governmental public health to not-for-profit and for-profit institutions, as well as in educational and healthcare institutions. There are approximately 500,000 public health professionals in the United States, and it is estimated that in coming years, there will be a substantial shortage.[5]

Public health is one of the last health fields to formalize educational and professional requirements and include a certifying examination. The recognition of public health as a distinct professional field with its own educational process has been formalized through accreditation of public health schools and programs by CEPH. Specific disciplines within public health, such as epidemiology and social and behavioral sciences, have provided recognition for specialized training through advanced degrees, such as the academically oriented doctor of philosophy (PhD) degree and the practice-oriented DrPH degree.

Specific technical areas have existed within public health for many years and have included competency examinations, especially in fields such as occupational and environmental health. Health educators in recent decades have formalized and standardized their education and increasingly taken on the structure of a profession, including examinations, certifications, and continuing education requirements.

Formal certification as a public health specialist has only been available since 2008, when the first certifying examination was given. **BOX 9.2** describes the current certifying examination.

## ▶ What Is the Education and Training Process for Physicians?

Physicians are a central part of what is called the practice of medicine. They can be categorized as allopathic or osteopathic physicians. Allopathic physicians graduate with a Doctor of Medicine (MD) degree, while osteopathic physicians graduate from osteopathic medical schools and receive a Doctor of Osteopathic Medicine (DO) degree. Graduates of both allopathic and osteopathic medical schools are eligible to apply for the same residency and fellowship programs for their postgraduate medical education. The number of osteopathic medical schools has grown rapidly in recent years and now totals over 30 nationwide. Allopathic medical schools number

---

**BOX 9.2** Certification in Public Health[6]

The National Board of Public Health Examiners administers the Certification in Public Health (CPH) examination as well as maintenance of certification programs to ensure that public health professionals have mastered the foundational knowledge and skills relevant to contemporary public health.

To be eligible to be certified, candidates must be enrolled in and complete a Council on Education in Public Health accredited master's program or have completed an undergraduate degree and have 5 years of relevant public health work experience.

The content areas tested as part of the CPH examination have recently been revised after an extensive "job task analysis" so that it reflects the tasks actually performed by the public health workforce. The new content areas, each of which will be of equal weight on the examination, are as follows:

- Evidence-Based Approaches to Public Health
- Communication
- Leadership
- Law and Ethics
- Public Health Biology and Human Risk
- Collaboration and Partnership
- Program Planning and Evaluation
- Program Management
- Policy in Public Health
- Health Equity and Social Justice

CPH certification is voluntary, but a growing number of jobs are expecting certification, and certification is becoming an important credential for those working in public health.

---

approximately 140 and in recent years have grown in size and number.[a]

Within medicine, specialties and subspecialties continue to emerge. For instance, hospice and palliative medicine has recently been added to the list of specialties. Subspecialty certification for **hospitalists**, those whose practice is entirely in the hospital, are being developed and implemented for both adult and pediatric hospitalists. **TABLE 9.1** outlines many of the current physician specialties and subspecialties.[7] **BOX 9.3** discusses the process of medical education and the changes that have occurred in recent years and continue to evolve.[8]

---

a Osteopathic and allopathic medical education curricula are quite similar today. The prerequisites for admission are similar, and both types of medical schools generally require the Medical College Admission Test (MCAT). However, osteopathic medical education retains its focus on manipulation of the muscular skeletal system and sees itself as providing a holistic approach to medicine, including a greater focus on prevention. A substantially higher percentage of DOs go into primary care as compared to MDs.

**TABLE 9.1** Selected Physician Specialties and Subspecialties

| Example of specialty area | Example of subspecialty area |
|---|---|
| Anesthesiology | Critical care medicine<br>Hospice and palliative medicine<br>Pain medicine |
| Emergency medicine | Hospice and palliative medicine<br>Medical toxicology<br>Pediatric emergency medicine<br>Sports medicine<br>Undersea and hyperbaric medicine |
| Family medicine | Adolescent medicine<br>Geriatric medicine<br>Hospice and palliative medicine<br>Sleep medicine<br>Sports medicine |
| Internal medicine | Adolescent medicine<br>Cardiovascular disease<br>Clinical cardiac electrophysiology<br>Critical care medicine<br>Endocrinology, diabetes, and metabolism<br>Gastroenterology<br>Geriatric medicine<br>Hematology<br>Hospice and palliative medicine<br>Hospital medicine<br>Infectious disease<br>Interventional cardiology<br>Medical oncology<br>Nephrology<br>Pulmonary disease<br>Rheumatology<br>Sleep medicine<br>Sports medicine<br>Transplant hepatology |
| Obstetrics and gynecology | Critical care medicine<br>Gynecologic oncology<br>Hospice and palliative medicine<br>Maternal and fetal medicine<br>Reproductive endocrinology/infertility |
| Orthopedic surgery | Orthopedic sports medicine<br>Surgery of the hand |
| Otolaryngology | Neurotology<br>Pediatric otolaryngology<br>Plastic surgery within the head and neck<br>Sleep medicine |
| PATHOLOGY<br>Anatomic pathology and clinical pathology<br>Pathology—anatomic<br>Pathology—clinical | Blood banking/transfusion medicine<br>Chemical pathology<br>Cytopathology<br>Dermatopathology<br>Forensic pathology<br>Hematology<br>Medical microbiology<br>Molecular genetic pathology<br>Neuropathology<br>Pediatric pathology |

| | |
|---|---|
| Pediatrics | Adolescent medicine |
| | Child abuse pediatrics |
| | Developmental-behavioral pediatrics |
| | Hospice and palliative medicine |
| | Medical toxicology |
| | Neonatal-perinatal medicine |
| | Neurodevelopmental disabilities |
| | Pediatric cardiology |
| | Pediatric critical care medicine |
| | Pediatric emergency medicine |
| | Pediatric endocrinology |
| | Pediatric gastroenterology |
| | Pediatric hematology-oncology |
| | Pediatric hospital medicine |
| | Pediatric infectious diseases |
| | Pediatric nephrology |
| | Pediatric pulmonology |
| | Pediatric rheumatology |
| | Pediatric transplant hepatology |
| | Sleep medicine |
| | Sports medicine |
| | Hospital medicine |
| Physical medicine and rehabilitation | Hospice and palliative medicine |
| | Neuromuscular medicine |
| | Pain medicine |
| | Pediatric rehabilitation medicine |
| | Spinal cord injury medicine |
| | Sports medicine |
| Plastic surgery | Plastic surgery within the head and neck |
| | Surgery of the hand |
| PREVENTIVE MEDICINE<br>Aerospace medicine<br>Occupational medicine<br>Public health and general preventive medicine | Addiction medicine<br>Clinical informatics<br>Medical toxicology<br>Undersea and hyperbaric medicine |
| Psychiatry<br>Neurology<br>Neurology with special qualifications in child neurology | Addiction psychiatry<br>Child and adolescent psychiatry<br>Clinical neurophysiology<br>Forensic psychiatry<br>Geriatric psychiatry<br>Hospice and palliative medicine<br>Neurodevelopmental disabilities<br>Neuromuscular medicine<br>Pain medicine<br>Psychosomatic medicine<br>Sleep medicine<br>Vascular neurology |
| RADIOLOGY<br>Diagnostic radiology<br>Radiation oncology<br>Radiologic physics | Diagnostic radiological physics<br>Hospice and palliative medicine<br>Medical nuclear physics<br>Neuroradiology<br>Nuclear radiology<br>Pediatric radiology<br>Therapeutic radiological physics<br>Vascular and interventional radiology |
| Surgery<br>Vascular surgery | Hospice and palliative medicine<br>Pediatric surgery<br>Surgery of the hand<br>Surgical critical care |
| Urology | Pediatric urology |

Data from American Board of Medical Specialties. Available at: http://www.abms.org/. Accessed July 21, 2017.

**BOX 9.3** Medical Education

Medical education in 19th- and early-20th-century America was built upon the apprentice system. Future physicians, nearly all men, worked under and learned from practicing physicians. Medical schools were often moneymaking enterprises and primarily used lectures without patient contact or laboratory experiences. That changed with the introduction of the European model of science-based medical education, hospital-based clinical rotations, and a 4-year education model.

The 1910 Flexner Report formalized these standards, which soon became universal for medical education in the United States, in what came to be called the Flexner era of U.S. medicine. This era extended into the 1980s, and at some institutions, into the 2000s. It led to the growth and dominance of specialties and specialists within particular medical fields. Hospital-based residency programs and fellowships leading to specialty and subspecialty training became the dominant form of clinical training. Emphasizing this trend, medical school education came to be called **undergraduate medical education**.

Medical school was traditionally formally or informally divided into 2 years of basic science or preclinical training, followed by 2 years of hospital-based clinical rotations in specialty areas including surgery, internal medicine, obstetrics and gynecology, and psychiatry. This division of medical education is reflected in the examinations of the National Board of Medical Examiners, which traditionally included Step 1 near the end of the second year of medical school, Step 2 prior to graduation, and Step 3 as part of the first-year residency, which is often called the "internship." Additional specialty and subspecialty board examinations were linked to completion of training that occurs after medical school.

Change began to accelerate in medical education during the mid-1980s with the increasing movement of health care outside of hospitals, the increased medical school enrollment of women and minorities, a broader view of what should be included in medical education, and a better understanding of how learning takes place. Specific changes have occurred in the last two decades at all stages of medical education, and new proposals for change continue to be formally reviewed and implemented. These can be outlined as follows, starting with the premed college years and continuing through residency and fellowship training:

- Premedical training in the Flexner era was largely restricted to majors in the physical and biological sciences, plus specific social sciences such as psychology. Beginning in the early 1990s, medical schools encouraged a wider range of majors, while usually retaining biology, chemistry, and physics courses as prerequisites. Medical schools are increasingly receptive to a wide range of preparation for medical education, encouraging completion of courses in behavioral and social sciences, including public health and epidemiology.

- The comprehensive review of the MCAT has resulted in changes to the MCAT. The changes include a new content section emphasizing the behavioral and social sciences to parallel the sections emphasizing the physical and biological sciences. A framework known as scientific inquiry and reasoning skills incorporates basic research methods and statistics into each of the content examinations.

- Admission to medical school was dominated by white males throughout the Flexner era. In the last 20–30 years, the percentage of women applicants has increased steadily. Today, the majority of medical students at many institutions are females. The number of minority applicants has increased slowly, paralleling the changes occurring in other aspects of U.S. education and society.

- The first 2 years of medical school in the Flexner era were dominated by lectures and laboratories. Basic sciences were the focus, with little or no patient contact. An important change in the last two decades includes widespread use of PBL. PBL is characterized by small-group, student-initiated learning centered on "cases," or patient-oriented problems. New curricula in medical education, including evidence-based medicine, interviewing skills, and ethics, have become a standard part of coursework. A new simulated patient interview and physical examination are now part of the certifying examination process.

- Changes in the third and fourth years of medical school began in the 1960s, the era of student activism. Since then, the fourth year of medical school has been dominated by electives. Fourth-year students may choose formal courses, elective clinical experiences, or a wide array of other options. These usually include options for laboratory or clinical research; international experiences; and clinical rotations at other institutions, often called "audition" rotations, designed to increase a graduate's potential for selection as a resident.

- The growing trend of patient treatment outside of the traditional hospital setting has increased the range of types and locations of clinical experiences available. Most medical schools now require primary care experiences, along with traditional specialty rotations.

- Residency training has paralleled the changes in medical school, with greater outpatient and less inpatient, or hospital-based, education. However, the payment systems still encourage hospital-based training. Fellowship training beyond residency is now a routine part of the process of specialization. The general move toward more and more specialization has led to longer postgraduate training. The rigors of residency training remain, but limits have now been placed on it by the Residency Review Committees, which govern graduate medical education. An average of 80 hours per week is now the maximum standard for residents.

Further changes in medical education and residency programs can be expected in the near future. The increasing recognition that health care is a group, and not an individual, enterprise is leading to a focus on interprofessional education and practice. An appreciation that evidence is central to improving quality and controlling costs should continue to encourage the critical reading of clinical research as part of evidence-based medicine in medical school and in journal clubs as part of postgraduate education. The use of computer-based information systems should increase the sharing and coordination of information, the ability to monitor and control health care, and the ways that physicians communicate with colleagues and patients. Technology is also likely to have continued unexpected impacts on the ways that medicine is taught, learned, and practiced.

Data from American Board of Medical Specialties. Available at: http://www.abms.org/. Accessed July 21, 2017.

Now let us take a brief look at the largest of the health professions—nursing.[9]

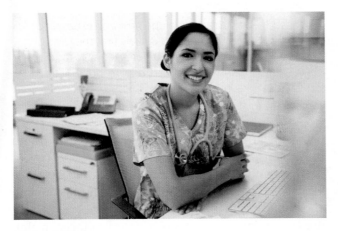

© Hero Images/Getty Images

## What Is the Education and Training Process for Nursing?

Nursing as a profession dates from the middle of the 1800s, when it began to be organized as a profession in England. Florence Nightingale is often associated with the founding of nursing as a profession. In the United States, the nursing profession grew out of the Civil War and the essential role played by women in this conflict, who performed what we today would call nursing functions. Nursing has long been organized as a distinct profession and is governed by its own set of laws, often referred to as the "nursing practice acts."

Today, there are a wide range of health professionals that fall under the legal definition of nursing.

Licensed practical nurses (LPNs), also called licensed vocational nurses in some states, provide a range of services often under the direction of registered nurses (RNs). An LPN's educational requirements vary widely from state to state, ranging from 1 year of education after high school to a 2-year associate's degree. Certified nursing assistants or nursing aides have usually completed a short-term certification program and are allowed to perform only the basic care of patients.

RNs are considered central to the nursing profession, and they are usually responsible for hospital-based services. Each state defines its own requirements for RN licensure. Traditionally, many nurses graduated with a diploma that was offered through hospital-based programs. The move toward integrating nursing into the formal degree system has resulted in nurses with associate's degrees, bachelor of science in nursing (BSN) degrees, as well as graduate degrees. Being an RN requires a state license that, depending on the state, may or may not require a BSN degree.

Advanced nursing degrees have been offered as a master of science in nursing, or as an academic research-based degree, the PhD. Recently, a clinical doctorate, the DNP is becoming central to graduate nursing education. The DNP is increasingly becoming the standard graduate degree for nursing, often replacing master's degrees.

Until recent years, there was little formal specialization within nursing, at least compared to physicians and other health professions. Nurse midwives and nurse anesthetists, however, are two traditional specializations within nursing. Graduate-level education and training of nurses has expanded rapidly in recent years. Nursing has added a series of advanced practice degrees, including NPs, as well as specialists such as pediatric, geriatric, and

---

**BOX 9.4** New and Expanding Roles for Nurses

The rapid aging of the population, expanded development and use of technology, increased complexity of our health system, and specialization by physicians have all contributed to the development of new roles for nurses. Examples of these new and expanded roles include:

- Infection control specialists are increasingly needed in hospitals, nursing homes, and other healthcare institutions to avoid the development of antibiotic resistant bacteria, control local outbreaks of infection, and manage the increasing number of immunologically compromised patients.

- Nurses have long served some of the functions now being called health navigation. Education in community health, the healthcare system, and the health insurance system, however, has been only a small portion of their formal education. This may change along with the growing need to help patients navigate the increasingly complex health system. New incentives such as those designed to avoid hospital readmission has provided new opportunities for nurses to incorporate health navigation into their practice responsibilities.

- Nurse case managers often work in hospitals to ensure timely provision of services, communications

between health professionals, and to expedite transitions to home or follow-up health facilities. Nurses are often well suited for these roles due to their experience working with patients, physicians, and administrators.

- Patient safety is now a priority in hospital and other health systems. Nurses often play key roles in investigating safety issues and identifying and implementing approaches to reducing the risk.

- Health information systems including electronic health records and administrative data systems span every aspect of the delivery and coordination of services. Nurses are increasingly playing important roles in designing, implementing, and evaluating health information systems.

- Disaster and emergency management is becoming increasingly important in healthcare institutions as well as in the community at large. Nurses can play important roles in preparation and response to disasters and emergencies.

These are only a sample of the new and expanding roles being played by nurses. It is likely that the roles of nurses will expand in new and unforeseen ways as our health system gains new abilities, new responsibilities, and increasing complexity.

---

intensive care nurses. The DNP degree is becoming standard for a range of specialty areas within nursing. Recent changes in nursing have opened up the option to pursue a bachelor's degree in a range of fields followed by a shorter accelerated degree program leading to a BSN.

The roles played by nurses in the public health and healthcare systems are expanding rapidly.[10] **BOX 9.4** discusses some of these new and expanding roles for nurses.

## ▶ What Roles Can Physicians, Nurses, and Other Clinical Health Professions Play in Public Health?

As we have seen, the aim of the initial schools of public health was to train physicians, nurses, and other professionals who sought to play lead roles in local and state health departments. Thus, for many years, public health education was often combined with other professions. **BOX 9.5** discusses the roles that clinicians still play in public health and what is increasingly

being called population health by the clinical health professions.

Remember that we have only touched on three basic types of health professionals: physicians, nurses, and public health professionals. There are several hundred other types of professions in the healthcare realm. As you think about a career in health, you should take a look at a range of health professions, using the concepts of education, training, and certification that we have discussed.

To understand the connections between the large numbers of diverse health professions, we need to look at how clinical care is organized into primary, secondary, and tertiary care.

## ▶ What Is Meant by "Primary, Secondary, and Tertiary Care"?

Primary, secondary, and tertiary care are traditional ways to categorize services delivered within the healthcare system.[12] **Primary care** traditionally refers to the first contact providers of care who are prepared to handle the great majority of common problems for which patients seek care. **Secondary care** often refers to

**BOX 9.5**  Traditional and New Roles of Clinicians in Public Health

Public health is often distinguished from the clinical health profession by its focus on populations rather than individuals, public service rather than individual service, and disease prevention and health promotion rather than disease diagnosis and treatment, and its broad perspective on the determinants of disease. However, at the professional level, individuals have commonly combined the two approaches or moved from one to the other.

Clinicians have always played key roles in public health. From the early years of formal public health training nearly a century ago, until the 1960s and 1970s, the MPH degree was aimed primarily at physicians and nurses who were expected to take up leadership roles in health departments. Today, public health professionals come from much more diverse backgrounds, many entering master's programs directly after receiving a bachelor's degree.

The role of clinicians in public health today is also far more varied. For instance, today's pharmacists—now educated as doctors of pharmacy or PharmDs—play an increasingly important public health role in providing education about drugs for patients and practitioners and controlling prescription drug abuse. Prevention of dental and gum disease and early detection of oral cancers have significantly improved due to the careful attention of dentists and dental assistants. The dental profession has been a long-standing advocate of fluoridation of public water systems and other population health interventions.

Primary care specialists, including allopathic and osteopathic physicians, NPs, and PAs, are on the front lines of clinical prevention. Their involvement in screening, behavioral counseling, immunization, and the use of preventive medication is key to the success of these efforts. Primary care clinicians, as well as specialty care clinicians, also have important roles to play in being alert to new diseases or changes in well-known diseases; reporting adverse effects of drugs, vaccines, and medical devices; and coordinating case-finding efforts with public health agencies.

Within medicine, the field of preventive medicine has a long history. Formal specializations exist in public health and general preventive medicine, occupational medicine, as well as aerospace medicine and the new subspecializations of addiction medicine and clinical informatics.

Finally, all clinicians have the right and often the responsibility to advocate for improvements in patient care and of the health system as a whole. A few clinical specialties, such as pediatrics, regard advocacy as a core responsibility of the profession. Their work has had major impacts on child health policies, ranging from the use of child car restraints, to advocacy for pediatric HIV/AIDS care, to universal coverage of childhood vaccinations, as well as the provision of comprehensive insurance coverage for children.

Collaboration between future clinicians, health administrators, and public health specialists is increasingly important as we move to connect the health care and public health systems as part of population health. The Interprofessional Education Collaborative[11] made up of over a dozen health professions educational association members has taken the lead in encouraging interprofessonal education efforts. Many of these health professions now require interprofessional education activities as part of their accreditation requirements. These increasing efforts to connect the professions should be of great benefit to the future of health care as well as public health.

specialty care provided by clinicians who focus on one or a small number of organ systems or on a specific type of service, such as obstetrics and gynecology or anesthesiology. **Tertiary care**, or subspecialty care, is usually defined in terms of the type of institution in which it is delivered, often academic or specialized health centers. Tertiary care may also be defined in terms of the type of problem that is addressed, such as trauma centers, burn centers, or neonatal intensive care units.

Primary care is widely seen as the foundation of a healthcare system, and a strong primary care system is viewed as a prerequisite for maximizing the potential benefits of health care. Traditionally, primary care was considered the domain of physicians. Today, a range of health professionals are involved in primary, as well as secondary and tertiary, care. In fact, the term "**medical home**" is becoming widely used, suggesting that primary care is increasingly viewed as a team effort.

Today, only about one-third of physicians in the United States practice primary care, and this proportion is shrinking. Increasingly, primary care is being delivered by PAs and nurse practitioners NPs, who in most states have authority to diagnose disease and prescribe medication either under the supervision of a physician (in the case of PAs) or under a nursing practice act (as in the case of NPs). A team approach to primary care is becoming standard practice. NPs now have greater ability to bill directly for services without going through a physician.

It is important to understand the ideals of primary care, as well as today's realities.[12] Primary care is key to the healthcare system because it is where most care is delivered, and it is often the entry point for subsequent specialty care. In addition, primary care is critical to the delivery of clinical preventive services and to the connections between health care and public

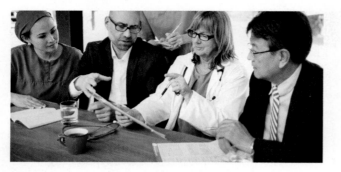

© Rawpixel.com/Shutterstock

health. Ideal primary care has been described using six Cs: contact, comprehensive, coordinated, continuity, caring, and community.

- "Contact" implies first contact with patients as they present for health care.
- "Comprehensive" refers to the ability of primary care practitioners or primary care teams to

completely or at least initially address most health issues.

- "Coordinated" relates to the concept that primary care teams should have the responsibility to ensure that the parts of the healthcare system work together for the good of patients.
- "Continuity" is the role that primary care teams see themselves playing to hold together the components of the system.
- "Caring" implies a personalized relationship with each patient.
- "Community" implies that primary care provides the link with the broader community, including with public health institutions and services.

Despite the fact that many primary care practitioners continue to see this model of primary care as a highly desirable way to deliver clinical care, the realities of today's healthcare system deviate substantially from this model. **TABLE 9.2** outlines the six Cs

| **TABLE 9.2** Ideals and Realities of Primary Care—the Six Cs | | |
|---|---|---|
| | **Primary care ideals** | **Realities** |
| Contact | The point of first contact with the healthcare system—the entry point | Patients enter the healthcare system through many disconnected points, including the emergency room, specialists, urgent care centers, nontraditional practitioners, etc. |
| Comprehensive | Primary care intends to be able to diagnose and treat the great majority of problems | Rapid increase in possible treatments and high-volume practices increase proportion of patient problems that are referred to specialists |
| Coordinated | Primary care intends to be the focal point for diagnosis and treatment, with coordination through referral to specialists for consultation and feedback | Primary care physicians increasingly being replaced by "hospitalists," who are full time in the hospital, provide care for inpatients, and direct patient access to specialists |
| Continuity | Patient followed over many years—continuous care provision | Patients increasingly required or encouraged to change physicians/providers for insurance purposes |
| Caring | Individualized care based on individual relationships | Primary care increasingly becoming an administrative entity without long-term individual relationships |
| Community | Primary care designed to connect the individual patient with community resources and community requirements (required examinations, reportable diseases, vaccinations, driver's licenses, etc.) | Healthcare professionals and public health have a long history of distant and—at times—contentious relationships |

Data from Institute of Medicine. Defining Primary Care: An Interim Report. Washington DC: National Academies Press; 1994.

and indicates ways that the current healthcare system differs from this primary care ideal.[12b]

Thus, there is a large gulf between the ideals of primary care and their execution in practice. Part of the reason for this and other realities of health care can be better understood by looking at how health professionals are rewarded and compensated.

## ▶ How Are Clinical Health Professionals Rewarded and Compensated for Their Services?

Physicians—and, increasingly, other health professionals—are compensated through a variety of mechanisms. Compensation levels depend on the site where care is delivered, the nature of the patient's insurance, and the type of institution in which the professional works or is employed.

Complicating the issues of coordination of services and continuity of care is the fact that patients can and are often encouraged to change insurance coverage on a yearly basis. Thus, clinicians now live in a complex, changing, and often confusing world in which issues of compensation can get in the way of quality care. Despite the best of intentions, many clinicians find themselves having to address compensation as another "C." **TABLE 9.3** outlines a number of methods of financial compensation to providers of health services and examines some of their advantages and disadvantages.

**TABLE 9.3** Method of Financial Compensation to Providers of Health Services

| Compensation method | Meaning | Examples | Advantages | Disadvantages |
|---|---|---|---|---|
| Fee-for-service | Clinician paid for each covered service | Physicians often paid for medical visits and procedure, but may not be paid for counseling for prevention | Reward linked directly to work performed    Encourages efficiency of delivery of services | May encourage delivery of unnecessary, as well as necessary, services |
| Capitation | Clinicians are paid a set amount per time period for each patient for whom they are responsible, regardless of level of use of services | Primary care physicians in health plans may be paid a set amount per patient per month and are expected to provide all primary care services | Discourages unnecessary care, may encourage preventive care, allows for predictable budgeting | May discourage necessary care, may encourage referral to specialists unless specialty care is financially discouraged |
| Episode of care | Institution or clinician is paid a set amount for providing comprehensive services, such as hospital treatment based on the patient's diagnosis | Medicare pays for hospital care based on diagnosis-related groups, allowing a defined number of days per condition | Encourages rapid and efficient delivery of care | May encourage discharge prior to ability to provide self-care |
| Salary | Set amount per time period | Governmental facilities generally pay clinicians on a seniority-based salary | May allow focus on quality | May discourage efficiency |

*(continues)*

b  A new approach, often called **concierge practice**, is attempting to provide primary care based upon many of these principles. Concierge practices often limit the number of patients they serve, provide more time for appointments, and guarantee same or next-day access to appointments. However, to provide these services, concierge practices often charge several thousand dollars per patient as a yearly charge, which is not covered by insurance. Thus, concierge practices have been limited to those who can afford to pay for these services.

**TABLE 9.3** Method of Financial Compensation to Providers of Health Services *(continued)*

| Compensation method | Meaning | Examples | Advantages | Disadvantages |
|---|---|---|---|---|
| Pay for performance "P4P" | Compensation adjusted based on measures of the quality of care delivered | Additional compensation for adherence to evidence-based guidelines New P4P being instituted as part of Medicare reimbursement | Links income with quality, providing strong incentive for quality | Difficult to measure quality, outcomes may be related to factors outside clinician's control |

In addition to the mechanism of payment for services, another key factor that affects health professionals is the number of people in the profession. Let us look at how the right number makes a difference.

## How Can We Ensure the System Has the Right Number of Healthcare Professionals?

Financial compensation is the fundamental market mechanism for regulating the supply of most professionals. This mechanism has not generally worked well in the health professions. The demand for positions in medical schools, for instance, far exceeds the supply. Thus, much of the control over the number of professionals who are trained has been made by the profession itself through policies that control the number and size of accredited degree-granting institutions.

This control has had limited success. For instance, in the 1980s, dentists determined that there was an oversupply of dentists. A number of dental schools were closed and new dental schools were limited. Today, there is an undersupply of dentists. Balancing the supply and demand for health professionals is a complex undertaking, as illustrated by the current shortage of nurses.[13] The nursing shortage is discussed in **BOX 9.6**.

We have now taken a look at the complex world of healthcare and public health professions, including the creation of health professions through education, training, and credentialing. We have also looked at issues of compensation and how we can try to ensure the right numbers of health professionals. Now, let us turn our attention to examining the institutions in which health care is delivered.

**BOX 9.6** The Nursing Shortage and What Is Being Done About It

Nursing is the largest of the health professions, with approximately 3 million RNs. Interest in nursing is growing rapidly, but nursing schools have not been able to keep up with the growing interest, turning down approximately one applicant for every two accepted. The number of U.S.-trained RNs has not kept up with demand.

The shortage of nurses, especially those who work in the increasingly technical hospital environment, continues to grow. The projected size of the shortage is controversial, but estimates of a shortage of 200,000 or more RNs in the coming years are commonly quoted. Everyone agrees that nursing is one of the most (if not the most) rapidly growing professions in terms of available job positions. The shortage is made worse by the fact that the average age of nurses is increasing, because until very recently, there was a decline in the number of newly trained nurses.

Why is there such a large shortage of nurses? A number of factors contribute to this problem, reflecting changes in nursing and the U.S. society. There is both a greater demand for nursing services and a supply that is not growing fast enough. Among the factors and what is being done about them are:

- *Technology*—The increased availability and use of technology has increased the need for technically skilled nurses. Many nursing programs now emphasize high-tech applications of nursing, but the number of recent graduates possessing these skills is still small compared to the demand.
- *More patients*—The aging baby boomer generation is expected to have a major impact on the need for nursing services. The large number of baby boomers born between 1946 and 1964 will need and expect increased nursing services. Increasingly, other health

professions are contributing to the community-based care of the elderly.

- *Image of nursing as a female profession*—Until recently nursing has been overwhelmingly a woman's profession, which has historically limited its attractiveness to men. The image of nursing as a male as well as a female profession is being encouraged by advertisements and recruitment efforts. In addition, many women leave the profession or practice part time, which may be accelerated by the increasingly stressful nature of the work, especially in hospitals. Flexible work scheduling may help counter some of these impacts.
- *Restrictions on entry*—Until recently, nursing education was self-contained—to become a nurse, you needed to complete an undergraduate nursing degree, and the only way to pursue a graduate nursing degree was to already have a bachelor's degree in nursing. This is changing rapidly as new options open up for accelerated BSN and graduate degree education.

- *Shortage of nursing faculty*—A shortage of nursing faculty and training facilities has also contributed to the shortage of nurses and the ability to rapidly expand the size of colleges of nursing. Nurse education has traditionally been restricted to doctoral-level nurses. Expanding the potential qualifications for nursing faculty may provide the ability to more rapidly increase the student bodies of schools of nursing.

A national effort is now under way to increase the number of nurses being educated. In the meantime a number of approaches are being used to deal with the realities of the nursing shortage. These include higher salaries, use of foreign trained and traveling nurses, and raising the status of nursing through a greater legally permitted scope of practice.

Progress is being made on addressing the nursing shortage, but it will be many years until the supply of qualified nurses meets the demand.

## Key Words

| | | |
|---|---|---|
| Accreditation | Hospitalist | Tertiary care |
| Certification | Licensure | Undergraduate medical |
| Concierge practice | Medical home | education |
| Credentialing | Primary care | |
| Health navigation | Secondary care | |

## Discussion Questions

Take a look at the questions posed in the following scenarios, which were presented at the beginning of this chapter. See now whether you can answer them.

1. Upon your arrival at the hospital, the nurse specialist examines you and consults with the radiologists, the gastroenterologist, and the general surgeon. Your medication is reviewed by the pharmacist and your meals by the clinical nutritionist. Throughout the hospitalization, you are followed by a hospitalist. Once you get back home, the home care team comes to see you regularly for the first 2 weeks, and the certified physician assistant (PAs) and the doctor of nursing practice (DNP) see you in the office. You realize that health care is no longer just about doctors and nurses. You ask yourself: What roles do all of these health professionals play in the healthcare system?

2. Jenna decides that after college, she wants to become a doctor and see patients and practice medicine. "I thought there was only one kind of doctor who could diagnose disease and prescribe medicine," she mentions at a career counseling meeting. "Not so, anymore," says her

advisor. "There are allopathic and osteopathic physicians. In addition, there are nurse practitioners (NPs) who are authorized to diagnose and prescribe medications, and there are PAs who do the same under a physician's supervision. The universe of 'doctors' now includes doctors of nursing practice, as well as other doctoral degree professionals, such as pharmacists, occupational therapists, and physical therapists." *Understanding careers in health care can be as difficult for students as it is for patients*, Jenna thinks to herself. Now she understands why her advisor asked: "What do you mean by 'practice'? What do you mean by 'doctor'?"

3. Sarah was about to begin medical school and was expecting 2 years of "preclinical" classroom lectures focusing on the basic sciences, followed by the study of clinical diseases. Then, as she had heard from her physician father, she expected 2 years of clinical hospital "rotations" and electives investigating specialties. She is surprised to find that medical school has changed. There are small-group, PBL sessions where she needs to be able to locate and read the research literature. There is contact with patients and their problems

right from the beginning. There is increasingly a 4-year approach instead of a preclinical and clinical approach to medical education. She wonders: Are these changes for the better? What else needs to be done to improve medical education?

4. You are interested in clinical care, as well as public health. *I need to make a choice*, you think to yourself. "Not necessarily," your advisor says. "There are many ways to combine clinical care with public health." After a little investigation, you find out that undergraduate public health education is increasingly seen as preparation for clinical education, and clinical prevention and population health are increasingly becoming part of clinical care. In addition, many careers, from health administration, to health policy, to health education, to clinical research, combine the individual orientation of clinical care with the population perspective of public health. So what is the best pathway to a public health career for you?

## References

1. Shi L, Singh DA. *Delivering health care in America: a systems approach.* Burlington, MA: Jones & Bartlett Learning; 2019.
2. Association of Schools and Programs of Public Health. Framing the future: The second hundred years of education for public health. http://www.aspph.org/educate/#educational -models. Accessed July 21, 2017.
3. Gebbie K, Rosenstock L, Hernandez LM. *Who Will Keep the Public Healthy? Educating Public Health Professionals for the 21st Century.* Washington, DC: National Academy Press; 2003: 144.
4. League for Innovation in the Community College. Community Colleges and Public Health Report. https://www.league.org /ccph. Accessed July 21, 2017.
5. Association of Schools and Programs of Public Health. ASPH Policy Brief. Confronting the Public Health Workforce Crisis. Executive Summary. http://www.healthpolicyfellows.org/pdfs /ConfrontingthePublicHealthWorkforceCrisisbyASPH .pdf. Accessed July 21, 2017.
6. National Board of Public Health Examiners. About NBPHE. https://www.nbphe.org/about/. Accessed July 21, 2017.
7. American Board of Medical Specialties. Specialties and subspecialties. http://www.abms.org Accessed July 21, 2017.
8. Ludmerer KM. *Time to Heal: American Medical Education from the Turn of the Century to the Era of Managed Care.* New York: Oxford University Press; 2005.
9. American Board of Nursing Specialties. Accredited Certification Programs. http://www.nursingcertification.org Accessed July 21, 2017.
10. Nursing.com. New and emerging roles for nurses. https:// www.nurse.com/blog/2013/02/11/new-and-emerging-roles -for-nurses-2/. Accessed July 21, 2017.
11. Interprofessional Education Collaborative. Connecting health professions for better care. https://www.ipecollaborative.org /about-ipec.html. Accessed July 21, 2017.
12. Institute of Medicine. *Defining Primary Care: An Interim Report.* Washington, DC: National Academy Press; 1994.
13. American Association of Colleges of Nursing. Nursing shortage. http://www.aacn.nche.edu/media-relations/fact-sheets/nursing -shortage. Accessed July 21, 2017.

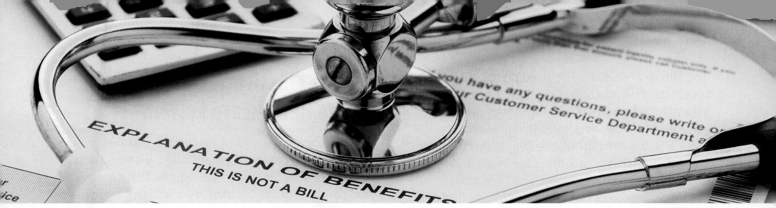

# CHAPTER 10

# Healthcare Institutions

George did not have health insurance and went to the emergency room whenever he needed care. They always treated him there, but then tried to get him connected to a primary care facility. He was not eligible for care at the Veterans Administration (VA) facilities, so they sent him to the local community health center, which they called the "safety net" provider. George did go there and they tried to treat his problems and get him his medicine. When he got sick, however, George went back to the emergency department. Even George agreed that it was not the best way to get care, but he wondered: What is needed to make the system work better?

Laura had breast cancer, and it had spread. Her medical records were on file at the hospital, at four doctors' offices, in two emergency rooms, and at an outpatient imaging facility. No one seemed to know how to put the system together. Whenever her old records were essential, they asked her to go get a copy of them and bring them to her next appointment. That worked for a while, but when she ended up in the emergency room, her records just were not available. Health care should be able to do better in the age of the Internet, Laura thought to herself. She wondered whether the system will work better as electronic health records become widely available.

Fred ended his walk one day at the emergency room. He seemed confused about how to get home. "It looks like we are dealing with Alzheimer's," his doctor told Fred's wife, Sonya, at their next appointment. Taking care of Fred at home was not easy. Home health aides and occasional weekend relief called "respite care" eased the burden for a while. The new assisted-living facilities looked attractive, but Fred's family just could not afford one. When Fred fell and broke his hip, he required hospitalization for surgery. The hospital discharge planner arranged for a skilled nursing home for rehabilitation services paid for by Medicare. After a few weeks there, the only alternative was long-term or custodial care in a nursing home paid for by Medicaid. The care at the nursing home was not what the family had expected. The staff did clean Fred up before the announced family visits, but once when the family arrived unannounced, they were shocked to see Fred lying half-naked in his wheelchair. The end came almost two years from the day they moved him to the nursing home. Looking back, the family asked: Can the healthcare system do better at addressing the needs of Alzheimer's patients?

Wanda, an experienced nurse, volunteers to transport a patient to radiology when no one else is available. As she is rolling the patient down the hall, the wheelchair hits a fire extinguisher on the wall. The patient falls out of the wheelchair and hits his head, suffering an internal bleed requiring emergency surgery. Wanda's supervisor gives her a written and verbal reprimand indicating that if she had been more careful the "adverse event" would not have happened. Wanda asks herself: Aren't these types of mistakes system problems rather than personal problems?

These are the types of situations faced by many patients as they try to navigate through the institutions that provide health care in the United States. Let us take a look at these different institutions.

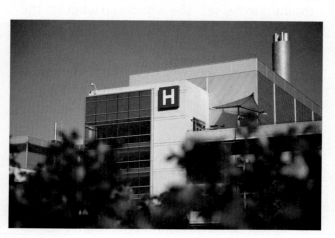

## ▶ What Institutions Make Up the Healthcare System?

The number and types of healthcare institutions are almost as diverse and complicated as the number and types of healthcare professionals. In recent years, the complexity has grown as a range of facilities have developed to serve new needs and new financial reimbursement approaches.[1,2] Nonetheless, it is possible to understand the scope of healthcare institutions by categorizing them as **inpatient facilities** and **outpatient facilities**, with inpatient facilities implying that patients remain in the facility for at least 24 hours.

Inpatient facilities include hospitals, skilled nursing and rehabilitation facilities, nursing homes, and institutional hospices. Outpatient facilities include those providing clinical services by one or more clinicians and those providing diagnostic testing or treatment. We will provide an overview of inpatient and outpatient facilities and then ask: Do these facilities together provide a coordinated system of care? Let us begin by looking at inpatient facilities.

## ▶ What Types of Inpatient Facilities Exist in the United States?

We can classify inpatient facilities as: (1) hospitals generally designed for short-term stays by patients, and (2) long-term care facilities. Let us first take a look at hospitals.

The history of hospitals in the United States goes back to the colonial period. However, prior to the middle of the 1800s, hospitals were generally institutions for those without other sources of care, which included the poor, the military, and those with communicable diseases. Hospitals generally provided little more than shelter and food and separated the sick—especially those with communicable diseases—from the healthy.[1]

Today, the U.S. hospital is usually a modern high-tech enterprise that lies at the center of the healthcare system educationally, structurally, and psychologically. You can often identify the hospital from far away because it is frequently the largest and most modern facility in town. The psychological hold that the hospital has on U.S. health care is symbolized by the term "house" and the concept of "house staff," or residents who practically live full time in the hospital during their training.[3,a]

Hospitals share some common features, including:

- Hospitals are licensed by the state and usually accredited by a national organization, such as The Joint Commission (formally called the Joint Commission on the Accreditation of Healthcare Organizations).
- Hospitals have an organized physician staff and provide 24-hour-a-day nursing services.
- The hospital is governed by a governing board separate from the medical and nursing staff that has overall responsibility for the operation of the hospital consistent with state and federal laws.

The several types of hospitals in the United States differ in their purposes and organizational structures. Hospitals can be categorized as general hospitals and specialty hospitals. General hospitals attempt to serve a wide spectrum of patients and problems, though they may concentrate on serving only children or only those who qualify for services, such as a VA hospital.

In the past, specialty hospitals sought to serve the needs of patients who could not be accommodated in general hospitals, such as those with tuberculosis or severe mental illness. Today, these conditions are usually addressed in general hospitals. Today's specialty hospitals are more a result of the specialization of medical services. Institutions focused on cancer, heart disease, psychiatric illness, ophthalmology, and orthopedics, for instance, are rapidly developing.

Hospitals are often categorized today by their funding source and financial arrangements. They can be divided into nonprofit and for-profit, or investor-owned, hospitals. Nearly 90% of the approximately 5,000 hospitals in the United States are nonprofits. These include the broad category of private nonprofit hospitals, hospitals run by the state or federal government, and hospitals run by institutions, such as universities.[b]

Approximately half of these 5,000 hospitals are private nonprofit hospitals, many of which have affiliations with religious denominations, but accept patients of all faiths. State and local governments run nearly 20% of hospitals, many of which are described—along with private nonprofit hospitals—as community hospitals. Federal medical institutions include the VA hospitals and the military hospital system. For-profit, or investor-owned, hospitals make up over 10% of all hospitals, many of which are owned by a small number of large corporations specializing in providing healthcare services.

Hospitals today are often more than an inpatient facility. The most rapidly growing component of most hospitals is the spectrum of outpatient services they provide. In addition to emergency departments, hospitals usually also provide outpatient surgical and medical services, including diagnostic and treatment services, and may provide facilities for routine office-type visits.

The hospital should no longer be viewed as one building. Hospital networks or systems are increasingly being created, some of which provide a range of services, including skilled nursing and rehabilitative services, as well as long-term care.

We have classified inpatient facilities as including hospitals and long-term care facilities. Today, there are a range of long-term care facilities, some of which are not primarily operated as healthcare facilities.[1,2] These facilities may include skilled nursing facilities, nursing homes, assisted living and dementia care, and, at times, hospice care. To fully understand the provision of long-term care, you also need to appreciate the types of services that are increasingly being provided in an individual's home.

It is important to distinguish between skilled nursing and rehabilitative services in contrast to nursing home or custodial services. Skilled nursing and rehabilitative services, like hospital services, are generally short term and aimed at accomplishing specific objectives, such as recovery from a stroke or injury. Though these services may continue for many months, they are not designed to provide long-term care beyond the point at which improvement can no longer be expected.

Nursing homes, on the other hand, are designed for long-term or custodial care, while also providing a limited amount of healthcare services. Individuals

---

a  The book *The House of God*, written in the 1960s, captured the mentality of the house staff of the era and has been unofficial required reading by subsequent generations of residents. It portrays house staff as having their own culture and portrays patients, as well as community physicians, in often disparaging ways.

b  Hospitals are also categorized as teaching and nonteaching hospitals. A teaching hospital is one that has one or more accredited residency programs. Today, many community hospitals, as well as federal and state hospitals, have residency programs. The designation **academic health center** implies a medical school, one or more other health professions schools, and an affiliated hospital.

in nursing homes usually require care because of their inability to perform what are called **activities of daily living**, such as dressing, feeding, and/or bathing themselves. Nursing homes may provide routine medical care and some acute care, but this type of facility is not primarily designed to improve the medical status of its residents.[c]

Nursing homes are generally operated according to a specific set of nursing home regulations determined by and enforced by the states. Federal minimal standards are set as part of the requirements to receive payment through the Medicare and especially the Medicaid system. Most nursing homes, like most hospitals, are run as private nonprofit institutions. However, for-profit, or investor-owned, nursing homes provide approximately 15% of the beds nationally.

There are over 16,000 nursing homes in the United States, with over 1.5 million residents. Most, but not all, residents are elderly. Over 80% need help with mobility, nearly 66% are considered incontinent, and nearly 50% require assistance with eating. Alzheimer's patients are the most rapidly growing population in the nursing home system of care.[1,2]

Assisted-living facilities increasingly provide long-term care for those who have less severe impairments. Assisted-living facilities are not organized as healthcare facilities, but may provide or coordinate health care as part of their services. Newer concepts, such as continuing care retirement communities, attempt to provide a range of options, including independent-living, assisted-living, and nursing home facilities.

Most elderly and disabled individuals are not residents in long-term care institutions; rather, they live on their own or with family members. Thus, much attention in recent years has been paid to providing and financing home healthcare services, including home health aides, health care delivered at home, and respite care. Respite care provides short-term time away for primary caregivers such as family members.

The hospice movement today can be viewed as part of the long-term care system. It is care designed for those with a life expectancy of six months or less as determined by a physician. The goal of hospice care is to provide comfort, emotional support, and palliation—not to increase longevity. In some cases, hospice care may occur in a separate institution, but today, it is more often provided in the patient's place of residence.

## What Types of Outpatient Facilities Exist in the United States?

The variety of types of outpatient facilities is even more diverse and complicated than that of inpatient facilities. The basic distinction between clinical facilities and diagnostic testing or therapeutic facilities helps define the types of services provided.

Clinical services were traditionally viewed as being provided in "the doctor's office." None of these words—"the," "doctor's," "office"—does a good job of describing the current organization of clinical services. "The" implies one. Today, clinical services are rarely organized around one doctor or clinician. Group practice and multispecialty practices have become the rule. "Doctors" (or physicians) are by no means the only health professionals to organize and provide clinical services. Physical therapists, nurse practitioners, audiologists, optometrists, clinical psychologists, and a long list of other health professionals often provide their own office services. Rather than "doctor," the term **provider** is increasingly used to encompass this growing array of health professionals. Even the term "office" is no longer appropriate. In addition to the traditional office setting, many clinicians now provide services in shopping centers and work places, and even make house calls.

The average American makes over three visits for clinical services per year. An increasing number of these visits are provided outside of "the doctor's office" in the traditional sense. These sites now include a growing network of community health centers designed to provide what is called the "safety net" services for those who cannot or do not wish to seek other types of clinical services. **BOX 10.1** provides an overview of community health centers.[4,5]

A key issue in the organization of health care is the delivery of quality services. Let us take a look at what we mean by "quality" and what mechanisms are being used to ensure the quality of healthcare services.

## What Do We Mean by the "Quality of Healthcare Services?"

The quality of healthcare services may mean different things to different people. Administrators may focus

---

c Some states, such as California, have developed an additional long-term care model that is not part of the "medical model." That is, limited or no nursing care is provided and the facility is not obligated to provide services if the individual's health status changes substantially. In addition these facilities do not generally accept Medicaid payments.

## BOX 10.1 Community Health Centers

Initially named neighborhood health centers, community health centers were established in 1965 as part of the Johnson administration's War on Poverty. The centers were designed based on a community empowerment philosophy that encouraged the flow of funds directly to nonprofit, community-level organizations, often bypassing state governments.

The Health Centers Consolidation Act of 1996 combined community health centers with healthcare services for migrants, the homeless population, and residents of public housing to create the consolidated health centers program under Section 330 of the Public Health Service Act. These centers are often called 330 grantees. To receive a 330 grant, a clinic must meet certain statutory requirements. It must:

- Be located in a federally designated medically underserved area or serve a federally designated medically underserved population
- Have nonprofit, public, or tax exempt status

- Provide comprehensive primary healthcare services, referrals, and other services needed to facilitate access to care, such as case management, translation, and transportation
- Have a governing board, the majority of whose members are patients of the health center
- Provide services to all in the service area regardless of ability to pay, and offer a sliding fee schedule that adjusts according to family income

Community health centers have undergone rapid expansion in recent years and now serve approximately 27 million individuals annually in approximately 10,000 communities in all 50 states and the District of Columbia. Most patients have low incomes, and the majority qualifies for Medicaid. According to an external review, "health centers have proven to be an effective investment of federal funds, have garnered sustained goodwill and advocacy in the communities they serve, and, as a result, generally have enjoyed broad, bipartisan support."[4]

---

on the structures, such as the availability of operating rooms or laboratory services. Clinicians may focus on the process, such as the technical competence of the practitioners. Patients may focus on different types of processes, like the personal relationships and their personal satisfaction. External reviewers may focus on the outcome—lives saved or disabilities prevented.

Quality can be assessed using what are called **structure, process, and outcome measures**. Structure focuses on the physical and organizational infrastructure in which care is delivered. Process concentrates on the procedures and formal processes that go into delivering care—for example, systems for ensuring credentialing of health professionals and procedures to ensure timely response to complaints. Outcome measures imply a focus on the result of care, from rates of infection to readmissions with complications.

Defining and measuring quality remains a controversial subject. However, the National Committee for Quality Assurance (NCQA) has developed a widely recognized general framework to assist with this challenge.[6] **TABLE 10.1** outlines this framework.[d]

The complexity of inpatient and outpatient services in the United States has made the delivery of quality healthcare services very challenging. The complexity of the system raises two closely connected questions:

- How can the pieces of the system be coordinated to provide integrated care?
- How can we improve and ensure the quality of health care?

The coordination and integration of healthcare delivery is often considered key to both the efficiency and the quality of health care. Let us begin by taking a look at how healthcare delivery can be coordinated among institutions.

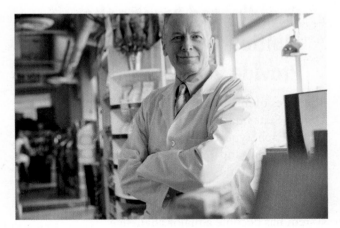
© Hero Images/Getty Images

---

d  Note that NCQA's framework emphasizes structure and process measures with little emphasis on the actual outcomes of care.

**TABLE 10.1** Characteristics of Healthcare Quality—National Committee for Quality Assurance

| Characteristic | Meaning | Examples | How is it measured? |
|---|---|---|---|
| Access and service | Access to needed care and good customer service | Enough primary care physicians and specialists<br>　Satisfaction of patients in terms of problems obtaining care | Patient satisfaction surveys, patient grievances and follow-up, interviews with staff |
| Qualified providers | Personnel licensed and trained and patients satisfied with services | System for checking credentials with sanctions<br>　Patient satisfaction with providers of care | Presence of system for checking credentials<br>　Patient satisfaction surveys |
| Staying healthy | Quality of services that help people maintain good health and avoid illness | Presence of guidelines for appropriate clinical preventive services<br>　Evidence that patients are receiving appropriate screening tests | Review of independently verified clinical records<br>　Review of responses from patients |
| Getting better | Quality of services that help people recover from illness | Presence of method for evaluating new procedures, drugs, and devices to ensure that patients have access to the most up-to-date care<br>　Providing specific services, such as smoking cessation | Review of independently verified clinical records<br>　Interviews with staff |
| Living with illness | Quality of services that help people manage chronic illness | Programs to assist patients to manage chronic conditions like asthma<br>　Provision of specific services, such as eye examinations for diabetics | Review of independently verified clinical records<br>Interviews with staff |

Data from NCQA Report Cards. Available at https://reportcards.ncqa.org/#/methodology. Accessed July 21, 2017.

## ▶ How Can Health Care Be Coordinated Among the Multiple Institutions That Provide Healthcare Services?

The types of institutions that deliver health care in the United States have continued to proliferate in recent years. Each type differs in its governance, finance, accreditation, and organizational structure. It is not surprising that most patients, policy makers, and even clinicians do not have a good overview of the system. Connecting the institutions to achieve an organized system has become a major challenge.

**Healthcare delivery systems** aim to connect inpatient and outpatient services, as well as short-term and long-term clinical services, to provide a coordinated system of care. The desire for an integrated healthcare delivery system is not a new idea. For many years, the concept of "the patient's doctor" was seen as the mechanism to hold together the system. The doctor provided all care or coordinated the care with other clinicians. The doctor "followed" the patient into the inpatient facility and provided the patient's "follow-up" care after he or she left.

Like the concept of "the doctor's office," the concept of "the patient's doctor" is no longer a reflection of reality. Once again "the" rarely reflects the reality of multiple providers of care. Primary care physicians are now far less likely to follow the patient and take care of the patient in the hospital or the nursing home and far less likely to be aware of the patient's multiple sources of care.

Efforts to integrate the system are under way. We will look at two basic approaches that are being used: the development of integrated healthcare delivery systems and the use of integrated electronic medical records. These approaches are likely to be used together and form the basis for a future integrated system of healthcare delivery. In order to understand the uses and potential of these two approaches, we first need to think about the types of coordination of care that we want to see occur and the purposes they serve.

## What Types of Coordination of Care Are Needed and What Purposes Do They Serve?

As we have discussed, the traditional approach to coordination of care revolved around the clinician–patient or doctor–patient relationship. Traditionally, the concepts of continuity of care and coordination of care have been almost synonymous. This approach assumed that the relationship between one doctor and one patient would provide the individualized knowledge, trust, and commitment that would ensure the coordination of care by ensuring the continuity of care. The concepts of primary care that we have discussed were built in large part upon this concept of one-to-one continuity.

Today, there is an increasing emphasis on ensuring coordination rather than one-to-one continuity.

Coordination is sought between institutions and settings where care is delivered. The approach that leaves continuity of information and continuity of responsibility for care to individual clinicians alone has often failed to produce the desired results. As we will see, efforts are underway to formally link institutions, services, and information between the various healthcare delivery sites and institutions.

Institutional coordination often relies on financial coordination. If services are covered by insurance in one setting but not another, the system is not likely to function efficiently or effectively. When services are not covered at all, patients may receive excellent care in one setting only to lose the benefits of that care when necessary preparation or follow-up is not paid for and not accomplished in another setting.

Coordination is not just an issue within the healthcare delivery system; it is also an issue that straddles healthcare delivery and public health functions. Communicable disease control and environmental protections, such as controlling antibiotic resistance and lead exposure, cannot be successful without effective and efficient coordination between healthcare and public health professionals and institutions. **TABLE 10.2** outlines these types of coordination, their intended function, and the types of challenges that commonly occur with their implementation.

**TABLE 10.2** Type of Coordination of Care, Intended Functions, and Challenges with Implementation

| Type of coordination | Intended function | Challenges with implementation |
|---|---|---|
| Clinician–patient relationship | Continuity as a mechanism for ensuring coordination<br><br>Development of one-to-one relationships built on knowledge and trust over extended periods of time | Multiple clinicians involved in care<br>Team rather than individual concept of primary care<br>Frequent changes in insurance coverage require change in health professionals |
| Institutional coordination | Coordination of individual's information between institutions needed to inform individual clinical and administrative decision making | Different structures and governance often lead to lack of coordination between inpatient facilities and between inpatient and outpatient facilities |
| Financial coordination | Implies that a patient has comprehensive coverage for services provided by the full range of institutions<br>Aims to maximize the efficiency of the care received and minimize the administrative effort required to manage the payment system | Lack of comprehensive insurance coverage often means that essential services cannot be delivered or cannot be delivered at the most efficient or effective institutional site |
| Coordination between health care and public health | Coordination of services between clinical care and public heath requires communication to ensure follow-up and to protect the health of others | Lack of coordination of services between public health services and clinical care is often based on lack of communications |

Let us take a look at the development of healthcare delivery systems as one approach to ensuring coordination of health care.

## What Types of Healthcare Delivery Systems Are Being Developed and How Can They Help Ensure Coordination of Health Care?

We will use the term "healthcare delivery system" to imply a linkage of institutions and healthcare professionals that together take on the responsibility of delivering coordinated care.[e]

In a nation such as the United States, in which health care is provided by a range of providers and institutions, holding together one delivery system is not easy. A wide range of efforts are under way to connect the pieces. Let us take a look at some successful examples.

Care coordination challenges have been quite successfully met in the emergency response system. Today, there is a network of institutions, including government agencies and private emergency medical services providers that cooperate with hospital emergency departments to facilitate and expedite the care of the seriously ill and injured. The emergency response system helps to quickly respond to emergencies, provide onsite assistance and information, and identify the healthcare institution that is best prepared to handle the emergency based on location, staffing, and capabilities. This system, while not perfect, demonstrates that coordination of care—at least urgent care—is possible.

Coordination of routine health care has proven to be a more difficult challenge. **Healthcare systems** are beginning to be developed, often based on common ownership or governance. These integrated systems are designed to provide a wide range of services, from outpatient clinical care, diagnostic testing, and treatment services, to inpatient, home health, skilled nursing, nursing home, and even hospice care.

Two of the longest standing and most developed healthcare systems are the Kaiser Permanente and VA systems.[7,8] These are discussed in **BOX 10.2**. Many more healthcare systems are being formed by caregivers, such as multispecialty group practices, and by institutions, such as university medical centers. The coming years are likely to produce a number of successful models that will become examples that others will try to replicate.

In addition to the development of comprehensive healthcare delivery systems, experimentation is under way to improve the functioning of existing systems such as Medicare. These demonstration programs are designed to improve performance and often focus on incentives for efficiency and coordination of care. **BOX 10.3** discusses a number of the Medicare demonstration programs that are now underway.[9]

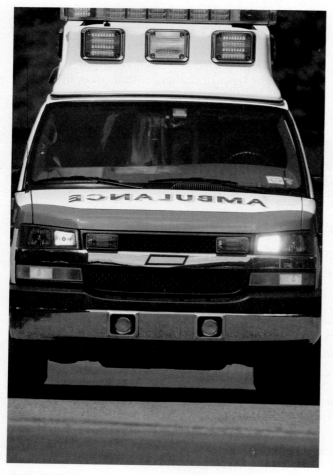

© Tetra Images/Getty Images

## How Can Electronic Medical Records Be Used To Facilitate Coordination of Care and Improve Quality?

There is widespread agreement that an electronic health record system could improve coordination

---

e   We will distinguish healthcare delivery systems, healthcare systems, and **health systems**. Healthcare delivery systems include the delivery of healthcare services to a defined population. A healthcare system also includes the financial arrangements needed to pay for the care. A health system, the broadest of the three terms, includes the public health system, as well as the healthcare system.

**BOX 10.2** Healthcare Delivery Systems: Kaiser Permanente and the Veterans Administration

The Kaiser Permanente and the VA healthcare systems are two of the largest organized healthcare systems in the United States. They have very different histories and philosophies, and they serve quite different populations. Nonetheless, they have both moved in the direction of developing an integrated set of healthcare delivery institutions linked together by an electronic health record and fostering evidence-based interventions. They share a common advantage in that they are financed by single sources, the Kaiser Permanente health plan and the federal government, respectively.

Kaiser helped introduce the concept of the health maintenance organization by offering a comprehensive package of preventive and curative services at a fixed monthly fee. The Kaiser Permanente health system has its roots in World War II, when employers offered health benefits when they were prohibited from raising wages. In the subsequent decades, Kaiser Permanente grew from its California base, enrolling over nine million individuals. It was created as a staff model prepaid health plan, enrolling patients who would receive all of their services directly from clinicians and institutions that were part of the plan. This allowed Kaiser Permanente to develop an integrated approach to healthcare delivery.

Kaiser, the management component, owns or contracts with hospitals, skilled nursing facilities, home healthcare systems, and a range of other institutions that provide care under their management. Permanente, the physician component, aims to provide an integrated set of inpatient and outpatient services. Kaiser Permanente competes actively in the market for healthcare services and often limits the amount and types of care that can be provided. Nonetheless, it has been able to develop an integrated healthcare delivery system, promote evidence-based interventions, and introduce an integrated electronic health record system.

The VA healthcare system began as an outgrowth of World War I, though its roots go back to the Revolutionary War. After World War II, the VA hospital system rapidly increased in size and developed strong relationships with medical schools and other health professional training schools for education and research. Today, the VA healthcare system is part of the cabinet-level Department of Veterans Affairs and serves over eight million patients each year.

For many years, the VA system was accused of poor quality care and lack of coordination of care because it emphasized inpatient services and patients often went back and forth between the VA and other healthcare delivery sites. In the mid-1990s, the VA health system underwent a major "systems reengineering," designed to improve quality. The changes included the development of an integrated electronic health record and an emphasis on evidence-based interventions for preventive, acute, and chronic care.

In recent years, the VA health system has been organized into a series of networks, including inpatient and outpatient facilities. Many of the networks aim to provide comprehensive outpatient and inpatient services, including skilled nursing and nursing home services, as well as outpatient and hospital services. Survey data collected a decade after the systems reengineering initiative began suggested that the VA health system provided an increasing quality of integrated care based upon evidence-based interventions.

The VA experience, however, demonstrates that adequate resources are required to maintain continuity and quality. In recent years the increased numbers of those eligible for care and the limited budgets have again made it difficult for the VA system to maintain continuity and quality.

The VA and Kaiser Permanente systems represent two of the largest healthcare systems in the United States. Both aim to serve a large number of patients and provide coordinated care utilizing evidence-based interventions and integrated healthcare records. These two quite different healthcare systems suggest that an integrated system of care, patient information, and financing is possible and can be widely applied to improve the quality of health care.

of care, as well as achieve a number of other quality objectives. The National Academy of Medicine outlined the following potential roles for an electronic health information system. These roles aim in large part to provide the cornerstone for coordination of healthcare delivery.

- *Health information and data*—laboratory and pharmacy data, as well as records of a patient's history and findings on examination, including past medical records

- *Results management*—integration of findings from multiple providers at multiple sites
- *Order entry/management*—electronic ordering of tests and prescriptions to maximize accuracy and speed implementation
- *Decision support management*—computer reminders and prompts to encourage timely follow-up and adherence to evidence-based guidelines
- *Electronic communication and connectivity*—facilitation of communications between providers and between providers and patients

## BOX 10.3 Medicare Demonstration Programs

The federal Centers for Medicare and Medicaid Services (CMS) has implemented a series of new demonstration programs. Key programs can be summarized as follows:

*Accountable Care Organizations (ACOs):* ACOs allow providers who voluntarily agree to work together to coordinate care for patients and providers who meet certain quality standards to share in any savings they achieve for the Medicare program. ACOs that elect to become accountable for shared losses have the opportunity to share in greater savings. ACOs coordinate and integrate Medicare services, with success being gauged by roughly 30 quality measures organized in four domains. These domains include patient experience, care coordination and patient safety, preventive health, and at-risk populations. The higher the quality of care providers deliver, the more shared savings their ACO may earn, provided they also lower growth in healthcare expenditures.

*Partnership for Patients:* This partnership is a demonstration designed to reduce hospital-acquired conditions and improve transitions in care, including reducing 30-day hospital readmissions. This public–private partnership supports the efforts of physicians, nurses, and other clinicians to make care safer and better coordinate patients' transitions from hospitals to other settings.

*Bundled Payments for Care Improvement:* The Bundled Payments for Care Improvement initiative seeks to improve patient care by fostering improved coordination through payments for multiple related services rather than for single services. Initial efforts have produced mixed results. Recent federal legislation has also allowed expanded use of a range of new Medicare payment systems including allowing physicians to choose between payment methods for routine Medicare payments.

*Comprehensive Primary Care Initiative:* In addition to regular fee-for-service payments, CMS is examining the impact on primary care practices of a monthly fee for clinicians to help patients with serious or chronic diseases follow personalized care plans; give patients 24-hour access to care and health information; deliver preventive care; engage patients and their families in their own care; and work together with other doctors, including specialists, to provide better coordinated care. The success of these initial efforts has led to an expanded program of Comprehensive Primary Care Plus.

The results of these experiments and demonstration programs are gradually becoming available. It is likely that these results will contribute to ongoing reform of the U.S. healthcare delivery system.

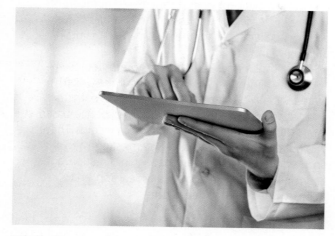

© Billion Photos/Shutterstock

- *Patient support*—tools for patient education and patient involvement in decision making
- *Administrative processes*—facilitation of scheduling, billing, and other administrative services to increase efficiency and reduce costs

- *Reporting and population health*—improvements in the efficiency and completeness of required reporting and the speed and completeness of public health surveillance

The National Academy of Medicine also concluded that electronic record systems have the potential for helping achieve quality and efficiency objectives as outlined in **BOX 10.4**.[10]

Efforts to implement a national system of electronic health records are under way. The process was kick started when nearly $20 billion was allocated as part of the 2009–2010 stimulus program. Recent efforts to include patients as direct users of their health information may spur more rapid acceptance of the electronic health records. The need for security of data and control by patients over who has access and for what purposes is critical to the acceptance and use of an electronic health records system. You should expect to see widespread use of electronic records and an increased role for patients in accessing and managing their own medical records.[f]

---

f  Despite the national commitment to implement electronic health records, the usage by U.S. physicians in their offices is still behind that of other developed countries. Financial incentives to utilize electronic medical records, however, are producing rapid changes in physician behavior, and electronic medical records are becoming widely available in the United States.

The National Academy of Medicine indicates that the electronic health record has the potential to improve the quality and efficiency of patient care in the following ways:

- *Improve patient safety.* Safety is the prevention of harm to patients. Each year in the United States, tens of thousands of people die as a result of preventable adverse events due to health care. Electronic records containing information on prescribed drugs and other treatments are expected to improve patient safety.
- *Support the delivery of effective patient care.* Effectiveness is providing services based on scientific knowledge to those who could benefit and at the same time refraining from providing services to those not likely to benefit. Only about one-half (55%) of Americans receive recommended medical care that is consistent with evidence-based guidelines. Reminder systems that require clinicians to accept or reject the recommendations of a clinical guideline are expected to increase the use of evidence-based guidelines.
- *Facilitate management of chronic conditions.* More than half of those with chronic conditions have three or more different providers and report that they often

receive conflicting information from those providers; moreover, many undergo duplicate tests and procedures, but still do not receive recommended care. Physicians also report difficulty in coordinating care for their patients with chronic conditions and believe that this lack of coordination produces poor outcomes. Electronic records can help inform clinicians of other care being given to their patients.

- *Improve efficiency.* Efficiency is the avoidance of waste—in particular, waste of equipment, supplies, ideas, and energy. Methods must be found to enhance the efficiency of healthcare professionals and reduce the administrative and labor costs associated with healthcare delivery and financing. Electronic records, if consistently and widely implemented in the healthcare arena, can be expected to reduce costs as they have in many other fields.

While there is widespread agreement that electronic medical records have the potential to improve health care, concerns have also been raised about privacy. In addition, the ease of ordering tests provided by many health information systems has raised concerns that these systems will result in additional ordering of costly and often unnecessary tests.

Electronic health records are only one of the many ways that technology is changing the delivery and quality of healthcare services in the United States.

## How Is Technology Being Used to Improve the Quality of Care?

The United States is among the leaders in adoption of new healthcare technologies, especially those that allow for technological approaches to disease diagnosis and treatment. In comparison with most other nations, the United States has more rapidly developed and accepted the use of medical technologies ranging from magnetic resonance imaging (MRI), to invasive cardiac procedures, to surgery for weight loss.

This country has generally relied on market mechanisms to develop, introduce, and disseminate or diffuse technology. This has resulted in extremely rapid innovation in areas with high levels of financial compensation and slower innovation in areas with less financial support. For instance, high-tech procedures ranging from heart surgery to hip replacements have been well compensated and have seen rapid

innovation and diffusion. Well-compensated preventive procedures, such as mammography, have likewise seen widespread use. Other technologies, like telemedicine, are likely to have widespread applications only after financial reimbursement is provided. This is beginning to happen and may dramatically affect the ability to provide home health care in the coming years.

Longer term innovations in technology have been fueled by the long-term U.S. investment in basic and applied research through the National Institutes of Health (NIH). The budget for the NIH was doubled during the 1990s, but has been relatively flat in recent years when adjusted for inflation. Ongoing efforts to limit or reduce the NIH budget may alter its ability to produce future innovations. The innovations in care and in technology pioneered by the NIH have often led to new approaches and new health-related industries. In recent years, the NIH has begun to focus on translational research or efforts to bring the benefits of new knowledge and new technologies to individual patients and whole communities.

Increased knowledge of the human genome has laid the groundwork for new diagnostic and

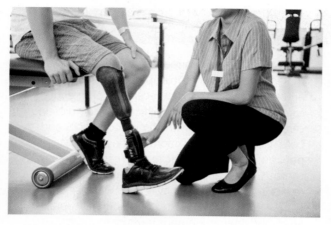

© JohnnyGreig/E+/Getty Images

therapeutic approaches, as well as a better under-standing of the causes of disease. Better under-standing of brain function and better technology for measuring changes in the brain are leading to new strategies for dealing with diseases ranging from Alzheimer's to depression. Advances in technology continue to provide hope and new challenges to improving health care.

We have now looked at how the development of integrated healthcare delivery systems and electronic health records and other technologies are being used to try to improve the quality and efficiency of health-care delivery. Now, let us take a look at mechanisms that are being developed to monitor and ensure qual-ity of care.

## ▶ What Mechanisms Are Being Used to Monitor and Ensure the Quality of Health Care in the United States?

There are a variety of methods, including accreditation of academic institutions and individual credentialing to help ensure that health professionals are well edu-cated and prepared for clinical practice. Increasing requirements for continuing education, recertification, and maintenance of licensure are being used to help ensure continued competence. Integrating financial compensation with quality of care through the use of pay-for-performance approaches is gaining momen-tum as an additional approach to ensuring quality.

In addition, there is a new emphasis on the use of evidence-based recommendations or clinical guidelines. Today, these recommendations are often available to clinicians in the form of protocols or step-by-step advice on approaches to the diagnosis and treatment of specific conditions. Computer sys-tems increasingly prompt clinicians to take actions or confirm their actions with an aim to implement evidence-based recommendations. The complexity of clinical practice and the limits of current research, however, mean that evidence-based recommenda-tions are available for only a small percentage of the problems that clinicians face on a daily basis.

In addition to these approaches, a series of other mechanisms attempts to address issues of quality. They include:

- Hospital privileges and approval to perform spe-cific procedures
- Accreditation of additional healthcare organiza-tions, including clinical practices
- Patient safety efforts
- Malpractice liability, not only for physicians, but increasingly for other health professionals

Hospital privileges imply that hospitals may set criteria for allowing clinicians to practice in their facil-ity. The criteria may include specialty and/or subspe-cialty boards. Approval to perform specific procedures implies the need to demonstrate competence either by training or experience or both.

Accreditation of hospitals and long-term care facilities has been a long-standing effort. It is often linked to reimbursement, and is thus essential to the survival of these institutions. Accreditation of clinical practices, especially large group practices, is a grow-ing trend. The NCQA and The Joint Commission are encouraging this process and providing specific qual-ity criteria that need to be met. While still a voluntary process, these new forms of accreditation are becom-ing a sign of quality that is useful when recruiting patients and dealing with insurance companies.

A new movement called the patient safety move-ment is rapidly gaining importance as a mechanism to improve the quality of care. **BOX 10.5** reviews the history and current efforts of the patient safety movement.

The U.S. healthcare delivery system has a unique body of law called **medical malpractice**. Medical malpractice is hailed by its supporters as the ultimate guarantor of quality. It is attacked by its detractors as leading to defensive medicine, increased costs, and shortages in vulnerable professions, such as obstet-rics. Regardless of your view of malpractice, it has come to have a major impact on the relationship between clinicians and patients. **BOX 10.6** examines the criteria for malpractice so you can understand what it means.[15]

## BOX 10.5  Patient Safety Movement

The patient safety movement began in the early years of the 21st century with the report of the National Academy of Medicine titled *To Err is Human: Building a Safer Health System*.[11] The report found that approximately 100,000 deaths per year in hospitals alone are the result of errors. Medication errors, equipment malfunctions, and interprofessional communication or "handoff errors" are among the most common errors leading to preventable adverse events. More recently an emphasis on diagnostic errors has become a focus as well.

The patient safety movement has shifted the focus from errors to safety. That is, it is built on the contention most adverse events are due to **systems errors** and are not a personal failure as the National Academy of Medicine wrote: "the biggest challenge to moving toward a safer health system is changing the culture from one of blaming individuals for errors to one in which errors are treated not as personal failures, but as opportunities to improve the system and prevent harm."[12]

The patient safety movement has developed a framework for what they call a "culture of safety." A culture of safety is built on the following three principles taken from the National Academy of Medicine report: Trust, accountability, and transparency. A recent patient safety movement summary of steps needed to build a culture of safety includes[13]:

- Achieving a culture of safety in a healthcare organization requires transformational change which is owned and led by the top leaders of the organization, including the board. Leaders cannot simply be "on board" with patient safety—they must own it.
- Transparency, both within and outside of the organization, drives improvement across the continuum of care.

- If patient harm results from a medical error: apologize in 30 minutes, pay for all care, seek a just resolution; provide a credit card for future care of survivor of harm.
- Creation of a reliable means to capture and analyze good catches/near-misses is the key to identifying and addressing unstable processes and systems.
- Both safety culture and patient outcomes require continual assessment: "What is measured gets managed."

The patient safety movement has benefited from the experience of complex non medical industries such as the airline industry that have evolved incident reporting systems which do the following[14]:

- focus on near misses
- provide incentives for voluntary reporting
- ensure confidentiality while bolstering accountability
- emphasize perspectives of systems in data collection, analysis, and improvement

The shift to reporting and investigating near misses has been especially important since it offers numerous benefits over investigating adverse events. These include:

- greater frequency of events allowing quantitative analysis
- limited legal liability
- ability to investigate recovery patterns that can be captured, studied, and used for improvement

The patient safety movement is now a full-fledged part of the healthcare system. It is beginning to have important impacts on the number of adverse events, the costs of health care, and the role of the malpractice system.

## BOX 10.6  Medical Malpractice

Medical malpractice is a body of state as well as federal law. It differs from state to state. It is part of the civil law, as opposed to criminal law, which means that a case may be decided by a jury based upon what is called the **preponderance of the evidence**. This implies that malpractice was more likely than not. Despite the differences that exist from state to state, malpractice law builds upon a tradition known as **negligence law**, which is intended to protect the individual from harm.

The occurrence of harm or a bad outcome resulting from health care is not the same as negligence or malpractice. Errors in judgment and unsuccessful efforts are only considered medical malpractice if the patient can establish all four of the following:

1. A duty was owed.
2. A duty was breached.
3. The breach caused an injury.
4. Damages occurred.

Let us look at each of these requirements.[a]

1. A duty was owed—This implies that a healthcare provider undertook the care or treatment of a patient. This duty may stem from services provided, ranging from a long-term relationship, a single visit, or a telephone call to a contractual relationship based upon an insurance agreement.

2. A duty was breached—This implies a failure of the healthcare provider to meet a relevant standard of care. The standard of care is defined in terms of the clinician's specialty. A healthcare provider is generally expected to possess the knowledge and skill and exercise the care and judgment expected of a reasonably competent clinician of the same specialty.

3. The breach caused an injury—The legal concept of causation is based on what is called proximal cause. In medical malpractice, responsibility for an injury lies with the last negligent act. **Proximal cause** asks whether the injury or other outcome would have occurred if the negligent act had not occurred. Causation can be divided among different "parties," including clinicians and institutions.

4. Damages occurred—Damages can be divided into direct, indirect, and punitive categories. Direct damages include lost earnings, as well as current and future medical expenses. Indirect damages may include pain and emotional distress. Punitive damages may be awarded when conduct is intentionally harmful or grossly negligent.[b]

Instructions to a jury in a medical malpractice case include efforts to convey the meaning of each of these components of malpractice law. However, juries have a great deal of latitude when interpreting their meaning. For example, the concept of proximal causation used in the law may not conform to the jurors' understanding of causation. For instance, assume a clinician refused to continue to provide prenatal care after the first 13 weeks. The jurors may decide based upon their own understanding of causation that the clinician's refusal was the cause of a subsequent birth defect.

Medical malpractice is a complex and changing field. Many factors affect whether or not a malpractice suit is brought. These include the extent and visibility of damages, the relationship between the patient and the healthcare provider, and the standards of practice of both medicine and law in the community.

---

a Physicians are not the only providers of health care who can be sued under malpractice laws. Other clinicians, such as pharmacists, may be sued, especially those who do not work directly under the authority of physicians. In addition, healthcare facilities as institutions may be sued and are often included as additional defendants in malpractice cases. In this section, we will refer to the defendant in a malpractice suit as a healthcare provider.

b Indirect damages may include what has been called a "loss of consortium," which includes services provided by a domestic partner, including companionship, homemaking, etc., and future reproductive capabilities of either sex. Gross negligence includes the intentional or wanton omission of care that would be proper to provide, or, alternatively, doing that which would be improper to do. Punitive damages are often justified as a method of deterring such conduct by other providers of care.

---

We have now examined the structure of the U.S. healthcare delivery system, including the types of services that are provided in the inpatient and the outpatient settings. We have seen the need for and difficulty in developing a coordinated system to provide continuity of care. We have also seen how the U.S. system is developing models of coordination linking institutions and providers in new ways. The use of technology is a major strategy used by the U.S. healthcare delivery system to hold the pieces together through electronic medical records and innovative approaches to diagnosis and treatment. The United States has a complicated and evolving system of quality assurance which includes accreditation of institutions and hospital privileges, patient safety efforts, and malpractice.

The development of the healthcare delivery system is closely tied to the way that health care is financed and services are paid for. Therefore, let us turn our attention directly to the issue of health insurance.

## Key Words

Academic health center
Activities of daily living
Health systems
Healthcare delivery systems
Healthcare systems

Inpatient facilities
Medical malpractice
Negligence law
Outpatient facilities
Preponderance of the evidence

Provider
Proximal cause
Structure, process, and
    outcome measures
Systems errors

## Discussion Questions

Take a look at the questions posed in the following scenarios, which were presented at the beginning of this chapter. See now whether you can answer them.

1. George did not have health insurance and went to the emergency room whenever he needed care. They always treated him there, but then tried to get him connected to a primary care facility. He was not eligible for care at the Veterans Administration (VA) facilities, so they sent him to the local community health center, which they called the "safety net" provider. George did go there and they tried to treat his problems and get him his medicine. When he got sick, however, George went back to the emergency department. Even George agreed that it was not the best way to get care, but he wondered: What is needed to make the system work better?

2. Laura had breast cancer and it had spread. Her medical records were on file at the hospital, at four doctor's offices, in two emergency rooms, and at an outpatient imaging facility. No one seemed to know how to put the system together. Whenever her old records were essential, they asked her to go get a copy of them and bring them to her next appointment. That worked for a while, but when she ended up in the emergency room, her records just were not available. Health care should be able to do better in the age of the Internet, Laura thought to herself. She wondered whether the system will work better as electronic health records become widely available.

3. Fred ended his walk one day at the emergency room. He seemed confused about how to get home. "It looks like we are dealing with Alzheimer's," his doctor told Fred's wife, Sonya, at their next appointment. Taking care of Fred at home was not easy. Home health aides and occasional weekend relief called "respite care" eased the burden for a while. The new assisted-living facilities looked attractive, but Fred's family just could not afford one. When Fred fell and broke his hip, he required hospitalization for surgery. The hospital discharge planner arranged for a skilled nursing home for rehabilitation services paid for by Medicare. After a few weeks there, the only alternative was long-term or custodial care in a nursing home paid for by Medicaid. The care at the nursing home was not what the family had expected. The staff did clean Fred up before the announced family visits, but once when the family arrived unannounced, they were shocked to see Fred lying half-naked in his wheelchair. The end came almost 2 years from the day they moved him to the nursing home. Looking back, the family asked: Can the healthcare system do better at addressing the needs of Alzheimer's patients?

4. Wanda, an experienced nurse, volunteers to transport a patient to radiology when no one else is available. As she is rolling the patient down the hall, the wheelchairs hits a fire extinguisher on the wall. The patient falls out of the wheelchair and hits his head suffering an internal bleed requiring emergency surgery. Wanda's supervisor gives her a written and verbal reprimand indicating that if she had been more careful the "adverse event" would not have happened. Wanda asks herself: Aren't these types of mistakes systems problems rather than personal problems?

## References

1. Shi L, Singh DA. *Delivering health care in America: a systems approach.* Burlington, MA: Jones & Bartlett Learning; 2019.
2. Sultz HA, Young KM. *Health Care USA: Understanding Its Organization and Delivery.* 6th ed. Sudbury, MA: Jones and Bartlett Publishers; 2009.
3. Shem S. *The House of God: The Classic Novel of Life and Death in an American Hospital.* New York: Delta Trade Paperbacks; 2003.
4. Taylor J. *The Fundamentals of Community Health Centers, National Health Policy Forum.* Washington, DC: The George Washington University; 2004:23.
5. National Association of Community Health Centers. About our Health Centers. http://www.nachc.org/about-our-health-centers/. Accessed July 21, 2017.
6. NCQA Report Cards. https://reportcards.ncqa.org/#/methodology. Accessed July 21, 2017.
7. Kaiser Permanente. Our history. http://xnet.kp.org/newscenter/aboutkp/historyofkp.html. Accessed July 21, 2017.
8. U.S. Department of Veterans Affairs. History of the Department of Veterans Affairs. http://www.va.gov/about_va/vahistory.asp. Accessed July 21, 2017.
9. Centers for Medicare and Medicaid Services. Accountable Care Organizations. http://www.cms.gov/Medicare/Medicare-Fee-for-Service-Payment/ACO/index.html?redirect=/aco. Accessed July 21, 2017.
10. Institute of Medicine Committee on Data Standards for Patient Safety. *Key Capabilities of an Electronic Health Record System: Letter Report.* Washington, DC: National Academies Press; 2004.
11. Kohn LT, Corrigan JM, and Donaldson MS. (Eds.). *To Err is Human: Building a Safer Health System (Vol. 6).* Washington, DC: National Academies Press; 2000.
12. Institute of Medicine Committee on Quality of Health Care in America. *Crossing the Quality Chasm: A New Health System for the 21st Century.* Washington, DC: National Academy Press; 2001.
13. Patient Safety Movement. Actionable patient safety solutions. Creating a culture of safety. http://patientsafetymovement.org/challenge/creating-a-culture-of-safety/. Accessed July 21, 2017.
14. Barach P., Small SD. Reporting and preventing medical mishaps: Lessons from non-medical near miss reporting systems. *British Medical Journal.* 2000;320(7237): 759–763.
15. MedicalMalpractice.com. Elements to prove in medical negligence cases. http://www.medicalmalpractice.com/resources/medical-malpractice/medical-negligence-lawsuits/4-elements-prove-medical-negligence. Accessed July 21, 2017.

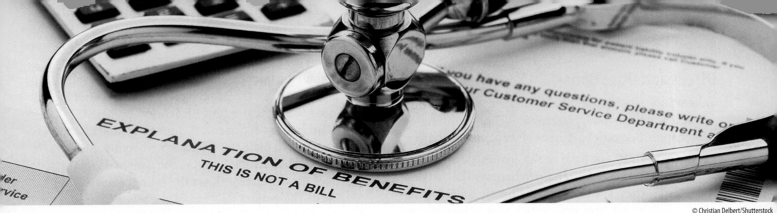

# CHAPTER 11

# Health Insurance and Healthcare Systems

## LEARNING OBJECTIVES

By the end of this chapter, the student will be able to:

- identify the largest governmental insurance systems in the United States, and explain the basic principles of their financing.
- describe the employment-based health insurance system in the United States, and discuss how fee-for-service insurance and capitated insurance options have evolved in recent years.
- describe other options for obtaining health insurance and the consequences of uninsurance.
- describe the basic structure and financing aspects of the healthcare systems in Canada and the United Kingdom, and compare them to those of the United States.
- identify and describe six sources of excess costs in the U.S. healthcare system.
- identify strategies for reducing the costs of health care in the United States.

You take a job right out of college and need to select from among your company's comprehensive healthcare options. The choices appear to be quite complicated, and none of them seems just right for you. You wonder: What are the key differences between comprehensive health insurance plans?

Jorge Rios's family is without health insurance. He works two jobs, neither of which provides health insurance. He earns a total income of slightly above the level which would make him eligible for Medicaid in his state. Jorge was born in the United States, but his brother, who lives with the family, is undocumented. Jorge is now trying to pay off the bills for his brother's treatment when he was recently seen in the emergency department. How

is this family affected by issues in the U.S. health insurance system?

Members of the Smith family live in the United States, Canada, and the United Kingdom. They have the same inherited disease. The recommended treatment is quite similar in the three countries and can be delivered as part of primary care. How might the delivery of care and the payment for care differ among the three countries?

You wonder how the United States ranks globally in terms of the performance of its healthcare system. You are surprised when you find out that its ranking is not number one, or even near the top. You ask yourself: Why is that?

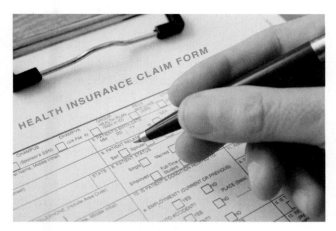

© tommaso79/Shutterstock

The politicians seem to agree that health care is too expensive. However, some argue for greater regulation, while others argue for less. You ask yourself: What are the options for controlling costs and what are the consequences?

Understanding healthcare systems requires us to understand the workforce and institutions that make up the system. It also requires us to examine the central measures of success: the issues of quality, access, and cost of health care.

In this chapter, we will take a look at questions of access to and the costs of health care. Both of these issues are closely tied to the availability of health insurance to pay for health care. In the United States, there is no comprehensive right to health care. The ability to access most health care is dependent on having health insurance. Thus, to better understand the U.S. healthcare system, we will begin by taking a look at the finances. We need to know how much money is spent and how it is spent. This will require us to look at the complicated U.S. health insurance system.

Then, we will look at the overall features of the U.S. healthcare system and compare them to features of the systems in Canada and the United Kingdom. Equipped with these understandings, we will see how health systems can be scored or graded and how the United States compares with other nations. Finally, we will examine the issue of controlling costs, while maintaining or improving healthcare quality—a major challenge facing the U.S. health system today. Let us start by looking at how much we currently spend on health care.

## How Much Money Does the United States Spend On Health Care?

The United States spends approximately $3 trillion per year on health care. That represents over 18% of the gross domestic product (GDP), or approximately $9000 per person per year. Dollars spent have been growing faster than inflation for over 40 years. At the current rate of growth, the United States is estimated to spend 20% of its GDP on health care in the coming years.[1]

Continuing that rate of growth takes money away from other activities, which makes it more difficult for the United States to compete globally or have discretionary resources to spend. Other developed countries, such as Canada, the United Kingdom, France, Germany, Japan, and Australia, spend about half as much per person and generally spend 10% or less of their GDP on health care.

To understand how we spend so much of our money on health care, it is critical to know more about the U.S. health insurance system. Much of the money spent on health care, whether by individuals, businesses, or government, pays for insurance coverage. The majority of the remaining funds are spent to fill in the holes in insurance coverage through direct payments by patients called **out-of-pocket expenses**.

Let us look at the basic types of insurance available in the United States. We start by examining government-financed insurance. We will then take a look at employment-based insurance. Finally, we will take a look at health insurance exchanges and the role that they are playing in the health insurance system. We will also examine the consequences of uninsurance and underinsurance. Before getting started, however, it is important to understand the language of health insurance. **BOX 11.1** defines some important insurance terms.

## What Types of Government-Supported Health Insurance Are Available?

The two largest government programs of insurance are **Medicare** and **Medicaid**.[2,3] Both programs began in the mid-1960s, but they have very different funding sources, coverage, and populations served.[a]

---

a  The federal government also provides health care through the Veterans Administration, military health systems, and the Indian Health Service. The Veterans Administration is required to provide health care for military service–related conditions, but may—contingent upon resources—also provide care to veterans for non-service-related conditions. The military healthcare system provides care directly or contracts for care through the TriCare system for all active duty military members and their families. American Indian and Alaskan Native members of federally recognized tribes are eligible for comprehensive health services, as well as public health services provided or funded through the Indian Health Service.

## BOX 11.1 Important Insurance Terms

**Cap**—A limit on the total amount that the insurance will pay for a service per year, per benefit period, or per lifetime.

**Copayment**—An amount that the insured is responsible for paying even when the service is covered by the insurance.

**Coinsurance**—In contrast to copayment, the percentage of the charges that the insured is responsible for paying.

**Covered service**—A service for which health insurance will provide payment or coverage if the individual is eligible—in other words, any deductible has already been paid.

**Customary, prevailing, and reasonable**—These standards were used in the past by many insurance plans to determine the amount that would be paid to the provider of services. Under many employer-based plans, the provider may bill patients above and beyond this amount. This is known as balance billing.

**Deductible**—The amount that an individual or family is responsible for paying before being eligible for insurance coverage.

**Eligible**—An individual may need to meet certain criteria to be able to enroll in a health insurance plan. These may include an income level for Medicaid, age and enrollment in the Social Security system for Medicare, or specific employment requirements for employer-based insurance.

**Medical loss ratio**—The ratio of benefit payments paid to premiums collected—indicating the proportion of the premiums spent on health services. Lower medical loss ratios imply that a larger amount of the premium is retained by the insurance company for administrative costs, marketing, and/or profit.

**Out-of-pocket expenses**—The cost of health care that is not covered by insurance and is the responsibility of the insured. These costs may be due to caps on insurance, deductibles, copayments, and/or balance billing.

**Portability**—The ability to continue employer-based health insurance after leaving a job—usually by paying the full cost of the insurance. A federal law, known as the Consolidated Omnibus Budget Reconciliation Act (COBRA), generally ensures employees 18 months of portability but requires the employee to pay the entire cost of the health insurance.

**Premium**—The price paid by the purchaser for the insurance policy on a monthly or yearly basis.

## Medicare

Medicare began as a program for persons 65 and older. It was expanded to include disabled persons eligible for Social Security disability benefits and those with end-stage renal disease. Today, nearly 50 million Americans are eligible for Medicare, and the number is expected to increase to over 60 million in the near future.

When Medicare began, it was designed primarily to cover hospital services and doctors' services. It did not cover drugs, most preventive services, or nursing home care. Drugs are now partially covered by Part D of Medicare. Covered preventive services have expanded in recent years. Skilled nursing or rehabilitative care, but not nursing home or custodial care, is covered by Medicare. Hearing aids and eyeglasses, perhaps the two most important medical devices for the elderly, are not generally covered by Medicare.

Medicare is a federal government program, which means that eligibility and benefits are consistent throughout the United States. Medicare is primarily funded by a payroll tax of 1.45% from employees and 1.45% from employers. There is no income limit on this tax, and high-income individuals pay a higher amount. Income from investments as well as employment is now taxed. Self-employed individuals pay the employer as well as the employee share.

Medicare is a complicated program because there are four different parts: A, B, C, and D. The following describes the current basic costs and coverage of Medicare. The details are expected to change in coming years.

Part A covers hospital care, skilled nursing care, and home health care after a hospitalization, as well as hospice care. It is paid for primarily by the payroll tax, and no premium is required. An annual deductible is required before receiving payments.

Part B is a voluntary supplementary insurance that covers a wide range of diagnostic and therapeutic services provided by physicians, emergency departments, and other outpatient services. For most people, about 75% of the cost of Part B is funded by general tax revenues and about 25% by a monthly premium, which starts at more than $100 per month. Those with higher incomes pay higher premiums, up to a maximum of approximately 80% of the cost of Part B. Those covered by Part B are still responsible for copayments of 20% for most services. There is also a deductible of approximately $150 per year. Health insurance policies called **Medigap** policies, which are offered by private insurance companies, are often obtained by individuals to cover all or most of the 20% copayment.

Part C is a special program designed to encourage Medicare beneficiaries to enroll in prepaid health plans.

Part D is the prescription drug coverage plan. It is a complicated plan that is open to those who are enrolled in Parts A and B of Medicare. It requires a monthly premium and an annual deductible. The exact terms depend on contracts through private plans that compete in part by offering lower costs or greater coverage. A gap, or "doughnut hole," in which no coverage is provided occurs but is being gradually eliminated over the next few years. Once an enrolled individual reaches a "catastrophic level" of total annual drug costs of about $5,000, Medicare pays 95% of the additional cost of drugs.

## Medicaid

Medicaid is a federal plus state program designed to pay for health services for specific categories of poor people and other designated categories of individuals. It is now the largest federal health insurance system covering nearly 50% of births in the United States, nearly 40% of children, and well over half of all custodial nursing home care.

In the basic program, the federal government pays a variable amount of the cost ranging from 50% to 83%, depending on the per capita income of the state. These funds are designed to match the funds provided by a state based on the state's Medicaid formula. All states have chosen to be part of the basic program and therefore must provide benefits for such groups as the disabled, children, and pregnant women based on the federal poverty level. The federal poverty level for a family of four is currently approximately $25,000 per year. Thus, there have been a substantial number of poor and near-poor individuals, especially men, who have not been eligible for the basic Medicaid program.

States at their discretion may include and receive federal matching funds for other categories of "medically needy" and may increase the eligible income level up to 185% of the federal poverty level. Most states cover custodial care in nursing homes for eligible individuals who have limited financial resources. As a result, Medicaid has become the largest source of insurance funds for nursing homes.[b]

In order to obtain federal matching funding through Medicaid, states that administer the program must provide basic services that include most inpatient and outpatient services, including preventive services. States may choose to offer other services, and the federal government will provide matching funds for a wide range of services including drugs, eyeglasses, and transportation services. Thus, for those who are eligible for Medicaid, the coverage is usually quite comprehensive. However, the reimbursement rates to clinicians are often comparatively low, and clinicians may choose not to participate in the Medicaid program.

A program begun in the late 1990s called the **State Child Health Insurance Program** provides additional funds that states may use to enhance the health care of children. This may include raising the income level for Medicaid eligibility, starting eligibility more rapidly, and ensuring longer periods of eligibility. In 2009, Congress expanded and made this program more flexible, utilizing funds from an increase in the tax on cigarettes.

Medicaid now covers over 70 million individuals, about half of whom are children. Funds spent on the elderly, who constitute less than 10% of Medicaid beneficiaries, exceed those spent on children. The rising costs and increasing number of individuals eligible for the Medicaid program have led many states to require that Medicaid enrollees become members of a Medicaid-managed care organization in an effort to reduce costs and improve continuity of care.

Changes in the Medicaid system are part of the national debate over health insurance. For an ongoing update on this debate and current legislation see Teitelbaum and Wilensky's Health Reform Update.

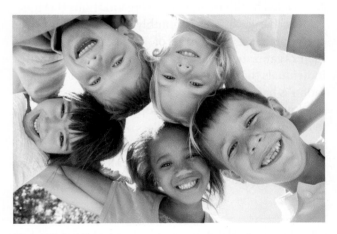

© Monkey Business Images/Shutterstock

---

b Medicaid requires that eligible individuals have very limited financial resources. Those with financial resources are generally expected to utilize most of these resources before becoming eligible. This process is known as "spending down." Complicated rules govern this process, including efforts to transfer the funds as gifts to others, including family members.

# ▶ What Types of Employment-Based Health Insurance Are Available?

Employment-based insurance is the largest single category of insurance coverage in the United States. Approximately 50% of all Americans have the option to purchase some form of this type of insurance.

Employment-based insurance is in large part an accident of history. During World War II, employers were prohibited from raising wages. Instead, they offered healthcare benefits. Employment-based insurance grew rapidly in the 1950s and 1960s based on a principle known as **community rating**. Community ratings implied that the cost of insurance was the same regardless of the health status of a particular group of employees. Community rating has since been replaced by what is called **experience rating** or medical underwriting. This concept means that employers and employees pay based on their groups' use of services in previous years.[c]

In the 1950s and 1960s and in many parts of the country well into the 1990s, employment-based insurance provided payments to clinicians and hospitals based almost entirely on **fee-for-service** payments, often using the customary, prevailing, and reasonable criteria. Fee-for-service, as its name implies, consists of charges paid for specific services provided, and as a payment system, it encourages the provision of as many services as possible. Thus, this system has been accused of increasing healthcare costs through overuse of services.

In 1973, the federal government began to encourage an alternative approach to employment-based insurance called health maintenance organizations (HMOs). HMOs charge patients a monthly fee designed to cover a comprehensive package of services. Clinicians or their organizations are paid based upon the number of individuals that enroll in their practice. Their compensation is based on what is called **capitation**, which is a fixed number of dollars per month to provide services to an enrolled member regardless of the number of services provided. Classic HMOs are traditionally "staff model" HMOs, like Kaiser Permanente, that directly or indirectly provide the entire package of services.

Capitation, as opposed to fee-for-service, has the potential for underuse of services in an effort to reduce costs. HMOs, in contrast to a fee-for-service system, generally cover preventive services and thus argue that they do a better job of keeping people healthy.[d]

Classic fee-for-service systems and classic staff model HMOs represent the two traditional models of employment-based health insurance in the United States. Beginning in the 1990s, both these systems began to change in ways that brought them closer together.

Fee-for-service systems often evolved into what are called **preferred provider organizations**, or **PPOs**. Staff model HMOs developed options for what are called **point of service plans (POSs)**. PPOs imply that the fee-for-service insurance system decides to work with only a limited number of clinicians, called preferred providers. These providers, who form the plan's network, agree to a set of conditions that usually includes reduced payments and other conditions. Patients may choose to use other clinicians in what is called out-of-network care, but if they do so, they typically will pay more out of pocket.

POS plans imply that patients in an HMO may choose to receive their care outside the system provided by the health plan. Like a PPO patient who goes out of network, patients who choose the POS option must expect to pay more out of pocket. PPOs and POSs are today the most common forms of employment-based insurance. They now come in a variety of forms and together can be called mixed models. An employer may offer its employees a number of complicated mixed model choices, as well as ones that are closer to the classic fee-for-service plus HMO staff model, or classic HMOs.

# ▶ What Mechanism Is Available to Obtain Insurance for Those Not Otherwise Eligible for Health Insurance?

**Health insurance exchanges** provide a mechanism to obtain health insurance for those who are not eligible for other forms of comprehensive health insurance. Health insurance exchanges provide an online marketplace—a service available in every state that

---

c  It has been argued that community rating is a form of health insurance that is closer to the social justice approach to health care because individuals and groups with better health subsidize those with poorer health and greater expenses. This implies that experience rating has moved the system toward a market justice approach. Note that mental health services are now treated the same as services directed at physical health under all types of health insurance plans.

d  It has been argued that the reason HMOs provide preventive services is related to the increased interest and use of these services by healthy individuals. Enrolling predominantly healthy individuals has been called **skimming**. By enrolling these individuals, HMOs can reduce their overall costs because healthy individuals are far less likely to require large amounts of health care.

helps individuals, families, and small businesses shop for and enroll in health insurance.

The aim of health insurance exchanges is to provide access to health insurance, at times subsidized by the federal government, for citizens and legal residents of the United States. The aim is to create a competitive marketplace to help increase access and control the costs of health insurance.

Access to the exchanges, subsidies for health insurance, types of health insurance offered, and the competitive nature of the health insurance offered have all been contentious issues in the national health insurance debate. For updated information on the health insurance exchanges see Teitelbaum and Wilensky's Health Reform Update.

Despite the multiple insurance systems in the United States a substantial percentage of the population still remains uninsured or underinsured. Let us take a look at the extent and consequences of uninsurance and underinsurance.

## ▶ What Are the Extent and Consequences of Being Uninsured and Underinsured in the United States?

Until 2010 over 15% of all Americans did not have any form of health insurance, and half of that number, or another 7.5%, were considered underinsured often facing bankruptcy when faced with major medical expenses. After the passage of the **Affordable Care Act** (ACA) in 2010 the percentage of uninsured was reduced to slightly less than 10%. The number of underinsured has been dramatically reduced by requiring insurance to cover **Essential Health Benefits**.

Essential Health Benefits are defined as healthcare services including all of the following 10 categories of health services:

1. Ambulatory patient services (outpatient services)
2. Emergency services
3. Hospitalization
4. Maternity and newborn care
5. Mental health and substance use disorder services, including behavioral health treatment
6. Prescription drugs
7. Rehabilitative and habilitative services (those that help patients acquire, maintain, or improve skills necessary for daily functioning) and devices

8. Laboratory services
9. Preventive and wellness services and chronic disease management
10. Pediatric services, including oral and vision care

It is important to understand what types of people have been uninsured and underinsured and to think about the consequences. Let us look first at the issue of the uninsured.

The uninsured can be classified into the following quite different groups:

- Healthy, often young, individuals who choose not to purchase insurance through their employer
- Poor or near poor individuals who do not qualify for Medicaid
- Self-employed persons or employees of small companies that despite substantial incomes decide not to purchase insurance

The ACA attempted to address the needs of each of these groups using different approaches. Young individuals were allowed to stay on their parents' insurance until age 26 and were allowed to purchase lower levels of coverage until age 30. The states were provided an option to expand eligibility for Medicaid. Self-employed individuals and those who worked for companies that did not provide comprehensive health insurance were permitted to purchase insurance through the health insurance exchanges, often subsidized for low and middle income participants. Under the ACA, all individuals were required to purchase health insurance that included the Essential Health Benefits or pay a substantial fine.

The consequences of being uninsured and underinsured can be very great. **BOX 11.2** outlines the consequences of lack of adequate health insurance.

## ▶ Are There Other Programs Available for Those Who are Disabled or Injured on the Job?

A complex system of federal and state programs are available for those who are injured on the job or have a disabling condition.[5] These programs can be categorized as:

- Worker's Compensation and Federal Programs for Workers
- Social Security Disability Insurance (SSDI) and Social Security Income (SSI)

**BOX 11.2** The Consequences of Lack of Adequate Health Insurance

The National Academy of Medicine[4] and the Henry J. Kaiser Family Foundation[4] have identified a series of consequences of a lack of adequate health insurance. Being uninsured harms individuals and families in at least the following ways:

- They receive less preventive care, are diagnosed at more advanced stages of disease, and receive less treatment once diagnosed.
- They are much less likely to have a usual source of health care and more likely to use the emergency department for routine care.
- They have an increased mortality rate with an estimated nearly 20,000 excess deaths per year.

Those without insurance can and often do use an Emergency Department to obtain care. Emergency Departments are required to provide care for life-threatening emergencies. However, after stabilizing an individual with a life-threatening emergency an Emergency Department is not required to hospitalize the patient or provide any continuing care. The Emergency Department may transfer the patient to another facility that provides care for those without insurance. For other conditions the uninsured and underinsured may delay care until it is too late to fully benefit. The National Academy of Medicine has described the care of the uninsured as too little and too late.[4]

When the uninsured and underinsured do seek health care, clinicians and healthcare institutions often bill the individual undiscounted prices for the healthcare services provided. When the uninsured or underinsured require substantial amounts of outpatient or inpatient health care, they often find themselves faced with large debts and often need to declare bankruptcy. When these individuals fail to pay their bills, the costs are often picked up by other patients with insurance thus raising the costs of health care for all those who purchase health insurance.

These programs are not designed to replace health insurance but do provide some assistance to those who are disabled including those injured on the job.

Workers Compensation or "workers comp" programs are state programs in the vast majority of the states which have existed since early in the 20th century when industrial era jobs became increasingly dangerous. Short-term assistance for traumatic injuries is covered by all workers compensation programs, but coverage of other conditions, long-term disability coverage, and coverage of off the job injuries varies from state to state.

Congress has also added disability assistance to cover specific populations and specific conditions. Federal workers are eligible for coverage for occupational injury and illness. The Department of Labor manages several employment focused disability programs including those for energy employees, longshore and harbor workers, and coal miners who suffer from black lung disease.

The Social Security Administration manages two sources of disability payments called SSDI and SSI both of which are designed to assist those with long-term disabilities preventing them from working. SSDI is designed for those who have paid into the social security system and their children. SSDI requires 12 months disability before applicants are eligible to apply and requires a complex disability determination process. Medicare is provided two years after the individual is determined to be eligible for SSDI.

SSI provides payments for disabled adults and children who meet income levels for eligibility regardless of their prior contributions to the social security system. Applicants have shorter waiting periods before being eligible to receive benefits and are enrolled in Medicaid immediately upon a determination of disability.

SSDI recipients receive payments comparable to other social security recipients, while SSI recipients receive lower payments often in the range of half of that received by SSDI recipients. Disability applications grew rapidly during the "great recession" to over 2 million applications and nearly 1 million accepted claims per year making it a part of the safety net. In recent years, the number of applicants has begun to fall even as employment has increased.

## ▶ How Does the United States' Health System Compare with Other Developed Countries?

In order to understand some of the options available to the United States as we continue to address issues of access, quality, and cost, let us take a look at how some other developed countries have addressed these issues.

First, let us look at a framework that we can use to describe and compare healthcare systems.

One approach to describing healthcare systems is to define their characteristics using the following categories:

- Method of financing
- Method of insurance and reimbursement
- Methods for delivering services

- Comprehensiveness of insurance
- Cost and cost containment
- Degree of patient choice
- Administrative costs

**TABLE 11.1** uses these categories to describe the complex U.S. healthcare system. The U.S. system is often compared to those of Canada and the United Kingdom. Despite the fact that these countries have much in common, their healthcare systems have evolved in very different ways.

## ▶ How Can We Describe the Healthcare Systems in Canada and the United Kingdom?

Let us use the same chart we used to describe the U.S. system to outline the features of the Canadian[6] and U.K.[7] healthcare systems. **TABLE 11.2** describes the Canadian healthcare system, and **TABLE 11.3** describes the healthcare system in the United Kingdom.

**TABLE 11.1** The U.S. Healthcare System

| Category | Description |
|---|---|
| Financing | Cost approximately 18% of GDP and rising rapidly<br>    Complicated mix of federal, state, employer, and self-pay |
| Type(s) of insurance and reimbursement | Employment-based insurance plus government insurance through Medicare and Medicaid provide most insurance. New exchanges provide options for individuals and small business employees<br>    Mix of fee-for-service, capitation, and salary with incentives are the most commonly used methods |
| Delivery of care | Mix of practice types with private practice dominant<br>    Physicians: ~1/3 primary care; ~2/3 specialists<br>    Primary care increasingly based upon nurse practitioners and physician assistants<br>    Hospitalists increasingly coordinate inpatient care<br>    Need for better continuity of care between institutions and between clinicians. New Accountable Care Organizations aiming to coordinate care for Medicare recipients |
| Comprehensiveness of insurance | Until recently, 15% uninsured plus half as many as that underinsured<br>    Health insurance with **cost sharing** offered through employment-based insurance and through health insurance exchanges, as well as government programs including Medicaid and Medicare<br>    Under the ACA, preventive services increased, insurance required coverage of approved preventive services and no copayments for approved preventive services; also generally requires coverage of Essential Health Benefits. Drug benefits provided through Medicare, Medicaid, exchange-purchased insurance, and most employment-based insurance |
| Cost and cost containment | Emphasis on competition as means of controlling costs, plus cost sharing by patients |
| Patient choice | Considerable choice of primary care and often direct access to specialty care<br>    Greatly increased access for those with comprehensive insurance with high levels of provider reimbursement |
| Administrative costs | High: 25%–30% of total costs, including administrative costs of health insurance, clinicians, and institutions, but this does not include administrative time spent by patients and their families |

**TABLE 11.2** The Canadian Healthcare System

| Category | Description |
| --- | --- |
| Financing | National policy to keep expenditures under 10% of GDP<br>    Combination of provincial and federal<br>    ~70% government through taxes<br>    ~30% private insurance payments by individuals |
| Type(s) of insurance and reimbursement | Government insurance for basic health services, individual policies with subsidies for the poor for most other services<br>    Negotiated fee-for-service reimbursement with single payer for basic services |
| Delivery of care | Mix of practice types with private practice dominant—emphasis on physicians in primary care<br>    Physicians 1/2 primary care and ~1/2 specialists<br>    Primary care physicians generally admit to the hospital and are responsible for continuity of care<br>    Concerns about limited access to high-tech procedures |
| Comprehensiveness of insurance | Three-tiered:<br>    Medically necessary basic services—universal coverage. Government funded and guaranteed to all without any cost sharing, including preventive services. No private insurance allowed for medically necessary services<br>    Private insurance and government-subsidized insurance for other medical services, including drugs, long-term care, home care with government payment for needy. Negotiated bulk purchasing of drugs on formulary keeps cost down<br>    Private insurance or self-pay for dental, vision, and many nonphysician services |
| Cost and cost containment | Capital purchases, such as of high-tech diagnostic equipment, are regulated and at times restricted<br>    Concern about waiting time for access<br>    Negotiated fees between providers and government with government as single payer having considerable negotiating power |
| Patient choice | Choice of primary care physician<br>    Referral often needed to see specialists |
| Administrative costs | Low—approximately 15% or less of total costs |

**TABLE 11.3** The U.K.'s Healthcare System

| Category | Description |
| --- | --- |
| Financing | Budget about 8% of GDP, has been rising. Does not include private insurance costs<br>    Tax-supported comprehensive and universal coverage through National Health Service<br>    Private insurance system with overlapping coverage purchased as additional coverage by ~15% of the population with perception of easier access and higher quality |
| Type(s) of insurance and reimbursement | National Health Service is single payer with capitation, plus incentives for general practitioners (i.e., physicians responsible for a panel of patients)<br>    Specialists generally salaried in National Health Service often earn substantial additional income through private insurance system |

| Category | Description |
|---|---|
| Delivery of care | Governmental system of healthcare delivery in National Health Service, including government-owned and administered hospitals<br>　　Emphasis on physicians<br>　　Primary care general practitioners ~2/3<br>　　Specialist physicians ~1/3<br>　　General practitioners generally do not admit to hospital |
| Comprehensiveness of insurance | National Health Service comprehensive with little cost sharing plus may cover transportation costs<br>　　Incentives to provide preventive services and home care |
| Cost and cost containment | Overall limit on national spending ("global budgeting")<br>　　Negotiated rates of capitation and salary with government as single payer with National Health Service having considerable negotiating power |
| Patient choice | National Health Service provides limited choice of general practitioners<br>　　Waiting lines for services in National Health Service, especially specialists and high-tech procedures<br>　　Referral to specialists generally needed<br>　　Greater choice with private insurance |
| Administrative costs | Greater than Canada, less than United States |

## ▶ What Conclusions Can We Reach from These Descriptions of the Healthcare Systems in the United States, Canada, and the United Kingdom?

These charts highlight key features of the three systems, while demonstrating substantial differences. When describing these characteristics, we can ask: On the spectrum of market justice versus social justice, where do the United States, Canada, and the United Kingdom lie?

It can be argued that the United States relies most heavily on market justice, while the United Kingdom places the greatest emphasis on social justice.

Canada lies somewhere in between. In describing these systems, it can also be useful to identify areas in which the United States has unique approaches and unique results. The following distinguish the U.S. healthcare system not only from that of Canada and the United Kingdom, but also from the healthcare systems of most other developed countries:

- The United States spends considerably more per person and as a percentage of GDP.
- The United States continues to have a higher percentage of uninsured individuals.
- The U.S. healthcare system is more complex for patients and providers of care and costs far more to administer.
- The U.S. healthcare system places more emphasis on specialized physicians and on nurse practitioners and physician assistants to provide primary care.
- The United States encourages rapid adoption of technology, especially for diagnosis and treatment when covered by insurance.
- The United States places greater emphasis on giving patients a wider choice of clinicians.
- The United States has a more complex system for ensuring quality and a unique system of malpractice law.

Equipped with all this information, we will now see if it is possible to grade or score the performance of the U.S. healthcare system compared to those of other developed countries.

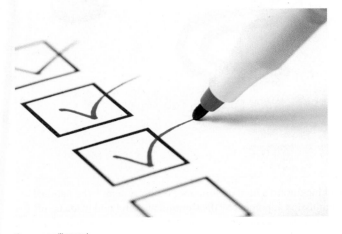

---

**BOX 11.3**    Criteria and Measurements Used in the Commonwealth Fund's Commission on a High Performance Health System

The Commission's scorecard measures the following five areas of health system performance:

- *Healthy lives:* National health outcomes using such measures as life expectancy, infant mortality, health-adjusted life expectancy (HALE) at age 60, limitations in activities among adults under 65, and missed school days by children due to illness or injury
- *Quality:* Quality of preventive, curative, and rehabilitative health care using such measures as adults and children receiving recommended preventive services; control of chronic diseases; availability of services (including mental health) after hours and on an urgent basis; hospital quality of care, including the ratio of observed to expected mortality; and preventive measures in nursing homes

- *Access:* Availability of care using such measures as insurance coverage, including the percentage of uninsured and underinsured, as well as the impact of the cost of insurance
- *Efficiency:* Inappropriate, wasteful, or fragmented care using such measures as emergency department use for routine care, hospital admissions for preventable conditions, short-term readmission rates, and costs of administration
- *Equity:* Disparities in health services and health outcomes by racial/minority status and income using such measures as access to preventive and acute services, control of chronic diseases, insurance coverage, and measures of healthy lives

The scores from each of these areas are added together to produce overall scores.

Data from The Commonwealth Fund. Commission on a high performance health system. Available at http://www.commonwealthfund.org/Publications/Fund-Reports/2011/Oct/Why-Not-the-Best-2011.aspx. Accessed June 27, 2017.

## ▷ How Can a Healthcare System Be Scored?

The Commonwealth Fund's Commission on a High Performance Health System (the Commission)[e] has developed the National Scorecard on the U.S. Health System (National Scorecard).[8] The national scorecard uses a standardized set of measurements to try to objectively measure performance in 19 developed countries. **BOX 11.3** outlines the criteria used to score these healthcare systems and the types of measurements that are used.

Let us take a look at how the United States scores in comparison with other developed countries based upon the national scorecard.

## ▷ Using the National Scorecard, How Does the United States' Healthcare System Perform Compared to Those of Other Developed Countries?

The Commission scored the performance of 19 developed countries, including the United States, 14 European nations, Canada, Japan, New Zealand, and

Australia. It set benchmarks high, but established realistic levels of performance for each area using the score of the top three countries as the highest standard. Thus, high but realistic performance is given a score of 100.

The Commission has scored the performance of these 19 countries three times, most recently in 2011. The scores in the United States changed very little over the period of 2006 to 2011.

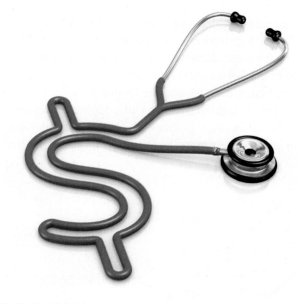

© Jan-Willem Kunnen/Shutterstock

---

e  The Commonwealth Fund describes itself as "a private foundation working toward a high performance health system."[9] The national scorecard on U.S. Health Systems Performance was developed by a commission appointed by the Commonwealth Fund made up of individuals who, according to the Commonwealth Fund, are "distinguished experts and leaders representing every sector of health care, as well as the state and federal policy arena, the business sector, professional societies, and academia."[10]

**TABLE 11.4** Performance of United States Compared to Best Performing Countries—2011

| Area of performance | U.S. score (out of 100) |
| --- | --- |
| Healthy lives | 70 |
| Quality | 75 |
| Access | 55 |
| Efficiency | 53 |
| Equity | 69 |
| Overall score | 64 |

Data from Commonwealth Fund. Why Not the Best? Results from the National Scorecard on U.S. Health System Performance, 2011. Available at: http://www.commonwealthfund.org/~/media/files/publications/fund-report/2011/oct/1500_wntb_natl_scorecard_2011_web_v2.pdf. Accessed December 4, 2017.

**TABLE 11.4** summarizes the performance of the United States on each of the criteria, as well as the overall score.

Perhaps the greatest negative aspect of the U.S. healthcare system is the issue of high and escalating costs. This is reflected in the U.S. score for efficiency of 53 on the Commonwealth score. Access has most likely improved in the United States since the adoption of the ACA. Let us complete our look at the U.S. healthcare system by examining the options for controlling costs.

## How Can the Costs of Health Care Be Controlled in the United States?

To understand the options for controlling costs, it is important to first understand the reasons that costs are increasing. The United States is not alone in facing increased costs for health care. There are a number of forces at work in most developed countries that increase and most likely will continue to increase the costs of health care, including the following:

- *The aging of the population*: The success of public health and healthcare efforts over the last century has produced a population that is living longer. Longer life is strongly associated with the development of chronic diseases, many of which require expensive care over many years or decades.
- *Technological innovations have greatly expanded treatment options*: A wide range of interventions are now possible, some of which can have dramatic impacts on longevity and the quality of life. However, many others produce very modest improvements at high costs. It may be difficult to distinguish these different types of results.
- *The successes of medical care over the last half century have raised the expectations of patients*: Greater expectations for access to technology, preventive interventions, individualized care, rapid access to care, privacy, and protection of confidentiality are now all possible, but often are quite expensive.

Nearly all developed countries face these forces to a greater or lesser extent. Many countries in Europe, as well as Japan, face an even more rapidly aging population than the United States. How the healthcare systems respond to these challenges will determine in large part the overall costs of health care in each country.

The United States, however, also faces some issues to a far greater extent than other developed countries. The United States healthcare system has a far more complex, diverse, and changing structure. The sheer complexity of the system has led to a need for multiple levels of administration, which are not required in most other countries, where care is often paid by one source called a **single payer**. In addition, patients in the United States are often expected to fill out and process complex insurance applications and claim forms. Clinicians are often required to bill for each service provided, justify the services provided, and, in many cases, obtain approval for payments prior to treating patients. Today, a clinician's office usually has more individuals involved in administering the system compared to those directly delivering care to patients.

The United States also has a far more complex and changing system of quality control. As we have seen, healthcare quality is monitored and maintained via a system that includes accreditation, certification, licensure, and malpractice, to name a few. The direct and indirect costs of this system may themselves contribute to the large and escalating cost of health care.

The National Academy of Medicine recently examined the excess costs that are built into the U.S. systems of delivering and paying for health care.[11] **BOX 11.4** describes its findings.

A variety of efforts are continuously being made to reduce costs in the United States. These include:

- *Cost control through reimbursement incentives*: The concept of capitation has been widely used as a mechanism for controlling or reducing costs. A special form of capitation, diagnosis-related groups (DRGs), has been successfully used to reduce the length of stay in hospitals. DRGs pay hospitals a set amount for a particular diagnosis, regardless of the length of hospital stay. However, reimbursement systems at times have moved the costs from

---

**BOX 11.4** Excess Costs of Health Care in the United States

The National Academy of Medicine has identified the following six categories of excess costs of health care. For each category, the institute indicates the types of excess costs that occur. In addition, it has estimated the potential annual savings from each of the six categories of excess costs.

*Unnecessary services and overuse*—beyond evidence-established levels—$210 billion

- Discretionary use beyond benchmarks
- Unnecessary choice of higher-cost services

*Inefficiently delivered services*—$130 billion

- Mistakes—errors, preventable complications
- Care fragmentation
- Unnecessary use of higher-cost providers
- Operational inefficiencies at care delivery sites

*Excess administrative costs*—$190 billion

- Insurance paperwork costs
- Insurers' administrative inefficiencies

- Inefficiencies due to care documentation requirements

*Prices that are too high*—$105 billion

- Service prices beyond competitive benchmarks
- Product prices beyond competitive benchmarks

*Missed prevention opportunities*—$55 billion

- Primary prevention
- Secondary prevention
- Tertiary prevention

*Fraud*—$75 billion

- All sources—payers, clinicians, patients

Together, these excess costs come to over $750 billion per year, or approximately 25% of the dollars the United States spends on health care. Efforts to reduce these costs provide great opportunities for controlling healthcare costs without jeopardizing quality or access.

Data from Institute of Medicine. The Healthcare Imperative: Lowering Costs and Improving Outcomes-Workshop Series Summary. Available at: http://iom.edu/Reports/2011/The-Healthcare-Imperative-Lowering-Costs-and-Improving-Outcomes.aspx. Accessed July 22, 2017.

---

one part of the system to another. Restrictions on payment for procedures may increase the number of procedures performed. Restriction on inpatient reimbursement may encourage an increase in outpatient or home care services.

- *Cost sharing*: This involves efforts to shift the costs of health care to individuals on the assumption that individuals will spend less when the costs are coming out of their pockets. Methods such as deductibles, copayments, and caps are all intended to reduce costs by shifting them to individual patients.

- *Regulation*: At times, efforts have been made to reduce costs by placing limits on how much care can be provided or how much compensation can be provided. Government-controlled health insurance, such as Medicare and Medicaid, is most easily targeted for these types of regulation. The national issue of rates of compensation for clinicians and hospitals has become part of the political process.

- *Restrictions on malpractice*: It has been argued that the U.S. malpractice system encourages clinicians to practice "defensive medicine"—that is, to perform unnecessary tests to protect themselves against lawsuits. The extent of the problem and the impact of changes in malpractice are controversial, but efforts are being made to reduce the number of lawsuits that reach the court system and to restrict the amount of compensation that can be awarded beyond actual damages.

A more general approach to reducing costs favored by many in the United States is to increase competition between providers of health services, including institutions and individual clinicians and groups of clinicians. To better understand the potential for competition to succeed and the changes that are occurring to encourage competition, take a look at **BOX 11.5**.[12]

## ▶ How Can Population Health Become a Mechanism for Controlling Costs?

The evolving view of population health as a mechanism for connecting traditional public health and the healthcare systems holds the potential for reducing costs as well as improving outcomes. More efficiently connecting prevention, treatment, and rehabilitation may reduce the costs and increase the effectiveness of health services.

Understanding the U.S. healthcare system is a challenge for patients, as well as those who work in the system. Understanding the roles of healthcare professionals, institutions, and the issues of quality, access, and cost help us understand the system as a whole.

A well-functioning healthcare system is essential to the public's health. An efficient system that works in concert with organized public health efforts and leaves adequate financial resources to invest in programs directed at the health of the entire population is

## BOX 11.5 Using Competition to Control Costs

The healthcare system in the United States is perhaps the most market-oriented system of any major nation. To successfully control costs through market mechanisms, a number of characteristics of a well-functioning market need to be in place. It has been argued that, until recently, the U.S. healthcare system has not reflected most of these characteristics. Advocates of a market approach often share these concerns, but argue that it is possible to modify the U.S. healthcare system so that it functions as a better market system.

Let us take a brief look at key features of a well-functioning market, examine the extent to which the U.S. healthcare system fulfills these conditions, and examine changes that are being made or considered to move the United States toward a more efficient market-based system.

■ *Informed purchaser:* An informed purchaser is a key requirement for a well-functioning healthcare market. In the U.S. healthcare system, the employer often serves an intermediary role in selecting the health plans from which their employees may choose. Until recent years, employers paid little attention to the details of the health plans that they offered. However, that habit is changing rapidly. Cost information is now widely available to both employees and employers, and quality measures are also becoming available. Employers often rely on accreditation standards, such as those of the National Committee for Quality Assurance, which now accredits a range of types of health plans and group practices. In addition, data on outcomes for surgical and medical procedures are increasingly available at the level of the hospital and group practice. In terms of purchasing health insurance through a health insurance exchange, the exchanges are required to provide an increasing amount of information.

■ *Purchasing power:* The second requirement of a well-functioning market is the ability of those who need the product to have the purchasing power to obtain it. The subsidies that are available for health insurance purchased through the exchanges are designed to provide purchasing power to a wide range of previously uninsured and underinsured consumers.

■ *Multiple competing providers:* Well-functioning markets give purchasers a choice of service providers. Consumers' choices then generally favor providers who offer the services at reduced costs and/or increased quality. The availability of choices for employed individuals has increased in some areas in recent years, especially for those whose employers pay a substantial portion of the premiums. Employees of some large firms and organizations may have a range of choices and can choose their health plan based on criteria including cost, quality, and/or convenience.

■ *Negotiation:* Negotiation is the key to putting information, purchasing power, and competition together. These negotiations increasingly take place through the employer. However, labor unions are becoming more involved in issues related to health benefits as well because health insurance constitutes an increasing percentage of employee's current, as well as future, benefits. The individual employee often has little negotiating power and needs to rely on his or her employee representatives and/or employers.

If the U.S. healthcare system continues to move in the direction of becoming a competitive healthcare market, it will need to ensure that these conditions are fulfilled as much as possible.

---

a key goal. The population health approach thus needs to pay considerable attention to the workings of the public and private healthcare system, as well as the workings of the public health system.

## Key Words

| | | |
|---|---|---|
| Affordable Care Act | Deductible | Out-of-pocket expenses |
| Cap | Eligible | Point of service plan (POS) |
| Capitation | Essential Health Benefits | Portability |
| Coinsurance | Experience rating | Preferred provider |
| Community rating | Fee-for-service | organization (PPO) |
| Copayment | Health insurance exchanges | Premium |
| Cost sharing | Medicaid | Single payer |
| Covered service | Medical loss ratio | Skimming |
| Customary, prevailing, and | Medicare | State Child Health Insurance |
| reasonable | Medigap | Program (SCHIP) |

## Discussion Questions

Take a look at the questions posed in the following scenarios, which were presented at the beginning of this chapter. See now whether you can answer them.

1. You take a job right out of college and need to select from among your company's comprehensive healthcare options. The choices appear to be quite complicated, and none of them seems just right for you. You wonder: What are the key differences between comprehensive health insurance plans?

2. Jorge Rios's family is without health insurance. He works two jobs, neither of which provides health insurance. He earns a total income of slightly above the level which would make him eligible for Medicaid in his state. Jorge was born in the United States, but his brother, who lives with the family, is undocumented. Jorge is now trying to pay off the bills for his brother's treatment when he was recently seen in the emergency department. How is this family affected by issues in the U.S. health insurance system?

3. Members of the Smith family live in the United States, Canada, and the United Kingdom. They have the same inherited disease. The recommended treatment is quite similar in the three countries and can be delivered as part of primary care. How might the delivery of care and the payment for care differ among the three countries?

4. You wonder how the United States ranks globally in terms of the performance of its healthcare system. You are surprised when you find out that its ranking is not number one, or even near the top. You ask yourself: Why is that?

5. The politicians seem to agree that health care is too expensive. However, some argue for greater regulation, while others argue for less. You ask yourself: What are the options for controlling costs and what are the consequences?

## References

1. The Henry J. Kaiser Family Foundation. Health care costs: A primer. http://kaiserfamilyfoundation.files.wordpress.com/2013/01/7670-03.pdf. Accessed July 22, 2017.
2. Shi L, Singh DA. *Delivering health care in America: a systems approach*. Burlington, MA: Jones & Bartlett Learning; 2019.
3. Sultz HA, Young KM. *Health Care USA: Understanding Its Organization and Delivery*. 6th ed. Sudbury, MA: Jones and Bartlett Publishers; 2009.
4. Institute of Medicine. *Hidden Costs, Value Lost: Uninsurance in America*. Washington, DC: National Academies Press; 2003.
5. Pozen A, Stimpson JP. *Navigating Health Insurance*. Burlington, MA: Jones and Bartlett Learning; 2018.
6. Health Canada. Health care system. http://www.hc-sc.gc.ca/hcs-sss/index-eng.php. Accessed July 22, 2017.
7. National Health Service History. Chapter 8. http://www.nhshistory.net/envoi1.html. Accessed July 22, 2017.
8. The Commonwealth Fund. Why not the best? Results from the national scorecard on U.S. health system performance, 2011. http://www.commonwealthfund.org/Publications/Fund-Reports/2011/Oct/Why-Not-the-Best-2011.aspx. Accessed June 27, 2017.
9. The Commonwealth Fund. A private foundation working toward a high performance health system. http://www.commonwealthfund.org. Accessed October 6, 2013.
10. The Commonwealth Fund. Commission on a high performance health system. http://www.commonwealthfund.org/~/media/Files/Annual%20Report/2012/2012_AR_Commission%201219.pdf. Accessed October 6, 2013.
11. Institute of Medicine. The healthcare imperative: lowering costs and improving outcomes—workshop series summary. http://iom.edu/Reports/2011/The-Healthcare-Imperative-Lowering-Costs-and-Improving-Outcomes.aspx. Accessed July 22, 2017.
12. CATO Institute. Health care needs a dose of competition. http://www.cato.org/pub_display.php?pub_id=5070. Accessed July 22, 2017.

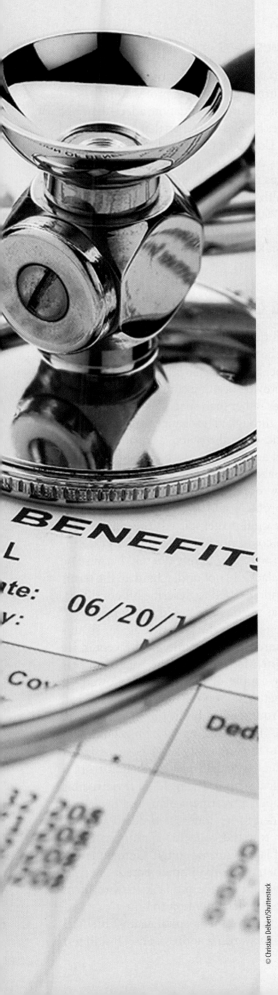
© Christian Delbert/Shutterstock

# Cases and Discussion Questions

## ▶ When Nursing Meets Medicine

Maureen felt she had no other choice but to let the hospital administrator know when a physician had repeatedly prescribed the wrong dose of medication. How many times could she double-check with Dr. George Ludwig just to be sure that she had understood his orders? *Orders, they still call them*, she thought to herself. *That is certainly what they want them to be.*

The days of obeying orders were over for Maureen. She had been through nursing school, and after five years working in the hospital, she went back to get her doctor of nursing practice degree to become a nurse specialist so she could work in an intensive care unit. Now she was doing the weekend 12-hour nursing shift to make ends meet and finish her doctoral degree. Nurses were in short supply, so she could now for the first time speak her mind without fear of losing her job. Nursing, she realized, was by its very name designed to nurture and take care of patients, but that did not apply to physicians. Their arrogance was so deep, she did not think they saw it.

Hospital policy required nurses to follow the orders after first checking with the head nurse and then double-checking with the physician who wrote the order. Complaints could be filed with the hospital quality assurance committee, but the process took months and the nurse who initiated the process could be reprimanded if the committee found his or her complaints to be unfounded or trivial. Trivial, this was not, but when she confronted the hospital administrator, he confided, "Do not put me in the middle of this." The pharmacist finally agreed to call the doctor and check on whether he preferred the "standard dose" of medication or the "unusual dose" he had first ordered. Dr. Ludwig agreed that the standard dose was "worth a try," so Maureen went ahead and followed the doctor's new orders.

Not too many months later, Maureen found herself confronted with new decisions in her first job as a nurse specialist in the intensive care unit. She now worked under "standing orders," which allowed her to make many decisions on her own. For the first time, she felt like she was calling the shots and making the decisions that made a difference for patients.

On one shift, late in the middle of the night, she was running from bed to bed covering the intensive care unit when she realized that she had given a patient the wrong medication. Fortunately, it was not a life-threatening mistake. She sighed with relief. Checking the chart carefully, however, she winced when her eyes fell upon the name of the attending physician, Dr. George Ludwig.

### Discussion Questions

1. How is Maureen's situation affected by the structure of the nursing profession?
2. How is Maureen's situation affected by the changes in roles of women that have occurred in the United States in the last 40 years?
3. How is Maureen's situation affected by the changes that have occurred in the delivery of health care over the last 10–20 years?
4. What changes do you think are needed in the healthcare system to prevent the types of mistakes illustrated in this case?

## ▶ Jack and Continuity of Care

Jack was told that he had high blood pressure and high cholesterol when he was in the army. Because the conditions did not bother him, Jack paid little attention to them. His job did not provide health insurance, so he decided to take his chances rather than spend his last dollar paying for insurance through an exchange. Anyway, he was strong and athletic. Over the years, Jack gained weight, exercised less, and developed a "touch of diabetes."

When the diabetes produced symptoms, he went to the emergency room, where they did a good job of diagnosing his problem and sent him off with a prescription and a few pills to get started. The pills seemed to help, but Jack could not afford to fill the prescription or follow up with his "family doctor" because he did not have one. Jack did not understand all the terms the doctors and nurses used to describe his condition, but he knew it was serious and could get worse.

It was not long before he was sick again, so this time, he sought care at a community health center. He did not qualify for Medicaid, but the treatment was affordable. For a couple of months, he followed up and was feeling better, but on the next scheduled visit, they told him, "You need to be in the hospital—you are getting worse." They got him to the hospital, where he was admitted to the university service and assigned to a young resident who had just graduated from a well-known medical school. The resident reviewed his condition, developed a treatment plan, and explained to Jack what needed to be done. He ordered a tuberculosis (TB) skin test and collected sputum to check for TB because of Jack's chronic cough. Unfortunately, before the treatment could be implemented, the resident rotated to another service and Jack's new resident did not seem to pay much attention to him.

Jack decided to leave the hospital against medical advice and left no forwarding address. His TB skin test was never read. When his positive sputum culture for TB came back, the laboratory alerted the local health department. Not knowing where Jack lived, the health department was not able to follow up.

Before he left, the hospital made sure that Jack had signed all the forms to receive Medicaid payments for the hospitalization. However, Jack did not complete the forms because he did not plan to get any more medical care. That changed one day when the pain was more than he could stand. He decided to try another emergency room. This time, the place was very crowded, and he had to wait hours to be seen. Once he was examined, the physicians and nurses tried to get information from him on his condition and treatment, but Jack could not provide much useful information.

He was prescribed pain medicine and sent home. He was told to follow up with a doctor in the next few days. By then, it was too late. One morning, as he was getting up, Jack's left leg was weak and numb and he lost his speech. He struggled to call 911. Despite the fact that he could not speak, the operator was able to send an ambulance by tracing his telephone location. The EMTs rushed to Jack's home and got him to the nearest hospital. Once again, the emergency room clinicians evaluated him, but this time, it was too late to be of much help. Jack was admitted for a stroke.

He stayed in the hospital for a week and made some improvement, but he needed help with the activities of daily living and could only speak a few words. The hospital was able to place him in a rehabilitation center because Jack, now 65, qualified for skilled nursing care under Medicare. He was transferred to the facility and received intensive rehabilitation services for the next month, until he no longer improved. At that point, Jack was no longer eligible for skilled nursing care. He was transferred to a Medicaid nursing home closer to his only relatives. The new facility had a large number of patients needing "custodial care." It provided all the services required by law, but Jack soon realized that he was just another stroke patient.

## Discussion Questions

1. How does this case illustrate the lack of institutional continuity?
2. How does this case illustrate the lack of continuity between the healthcare and public health systems?
3. How does this case illustrate the lack of financial continuity?
4. What role does the lack of information play in this case? How can information technology serve to reduce or eliminate these lapses in continuity?
5. Which lapses in continuity require other types of interventions?

## ▶ Donna's Doctor—To Err Is Human

Donna's heart was racing again, and there just did not seem to be a reason for it. She was not upset and had not been exercising. She was only 48, and no one seemed to take her seriously when she told everyone that something was wrong with her heart. She knew it was more than her recent divorce and raising a couple of teenagers. Not even the diagnosis of menopause satisfied her.

She decided to change primary care doctors, having heard that Dr. Stein actually listened. He did listen and examined her carefully, but did not find anything. He ordered a 24-hour test to monitor her heart. Donna did her usual activity, and the portable device recorded a basic electrocardiogram. She had one brief episode of racing heart. She recorded the time and length of the episode just as requested.

A week later, Donna got the results—episodes of atrial fibrillation. The upper chambers of her heart, called the atria, were beating very rapidly. Her lower chambers, called the ventricles, which pump the blood out of the heart, were doing just fine, so she was not in immediate danger.

"The real danger is blood clots and potentially a stroke," Dr. Stein told her, "and we should thin, or anticoagulate, your blood."

The thought of a stroke was enough to convince Donna to go ahead.

Anticoagulation can be done economically using a drug called Warfarin, often known by the brand name Coumadin, she was told, but it has to be done carefully. It can cause bleeding if it is not checked often. Taking Coumadin, Donna felt protected. She went back for the tests to adjust the dose. She felt better and now had lots of energy, but she still had some of those episodes of rapid heart rate.

When the hot flashes began, she knew that menopause had in fact arrived, but she felt better than ever and found herself skipping her blood tests because she wanted to be sure that she had time for her exercise routine. She did not realize that anything was wrong until she fell off her bike one day, hitting her head. Fortunately, she was wearing a helmet, so the injury did not seem too bad. However, she did feel dizzy afterward. And then a few hours later, her son told her that her speech was slurred.

"Have you been drinking, Mom?" he asked.

The look of disdain on his mother's face was enough to worry her son, who now insisted on taking her to the emergency room.

Dr. Stein met Donna and her son in the emergency room. He arranged an emergency MRI scan, which showed evidence of a small bleed, and the blood test showed her anticoagulation level was too high. The doctors rapidly reversed the level, and over the next few days, Donna's mental state returned to normal.

*What a relief*, she thought, *but there has to be a better answer than going back to anticoagulation.* Her doctors in the hospital asked for a consultation. First, the medical student, then the resident, and finally the professor came to look her over, examined her carefully, and then talked about her just outside her door, where she could hear bits and pieces of their conversation. "Dr. Stein sure missed the diagnosis"…"If she had only been compliant, none of this would have happened"…"An obvious case of hyperthyroidism"…"No need for Coumadin."

"The blood tests confirm overactivity of your thyroid, which is a condition called hyperthyroidism," the resident told her. "This caused your atrial fibrillation and your increased energy. You need treatment, but we do not do that here—we will give you a referral."

Donna could hardly absorb everything and did not get a chance to even ask questions.

She went back to Dr. Stein, who told her how badly he felt about missing the hyperthyroidism—he too had learned a lesson, and he apologized for what had happened. He told her that there was very good treatment for hyperthyroidism, and he would be pleased to take care of her after consultation with a specialist. Donna knew that doctors make mistakes, but she did not know that they admitted them. She knew that Dr. Stein was a good doctor and that he would pay extra attention to her. Donna hoped that things would go well and was confident that she was in good hands with Dr. Stein.

## Discussion Questions

1. Did Dr. Stein's care fulfill the duty, breach, causation, and damages criteria for medical malpractice?

2. What additional aspects of Dr. Stein's care affected whether a malpractice case resulted?

3. What role do you think the disclosure of error played in preventing a malpractice suit?

4. What attitudes toward decision-making in health care on the part of Donna influenced the approach she took to her health care?

## ▶ Health Care in the United States—For Better or Worse?

The final hours came as no surprise to his wife and family, who made daily visits to the hospital where Sam had been treated on and off for the final year of his life. His doctor had spared no expense to give him the most effective treatments available.

*But wouldn't it have been nice if he could have died at home?* they thought to themselves as they gathered at the funeral. *At least he held out until after the baby was born.*

Sam's diagnosis of colon cancer did not shock him. His father had died of colon cancer, and he had been thinking for some time that it was time to be checked. Surgery went well and he and his doctor were optimistic about the future. The surprise came about 18 months later, when during a follow-up examination, he was told that there might be a recurrence.

Chemotherapy seemed to do more harm than good. There did not seem to be a good answer. Sam's physician sought out the newest treatment, but it did not seem to help. The final shock to his system came after he received a dose of the wrong medicine administered by a nurse who was new to the unit. She was hired in response to the recent accreditation review, which criticized the hospital for understaffing.

Though his death was no surprise, the bills from the hospital and physician were an unexpected burden in the months and years that followed. The health insurance that was offered through Sam's employer did not pay for screening for the colon cancer that killed him. In addition, its loopholes, caps, and copayments left the family with bills that would require years to repay. It was not just the uncovered expenses that they had to pay out of pocket; it was the mountains of paperwork that arrived in the mail.

Nonetheless, the family understood. The doctors had done everything possible, treated Sam and them with respect, and responded quickly to their calls and continuous questions. Maybe things were not ideal, they concluded, but at least they did everything they could.

## Discussion Questions

1. What strengths of the U.S. healthcare system are illustrated in this case?

2. What limitations of the U.S. healthcare system are illustrated in this case?

3. How would the Affordable Care Act affect the services provided in this case?

4. What steps would you recommend to improve the delivery of preventive and curative services to better serve patients like Sam?
5. How might Sam's health care have been different in other developed countries, such as Canada and the United Kingdom? In what ways might it have been better and in what ways might it have been worse?

## ▶ Excess Costs—How Much Can Be Saved?

Doris, an 80-year-old white female, had been previously healthy. Her mother had a history of hip fracture. Doris was told to take extra calcium to prevent osteoporosis, but she was never tested or prescribed any treatment.

One Saturday morning, Doris fell in her home and landed on her hip. She lay in pain for about an hour before she was able to reach the telephone and call for help. The ambulance took her to the nearest hospital rather than the hospital she had requested. The doctors at the hospital had none of her medical records and did not realize that she was allergic to penicillin, which they prescribed because of the deep skin abrasions she suffered in the fall. Within minutes after receiving a shot of penicillin, she experienced anaphylaxis, a severe allergic reaction, and required an emergency team to be called to provide immediate resuscitation.

Doris was admitted to the intensive care unit on a Friday night. She underwent X-rays and was seen by five teams of doctors over the weekend. The doctors determined that she had a hip fracture and needed surgery as soon as possible. No surgeons were available to see her until Monday morning, at which time surgery was scheduled for Wednesday morning.

While Doris was in the hospital, the physicians decided to do a work-up for gallbladder disease because gallbladder disease is very common in her age group. The scans did show gallstones, and she was initially advised to have surgery for her gallstones. A consult recommended that rather than surgery, she seek health care if she ever had pain in the area of the gallbladder.

The physicians who took care of Doris in the hospital decided to treat her aggressively for osteoporosis using the newest and most expensive medication. The medication was covered by Medicare because Doris was in the hospital. The medication could be given by an injection and lasted for a year.

After discharge, Doris was supposed to receive physical therapy to be sure that she was ambulatory and did not develop blood clots in her legs. Unfortunately, the wrong telephone number and address were provided to the physical therapy team, and it took a week before the physical therapists were able to locate Doris to begin physical therapy.

Doris began the therapy, but on the second day in the middle of the treatment, she became short of breath. The physical therapist recognized the signs of a pulmonary embolism, or a blood clot traveling to the lungs. She immediately called the ambulance, which took Doris to the same hospital where she stayed before.

The hospital staff recognized that Doris had been discharged less than one month earlier and were concerned that Medicare might not pay the bills for her readmission. They decided to transfer her to the hospital that she had originally requested. She was successfully treated for pulmonary emboli and was followed up as an outpatient on a weekly basis for several months.

Doris received over 40 mailings related to the billing for her hospitalization, many of which said, "This is not a bill." She did receive 10 separate bills, including ones from the two hospitals, three laboratories, the physical therapy group, and four different doctor groups. The bills for her care totaled $215,000, $212,000 of which was covered by Medicare or her Medigap policy. The bills included a $50,000 bill for the orthopedic surgery, which was fully covered, and a $1000 bill for transportation to the second hospital, which was not covered by Medicare.

When Doris inspected the 10-page bill from the hospital, she noticed a bill to Medicare for equipment for three blood transfusions. "No one told me about that," she said to herself, so she called the hospital to confirm whether she in fact had had blood transfusions. The billing clerk checked with the hospital administration, let Doris know that this was a mistake, and apologized. A week later, Doris read in the newspaper that a large number of Medicare patients were being charged for equipment for blood transfusions they never received.

## Discussion Questions

1. Identify ways that each of the National Academy of Medicine categories of excess costs played a role in this case.
2. Identify ways that excess costs could be reduced in this case.
3. Discuss ways in which a reduction in the costs of health care in the United States could affect the quality of health care favorably.
4. Discuss ways in which a reduction in costs of health care in the United States could affect the quality of health care unfavorably.

# ▶ Navigating the Health System

Sylvia knew that things had not gone well as she lay in her hospital bed thinking back on how she ended up in the hospital with stage 4 breast cancer and tubes coming and going from almost everywhere. Her mind was clear even though her body was failing. She often wondered how she got to this point. She felt like she was in it on her own not understanding the complexities of the U.S. health system. "They couldn't have invented a more complicated system if they had tried," she thought to herself.

Sandra, the woman in the next bed was there to have breast cancer surgery too, but it was early, and she kept talking about Bonnie who she called her "health navigator." What was health navigation, Sylvia wondered. Sandra was ready and willing to fill her in.

The U.S. health system, both preventive and therapeutic, is a complicated system not designed to be easily navigated even by those with a health background. The need for help navigating the health system has existed for decades. The need has been partially filled by nurses, medical social workers, and a range of other health professionals who have seen the need and extended their efforts beyond their formal professional responsibilities. Despite the complexity of the health system, however, it has not been anyone's responsibility to see that the average person makes it through the maze.

The people needing health navigation today range from those with limited English to those with limited health literacy; from those with complex diseases such as advanced cancer and HIV to those with complex social-economic problems; from those with no or with limited health insurance to those without an understanding of how to utilize their health insurance. In fact, it is increasingly difficult to find anyone who would not benefit from some help getting through the system.

Health navigation is beginning to emerge as a health profession as part of the development of a comprehensive health system. The field today includes paid positions and a confusing mix of job titles. Three areas of focus, and associated job titles, have begun to emerge: Community Health Worker, Patient Navigator, and Health Insurance Navigator.

As the names imply, Community Health Workers are usually outpatient based and help patients obtain services in their home or community. Patient Navigators are often institution based, often hired by a hospital, to assist patients navigating a large institution, including preventing unnecessary readmissions. Health Insurance Navigators help the sick and the healthy identify and utilize available health insurance.

Most individuals at some point in their lives need all three of these types of services. Therefore, the term "health navigator" or "health navigation professional" is increasingly used to refer to all three types of these emerging health professions. To fill these needs health navigation professionals need to know about prevention and community health, the U.S. healthcare system as well as its health insurance system. They also need to be able to access and analyze health information, have health communication skills, and have hands-on experience serving as a health navigation professional. Realizing the potential of health navigation still requires full acceptance of health navigators as part of the healthcare team and efforts to make their work cost-effective.

Nurses whose education is enhanced by additional knowledge of community health, the U.S. healthcare system, and the U.S. health insurance system can become excellent health navigation professionals. Therefore, it is not surprising that nursing programs are beginning to teach the special skills and knowledge needed for health navigation.

After a few minutes of silence Sylvia said to Sandra "so what could a health navigator have done for me?" "Are you ready? This might be painful" Sandra said, "I'll tell you all about it" and she did.

Sandra told Sylvia, "Health navigation professionals in the community often focus on ensuring that people like you get preventive services. Mammography—as well as a wide range of preventive services—are now covered by nearly all health insurance, so why not take advantage of this and detect the disease early. Health navigation professionals often encourage screening, arrange for appointments, and ensure that patients follow-up. There is growing evidence that health navigation increases the rates of screening and early diagnosis."

Sandra went on, "That's not all that health navigators do, they help patients access and coordinate care. This is especially important for patients like you who have complex problems and need to coordinate care both before and after hospitalization. Hospitals are increasingly recognizing this and Medicaid has helped by creating a 30-day readmission rule that penalizes hospitals when patients are readmitted within 30 days for the same diagnosis.

Helping the sick and the healthy get the right health insurance and maximizing its benefits is becoming an important part of the work of health navigators. Health navigators potentially help people with individual health insurance as well as Medicare, Medicaid, and even employment-based health insurance. They are also increasingly employed by Community Health Centers where they reach out to the community to bring the uninsured into the health system and get them insurance if possible.

There is increasing evidence that health navigation increases patient satisfaction and improves their engagement in self-care, an increasingly important part of health care."

"OK I got it, so what's the bottom line?" Sylvia asked. "Will health navigation cure the U.S. health system? Will it improve quality without increasing costs?" "I wish I knew," Sandra said.

Only time will tell how well health navigation works as a key component of a comprehensive patient oriented health system. The answer may depend on how well health navigators are accepted by patients and clinicians as well as by the health insurance system. For Sandra, however, the answer was already in.

1. Who do you think should be eligible for health navigation services? Explain.
2. What do you think is needed to fully integrate health navigation into the public health and healthcare systems? Explain.
3. Should future health navigation professionals have a formal degree or academic certificate? Should they be certified or licensed? Explain.
4. Should nurses or other clinical health professionals be encouraged to also serve as health navigators? Explain.
5. How should health navigators be paid? As employees of clinicians or hospitals, directly from health insurance, from tax dollars, etc.? Explain.

## ▶ Influenza in Middleburg and Far Beyond

"New strain of influenza A found in Middleburg" read the headlines in Middleburg, a medium size Midwestern community. The local, national, and even world-wide twitter accounts went wild with doomsday scenarios, and Facebook pages were filled with stories on how to hide and histories of relatives who died in the 1918 and 1958 influenza pandemics which killed more people than any other disease of the 20th century.

Within days, doctor's offices, nurse-run clinics, and emergency rooms in Middleburg were filled with patients with coughs who were convinced they had a deadly disease. Pharmacists were bombarded with questions about what they could do to prevent the disease and what they could do if they had the early signs. Fortunately only a few cases of the new

strain appeared near the end of influenza season and calm soon returned. The new strain did pose a danger for the coming season but not an immediate threat.

It was ironic that the new strain of influenza A should appear just as Middleburg and the United States were completing the most successful efforts yet to prevent, control, and limit the impact of seasonal influenza which in the past had taken 25,000 to 50,000 lives a year during flu season. Within days, an inter-agency federal task force including the Centers for Disease Control and Prevention (CDC), Food and Drug Administration, and the National Institute of Health was at work developing a plan to address this new threat. They began by looking at what could be learned from the progress that had been made in reducing the number of deaths from seasonal influenza in the United States to below 10,000 and what was needed to confront the potential epidemic to come.

The Task Force found that the work of public health professionals, physicians, physician assistants, nurses, and nurse practitioners along with pharmacists and pharmaceutical professionals as well as health administrators had all played a role in this success story and they needed to be fully engaged to minimize the impact of the new strain. They also found a need for expanded engagement of the broader community.

They identified specific examples of changes in recent years which have most likely contributed to the reduced impacts of influenza including:

- Better public health surveillance was occurring for changes in influenza strains enabling but not ensuring better matches between the antigens included in seasonal influenza vaccines and the dominant circulating viruses.
- New vaccines have been developed by pharmaceutical companies with U. S. governmental support. Some vaccine modifications have already been widely adopted including those that produce higher antibody levels in those 65 and older; an intradermal vaccine requiring fewer antigens; and a four component influenza vaccine providing greater protection against influenza B.
- Vaccine effectiveness studies have shown that the intranasal influenza vaccine has not been effective in recent years and has been discontinued based on recommendations of the CDC's Advisory Committee on Immunization Practices which includes public health and medical professionals with formal relationships including nursing, physician assistants, health administrators, and pharmacists.

- Increased levels of vaccination resulting from widespread vaccine administration in pharmacies, nurse-run clinics, as well as school-based and community-based vaccine administration.
- Selected use of antiviral drugs for prevention and control have helped, especially in nursing homes, to prevent and control outbreaks. Use of antiviral drugs early in the course of influenza may have helped to shorten the course of the disease and modestly reduce its spread. Selective use of new rapid diagnostic tests may help in implementing this process though false negatives are still frequent.
- Better workplace precautions and school-based education to reduce the local spread of influenza.
- Greater insurance coverage for influenza vaccine in a wide-range of types of health insurance.

The Task Force report concluded that next flu season the United States may be faced with an epidemic or even a pandemic from the new influenza strain, but coordinated efforts to prevent, control, and minimize the impact can save thousands of lives and improve population health.

The Task Force recommended that current efforts need to continue and be expanded even further in the face of the new influenza strain. They recommended the use of the following additional efforts by the health and broader community including:

- Aggressive use of recently approved vaccine technology including cell-based vaccines and recombinant vaccines which may be more effective, can be produced more rapidly, and in the case of recombinant vaccines does not use eggs in its production. These new types of vaccines have recently been shown to be safe and have efficacy in clinical trials.
- Early efforts to vaccinate high-risk populations including healthcare professionals and nursing home residents.

- Development of community-based planning for hospital "surge capacity" and triage procedures including preparation for a large increase in the need for intensive care.
- Planning by local governments, businesses, schools, and healthcare organizations to implement phased-in efforts to reduce spread such as school closings, increased telecommuting and widespread use of tele-medicine.
- A coordinated governmental and private communications system needs to be in place to rapidly get accurate information out to the public and address rumors and false information.

The leadership and citizens of Middleburg took these recommendations to heart and took action. With an unusual consensus among community leaders, the citizens of Middleburg were cautiously optimistic that they were ready for what might come their way next year.

## Discussion Questions

1. Identify types of health professionals needed to reduce the impacts of influenza and the role(s) they need to play.
2. Discuss the roles played by non health professionals and organizations in a successful effort to control seasonal or epidemic influenza.
3. Using this influenza case identify different approaches to population health including focusing on high-risk populations and providing broad levels of population protection.
4. Discuss the types of communication that are needed between health professionals and the community to minimize the impact of influenza.

# SECTION V

# Public Health Institutions and Systems

Now that we have taken a look at the U.S. healthcare institutions and healthcare system, we need to turn our attention to the public health system. Treating healthcare and public health systems as separate systems is artificial because they have many points of overlap and collaboration. However, historically, public health institutions and systems have developed from different philosophies, have different goals, and have organizational structures and lines of accountability different from those of the healthcare system.

We will begin by outlining the current goals and roles of public health agencies. Then we will look at the current system of local/state, federal, and global public health institutions and examine how they are organized. We will explore why public health agencies need to coordinate with each other to achieve the goals of public health.

We will then return to our definition of population health—the totality of all evidence-based public and private efforts throughout the life cycle that preserve and promote health and prevent disease, disability, and death. This broad 21st-century definition requires public health agencies and professionals to collaborate with a range of government agencies and healthcare professionals and institutions.

After getting an overview of what public health agencies do, we will focus in on one especially important and rapidly changing area of public health: foods and drugs. In Chapter 13, we will look at food and drugs as public health issues. Concerns about food and drugs have played an important role in forming today's approaches to population health and continue to play important roles in our thinking about the future.

Finally, we will take a look in Chapter 14 at a relatively new and increasingly important part of population health known as systems thinking. Systems thinking helps us put together the pieces and think about how they can and need to work together to address today and tomorrow's complex health challenges. We will end with a detailed look at the **One Health** concept. One Health can be viewed as the broadest of all examples of systems thinking since it encompasses the relationships between human health, animal health, and ecosystem health. Let us now turn our attention in Chapter 12 to the current public health institutions and public health systems.

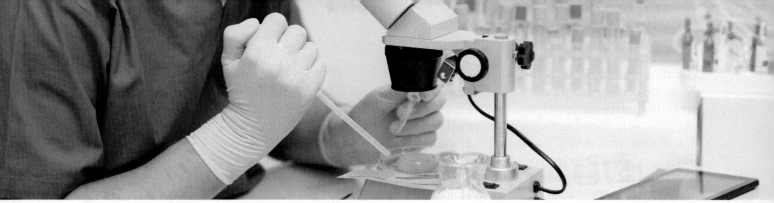

# CHAPTER 12

# Public Health Institutions and Systems

## LEARNING OBJECTIVES

By the end of this chapter, the student will be able to:

- identify goals of governmental public health.
- identify the 10 essential services of public health.
- describe the foundational public health services.
- describe basic features of local, state, and federal public health agencies in the United States.
- identify global public health organizations and agencies, and describe their basic roles.
- identify roles in public health for federal agencies not identified as health agencies.
- illustrate the need for collaboration by governmental public health agencies with other governmental and nongovernmental organizations.
- describe approaches to connecting public health and the healthcare system.

A young man in your dormitory is diagnosed with tuberculosis (TB). The health department works with the student health service to test everyone in the dorm, as well as in his classes, with a TB skin test. Those who are positive for the first time are advised to take a course of a medicine called Isoniazid (INH). You ask: Is this standard operating procedure?

You go to a public health meeting and learn that many of the speakers are not from public health agencies, but from the Departments of Labor, Commerce, Housing, and Education. You ask: What do these departments have to do with health?

You hear that a new childhood vaccine was developed by the National Institutes of

Health (NIH), approved by the Food and Drug Administration (FDA), endorsed for federal payment by the Centers for Disease Control and Prevention (CDC), and recommended for use by the American Academy of Pediatrics. You ask: Do all these agencies and organizations always work so well together?

A major flood in Asia leads to disease and starvation. Some say it is due to global warming, others to bad luck. Coordinated efforts by global health agencies, assisted by nongovernmental organizations (NGOs) and individual donors, help get the country back on its feet. You ask: What types of cooperation are needed to make all of this happen?

A local community health center identifies childhood obesity as a problem in the community. They collect data demonstrating that the problem begins as early as elementary school. They develop a plan that includes clinical interventions at the health center and also at the elementary school. They ask the health department to help them organize an educational campaign and assist in evaluating the results. Working together, they are able to reduce the obesity rate among elementary school children by 50%. This seems like a new way to practice public health. What type of approach is this?

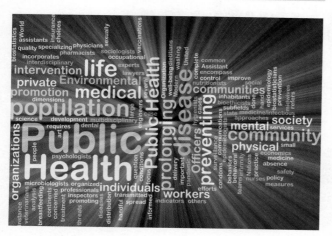

© Kheng Guan Toh/Shutterstock

These cases all reflect the responsibilities of public health agencies at the local, federal, and global levels. They illustrate public health working the way it is supposed to work. Of course, this is not always the case. Let us start by taking a look at the goals and roles of public health agencies.

## ▶ What Are the Goals and Roles of Governmental Public Health Agencies?

Public health is often equated with the work of governmental agencies. The role of government is only a portion of what we mean by "public health," but it is an important component. It is so important, in fact, that we often define the roles of other components in terms of how they relate to the work of governmental public health agencies. That is, we may refer to them as nongovernmental public health.

In 1994, the United States Public Health Service (PHS) put forth the Public Health in America statement, which provided the framework that continues to define the overall goals and services of governmental public health agencies.[1] These goals should already be familiar to you. They are:

- To prevent epidemics and the spread of disease
- To protect against environmental hazards
- To prevent injuries
- To promote and encourage healthy behaviors
- To respond to disasters and assist communities in recovery
- To ensure the quality and accessibility of health services

These are ambitious and complicated goals to achieve. To be able to successfully achieve them, it is important to further define the roles that governmental public health agencies themselves play, and by implication, the roles that other governmental agencies and NGOs need to play to achieve these goals.

The Public Health in America statement built upon the National Academy of Medicine's 1988 report called *The Future of Public Health*.[2] The National Academy of Medicine defined three **core public health functions** that governmental public health agencies need to perform. The concept of "core function" implies that the responsibility cannot be delegated to other agencies or to nongovernmental organizations. It also implies that the governmental public health agencies will work together to accomplish these functions because as a group they are responsible for public health as a whole—no one agency at the local, state, or federal level is specifically or exclusively responsible for accomplishing all the essential public health services.[a]

The core functions defined by the National Academy of Medicine are: (1) assessment, (2) policy development, and (3) assurance.[2]

- **Assessment** includes obtaining data that defines the health of the overall population and specific groups within the population, including defining the nature of new and persisting health problems.
- **Policy development** includes developing evidence-based recommendations and other analyses of options, such as health policy analysis, to guide implementation, including efforts to educate and mobilize community partnerships.
- **Assurance** includes governmental public health's oversight responsibility for ensuring that key

---

a This does not imply that components of the work cannot be contracted to nongovernmental organizations. This activity is increasingly occurring. The concept of core function, however, implies that public health agencies remain responsible for these functions even when the day-to-day work is conducted through contracts with an outside organization.

components of an effective health system, including health care and public health, are in place even though the implementation will often be performed by others.

The three core functions, while useful in providing a delineation of responsibilities and an intellectual framework for the work of governmental public health agencies, were not tangible enough to provide a clear understanding or definition of the work of public health agencies. Thus, in addition to the goals of public health, the Public Health in America statement defined a series of 10 **essential public health services** that build upon the National Academy of Medicine's core functions, guide day-to-day responsibilities, and provide a mechanism for evaluating whether the core functions are fulfilled. These 10 services have come to define the responsibilities of the combined local, state, and federal governmental public health system.

## ▶ What Are the 10 Essential Public Health Services?

**TABLE 12.1** outlines the 10 essential public health services and organizes them according to which National Academy of Medicine core function they aim to fulfill.[1] A description of each service is presented in the second column, and examples of these essential services are listed in the third column.

**TABLE 12.1** Ten Essential Public Health Services

| Essential service | Meaning of essential service | Examples |
|---|---|---|
| **Core function: assessment** | | |
| Monitor health status to identify and solve community health problems | This service includes accurate diagnosis of the community's health status; identification of threats to health and assessment of health service needs; timely collection, analysis, and publication of information on access, utilization, costs, and outcomes of personal health services; attention to the vital statistics and health status of specific groups that are at a higher risk than the total population; and collaboration to manage integrated information systems with private providers and health benefit plans. | Vital statistics<br>Health surveys<br>Surveillance, including reportable diseases |
| Diagnose and investigate health problems and health hazards in the community | This service includes epidemiologic identification of emerging health threats; public health laboratory capability using modern technology to conduct rapid screening and high-volume testing; active communicable disease epidemiology programs; and technical capacity for epidemiologic investigation of disease outbreaks and patterns of chronic disease and injury. | Epidemic investigations<br>CDC's Epidemic Intelligence Service<br>State public health laboratories |
| **Core function: policy development** | | |
| Inform, educate, and empower people about health issues | This service includes social marketing and media communications; providing accessible health information resources at community levels; active collaboration with personal healthcare providers to reinforce health promotion messages and programs; and joint health education programs with schools, churches, and worksites. | Health education campaigns, such as comprehensive state tobacco programs |
| Mobilize community partnerships and action to identify and solve health problems | This service includes convening and facilitating community groups and associations, including those not typically considered to be health-related, in undertaking defined preventive, screening, rehabilitation, and support programs; and skilled coalition-building to draw upon the full range of potential human and material resources in the cause of community health. | Lead control programs: testing and follow-up of children, reduction of lead exposure, educational follow-up, and addressing underlying causes |

*(continues)*

**TABLE 12.1** Ten Essential Public Health Services *(continued)*

| Essential service | Meaning of essential service | Examples |
|---|---|---|
| Develop policies and plans that support individual and community health efforts | This service requires leadership development at all levels of public health; systematic community- and state-level planning for health improvement in all jurisdictions; tracking of measurable health objectives as a part of continuous quality improvement strategies; joint evaluation with the medical/healthcare system to define consistent policy regarding prevention and treatment services; and development of codes, regulations, and legislation to guide public health practice. | Newborn screening and follow-up programs for phenylketonuria (PKU) and other genetic and congenital diseases |
| *Core function: assurance* | | |
| Enforce laws and regulations that protect health and ensure safety | This service involves full enforcement of sanitary codes, especially in the food industry; full protection of drinking water supplies; enforcement of clean air standards; timely follow-up of hazards, preventable injuries, and exposure-related diseases identified in occupational and community settings; monitoring quality of medical services (e.g., laboratory, nursing home, and home health care); and timely review of new drug, biological and medical device applications. | Local: Fluoridation and chlorination of water<br>State: Regulation of nursing homes<br>Federal: FDA drug approval and food safety |
| Link people to needed personal health services and ensure the provision of health care when otherwise unavailable | This service (often referred to as "outreach" or "enabling" services) includes ensuring effective entry for socially disadvantaged people into a coordinated system of clinical care; culturally and linguistically appropriate materials and staff to ensure linkage to services for special population groups; ongoing "care management"; and transportation. | Community health centers |
| Ensure the provision of a competent public and personal healthcare workforce | This service includes education and training for personnel to meet the needs of public and personal health services; efficient processes for licensure of professionals and certification of facilities with regular verification and inspection follow-up; adoption of continuous quality improvement and lifelong learning within all licensure and certification programs; active partnerships with professional training programs to ensure community-relevant learning experiences for all students; and continuing education in management and leadership development programs for those charged with administrative/executive roles. | Licensure of physicians, nurses, and other health professionals |
| Evaluate effectiveness, accessibility, and quality of personal and population-based health services | This service calls for ongoing evaluation of health programs, based on analysis of health status and service utilization data, to assess program effectiveness and to provide information necessary for allocating resources and reshaping programs. | Development of evidence-based recommendations |
| *All three National Academy of Medicine core functions* | | |
| Research for new insights and innovative solutions to health problems | This service includes continuous linkage with appropriate institutions of higher learning and research and an internal capacity to mount timely epidemiologic and economic analyses and conduct needed health services research. | NIH, CDC, Agency for Healthcare Research and Quality (AHRQ), other federal agencies |

Data from The Public Health System and the 10 Essential Public Health Services. Available at https://www.cdc.gov/nphpsp/essentialservices.html. Accessed July 22, 2017.

We have now looked at the core public health functions and the 10 essential services of public health agencies. **FIGURE 12.1** puts these together to allow you to see the connections.

Public health services are delivered through a complex web of local and federal agencies, as well as via increasing involvement of global organizations. Let us take a look at the work of public health agencies at each of these levels.

**FIGURE 12.2** provides a framework to guide our review of the delivery of public health services. It diagrams the central role of governmental public health agencies and the complicated connections required to accomplish their responsibilities. We will begin by taking a look at the structure and function of governmental public health agencies at the local/state, federal, and global levels. Then we will examine the key connections with other governmental agencies, community organizations, and private organizations, and finally the connections with the healthcare delivery system as a whole.

## What Are the Roles of Local and State Public Health Agencies?

The U.S. Constitution does not mention public health. Thus, public health is first and foremost a state responsibility. States may retain their authority, voluntarily request or accept help from the federal government, or delegate their responsibility and/or authority to local agencies at the city, county, or other local levels.[b]

**BOX 12.1** describes a brief history of public health agencies in the United States. It is a complex history and has resulted in more structures than there are states—more because large cities often have their own public health systems.[3] In addition, the District of Columbia and several U.S. territories have their own systems and often have the authority to make public health system decisions as if they were states.

To understand the role of local health departments, it is useful to think of two models.[4] In the first model, which we will call the **home rule** or local autonomy model, authority is delegated from the state to the local health department. The local health department, or the local government, has a great deal of autonomy in setting its own structure and function and often raising its own funding.

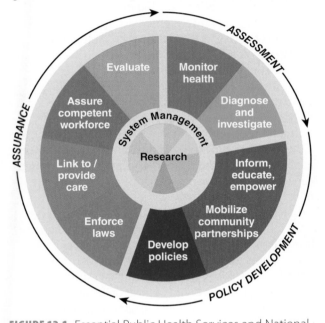

**FIGURE 12.1** Essential Public Health Services and National Academy of Medicine Core Functions

Reproduced from Centers for Disease Control and Prevention. The Public Health System and the 10 Essential Public Health Services. Available at https://www.cdc.gov/nphpsp/essentialservices.html. Accessed April 27–July 22, 2017.

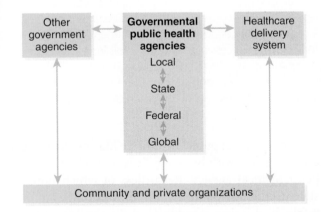

**FIGURE 12.2** Framework for Viewing Governmental Public Health Agencies and Their Complicated Connections

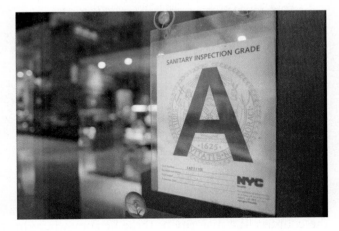

© Sorbis/Shutterstock

---

b  This delegation may occur at the discretion of the state government or it may be included in the state's constitution, providing what is called home rule authority to local jurisdictions. In general, jurisdictions with home rule authority exercise substantially more autonomy.

**BOX 12.1** Brief History of Public Health Agencies in the United States

An understanding of the history of U.S. public health institutions requires an understanding of the response of local, state, and federal governments to public health crises and the complex interactions between these levels of government.

The colonial period in the United States saw repeated epidemics of smallpox, cholera, and yellow fever focused in the port cities. These epidemics brought fear and disruption of commerce, along with accompanying disease and death. One epidemic in 1793 in Philadelphia, which was then the nation's capital, nearly shut down the federal government.

These early public health crises brought about the first municipal boards of health, made up of respected citizens authorized to act in the community's interest to implement quarantine, evacuation, and other public health interventions of the day. The federal government's early role in combating epidemics led to the establishment in 1798 of what later became known as the U.S. PHS.

Major changes in public health happened in the last half of the 1800s, with the great expansion of understanding of disease and the ability to control it through community actions. The Shattuck Commission in Massachusetts in 1850 outlined the roles of state health departments as responsible for sanitary inspections, communicable disease control, food sanitation, vital statistics, and services for infants and children. Over the next 50 years, the states gradually took the lead in developing public health institutions based upon delivery of these services.

Local health departments outside of the largest cities did not exist until the 1900s. The Rockefeller Foundation stimulated and helped fund early local health departments and campaigns in part to combat specific diseases, such as hookworm. There was no standard model for local health departments. Local health departments developed in at least 50 different ways in the 50 states and were chronically underfunded.

The federal government played a very small role in public health throughout the 19th century and well into the 20th century. An occasional public health crisis stimulated in part by media attention did bring about federal action. The founding of the Food and

Drug Administration in 1906 resulted in large part from the journalistic activity known as "muckraking," which exposed the status of food and drug safety. The early 20th century set the stage for expansion of the federal government's role in public health financed as the result of the passage of the 16th Amendment to the Constitution, which authorized federal income tax as a major source of federal government funding.

The Great Depression, in general, and the Social Security Act of 1935, in particular, brought about a new era in which federal funding became a major source of financial resources for state and local public health departments and nongovernmental organizations. The founding of what was then called the Communicable Disease Center (CDC) in 1946 led to a national and eventually international leadership role for the CDC, which attempts to connect and hold together the complex local, state, and federal public health efforts and integrate them into global public health efforts.

The Johnson administration's War on Poverty, as well as the Medicare and Medicaid programs, brought about greatly expanded funding for healthcare services and led many health departments to provide direct healthcare services, especially for those without other sources of care. The late 1980s and 1990s saw a redefinition of the roles of governmental public health, including the National Academy of Medicine's definition of core functions and the development of the 10 essential public health services. These documents have guided the development of a broad population focus for public health and a move away from the direct provision of healthcare services by health departments.

The terrorism of September 11, 2001, and the subsequent anthrax scare moved public health institutions to the center of efforts to protect the public's health through emergency response and disaster preparedness. The development of flexible efforts to respond to expected and unexpected hazards is now a central feature of public health institutions' roles and funding. The success of these efforts has led to new levels of coordination of local, state, federal, and global public health agencies utilizing state-of-the-art surveillance, laboratory technology, and communications systems.

In the second model, which we will call the branch office model, the local health department can be viewed as a branch office of the state agency with little or no independent authority or funding. There are several thousand local health departments across the country. The majority of these lie somewhere in between these two extreme models; however, these models provide a framework for understanding the many varieties of department structures. Thus, when

we speak of local public health, we may be speaking of a state agency with branch offices or a relatively independent local agency. Regardless of which model a state uses, many public health responsibilities of local public health departments are quite similar, and they usually have authority and responsibility for at least the following:[4]

■ Immunizations for those not covered by the private system

- Communicable disease surveillance and initial investigation of outbreaks
- Communicable disease control, often including at a minimum tuberculosis and syphilis case finding and treatment
- Inspection and licensing of restaurants
- Environmental health surveillance
- Coordinating public health screening programs, including newborn and lead screenings
- Tobacco control programs
- Public health preparedness and response to disasters

Health departments in many parts of the United States have also served as the healthcare provider for those without other sources of health care. This has been called the **healthcare safety net**. In recent years, many health departments have reduced or discontinued these services, often transferring them to the healthcare system or integrating their efforts into community health centers. The concept of core functions holds that while these activities can be performed by other organizations or agencies, the public health agencies still retain responsibility for ensuring access to and the quality of these services.

The work of local public health agencies cannot be viewed in isolation. The state health department usually retains important roles even in those states where the local departments have home rule authority. These responsibilities often include collecting vital statistics, running a public health laboratory, licensing health professionals, administering nutrition programs, and regulating health facilities, such as nursing homes. In addition, drinking water regulation, administration of the state Medicaid program, and the office of the medical examiner may also fall under the authority of the state health department.

## ▶ Is There a Process of Accreditation of Health Departments?

Until recently there was no accreditation process for state or local health departments. The 2003 National Academy of Medicine report *The Future of the Public's Health in the 21st Century*[5] recommended the development of a national accreditation process. Over the last decade the Public Health Accreditation Board[6] has developed a widely accepted accreditation process. Accreditation is voluntary, but health departments that serve over 75% of the U.S. population have now been accredited or in the process of being reviewed for accreditation.[7]

The accreditation criteria utilize the Essential Public Health Services. In addition a series of Foundational Public Health Services has been defined. To learn more about this new concept see **BOX 12.2**.

Today, the federal government has a great deal of involvement in national and global issues of public health and often works closely with local agencies. Let us take a look at the structure and role of the federal government in public health.

## ▶ What Are the Roles of Federal Public Health Agencies?

The federal government's role in public health does not explicitly appear in the U.S. Constitution. It has been justified largely by the Interstate Commerce clause, which provides federal government authority to regulate commerce between the states. Federal public health authority often rests on the voluntary acceptance by the states of funding provided by the federal government. This may come with requirements for state action in order to qualify for the funding.

The Department of Health and Human Services (HHS) is the central public health agency of the federal government. It includes operating agencies, each of which report directly to the cabinet-level secretary of HHS. **TABLE 12.2** outlines many of these agencies, their roles and authority, and their basic public health structure and activities.[9]

The NIH is far and away the largest agency within HHS, with a budget of over $30 billion—as much as all the other six agencies' budgets combined. However, most of its efforts are devoted to basic science research and the translation of research into clinical practice. Some of the federal agencies, such as the Health Resources and Services Administration (HRSA), Substance Abuse and Mental Health Services

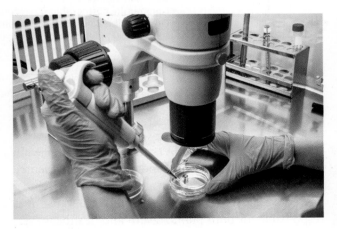

© Viacheslav Lopatin/Shutterstock

**BOX 12.2** Foundational Public Health Services

The Public Health Leadership Forum of the Institute of Medicine with the support of the Robert Wood Johnson Foundation has defined what they call **Foundational Public Health Services** which are the skills, programs, and activities that must be available in state and local health departments system-wide. The Foundational Public Health Services include "foundational capabilities" and "foundational areas" which have been defined as follows:[8]

**Foundational Capabilities** are cross-cutting skills that need to be present in state and local health departments everywhere for the health system to work anywhere. They are the essential skills and capacities needed to support the foundational areas, and other programs and activities, key to protecting the community's health and achieving equitable health outcomes. Examples of these skills include organizational competencies such as leadership, governance, quality management, and health equity; all hazards preparedness and emergency response; assessment; and others.

**Foundational Areas** are those substantive areas of expertise or program-specific activities in all state and local health departments also essential to protect the community's health. Examples of foundational areas include communicable disease control; chronic disease and injury prevention; and environmental public health inspections and monitoring, among others.

The Public Health Leadership Forum has displayed these Foundational Public Health Services as well as the Foundational Capacities and Foundational areas as depicted in **FIGURE 12.3**:[8]

The Foundational Public Health Services have been defined in detail allowing a health department and their governing authority to estimate the costs of these services and include them in their budget. The Foundational Public Health Services are being used along with the Essential Public Health Services as part of the health department accreditation process.

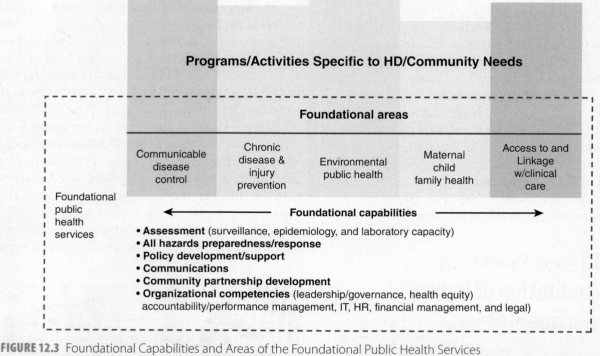

**FIGURE 12.3** Foundational Capabilities and Areas of the Foundational Public Health Services

Reproduced from RESOLVE, Public Health Leadership Forum. Defining and Constituting Foundational "Capacities" and "Areas." Available at http://www.resolv.org/site-healthleadershipforum/files/2014/03/Articulation-of-Foundational-Capabilities-and-Foundational-Areas-v1.pdf. Accessed July 22, 2017. Courtesy of RESOLVE.

Administration (SAMHSA), and the Indian Health Service (IHS), provide or fund individually oriented health services in addition to population-oriented preventive services. The IHS is unique because it is responsible for both public health and healthcare services for a defined population.

The CDC is perhaps the agency most closely identified with public health at the federal level. Since its establishment over 70 years ago, the CDC has become a national and global resource conducting research and epidemiologic investigations. It works closely with states to monitor and prevent disease through

**TABLE 12.2** Key Federal Health Agencies of the Department of Health and Human Services

| Agency | Roles/authority | Examples of structures/activities |
|---|---|---|
| CDC and the Agency for Toxic Substances and Disease Registry (ATSDR) | The CDC is the lead agency for prevention, health data, epidemic investigation, and public health measures aimed at disease control and prevention.<br><br>The CDC administers the ATSDR, which works with the Environmental Protection Agency (EPA) to provide guidance on health hazards of toxic exposures. | The CDC and ATSDR work extensively with state and local health departments.<br><br>The CDC's Epidemic Intelligence Service (EIS) functions domestically and internationally at the request of governments. |
| NIH | Lead research agency; also funds training programs and communication of health information to the professional community and the public. | 17 institutes in all—the largest being the National Cancer Institute. The National Library of Medicine is part of NIH Centers, which also include the John E. Fogarty International Center for Advanced Study in the Health Sciences.<br><br>NIH is the world's largest biomedical research enterprise, with intramural research at NIH and extramural research grants throughout the world. |
| FDA | Consumer protection agency with authority for safety of foods and safety and efficacy of drugs, vaccines, and other medical and public health interventions. | Divisions responsible for food safety, medical devices, drug efficacy, and drug safety pre- and post-approval. |
| HRSA | Seeks to ensure equitable access to comprehensive quality health care. | Funds community health centers, HIV/AIDS services, scholarships for health professional students. |
| AHRQ | Research agenda to improve the outcomes and quality of health care, including patient safety and access to services. | Supports U.S. Preventive Services Task Force, evidence-based medicine research, and Guidelines Clearinghouse. |
| SAMHSA | Works to improve quality and availability of prevention, treatment, and rehabilitation for substance abuse and mental illness. | Research, data collection, and funding of local services. |
| IHS | Provides direct health care and public health services to federally recognized tribes. | Services provided to approximately 550 federally recognized tribes in 35 states.<br><br>Only comprehensive federal agency responsibility for healthcare plus public health services. |

Data from United States Department of Health and Human Services. Organizational chart. http://www.hhs.gov/about/orgchart. Accessed July 25, 2017.

health surveillance, assisting in program implementation, and maintaining health statistics through the National Center for Health Statistics, which has been a part of the CDC since 1987.

**BOX 12.3** describes the first 50 years of the CDC, from 1946 to 1996, in a reprint of its official history first published in the *Morbidity and Mortality Weekly Report* (*MMWR*), a weekly publication of the agency.[10]

The CDC's role in connecting federal, state, and local governmental public health efforts is central to the success of the system. Approximately half of the CDC's over $10 billion total budget is channeled to state and local health departments. A key function

of the CDC is to provide national leadership and to coordinate the efforts of local/state and federal public health agencies.

To understand the local/state and federal public health system, it is important to appreciate that less than 5% of all health-related expenditures in the United States goes to governmental public health agencies, and of that, less than half goes to population-based prevention as opposed to providing healthcare services as a safety net for individuals.

In addition, the role of governmental public health is limited by social attitudes toward government. For instance, we have seen that there are

**BOX 12.3** History of the CDC

The Communicable Disease Center was organized in Atlanta, Georgia, on July 1, 1946; its founder, Dr. Joseph W. Mountin, was a visionary public health leader who had high hopes for this small and comparatively insignificant branch of the PHS. It occupied only one floor of the Volunteer Building on Peachtree Street and had fewer than 400 employees, most of whom were engineers and entomologists. Until the previous day, they had worked for Malaria Control in War Areas, the predecessor of CDC, which had successfully kept the southeastern states malaria-free during World War II and, for approximately 1 year, from murine typhus fever. The new institution would expand its interests to include all communicable diseases and would be the servant of the states, providing practical help whenever called.

Distinguished scientists soon filled CDC's laboratories, and many states and foreign countries sent their public health staffs to Atlanta for training.... Medical epidemiologists were scarce, and it was not until 1949 that Dr. Alexander Langmuir arrived to head the epidemiology branch. Within months, he launched the first-ever disease surveillance program, which confirmed his suspicion that malaria, on which CDC spent the largest portion of its budget, had long since disappeared. Subsequently, disease surveillance became the cornerstone on which CDC's mission of service to the states was built and, in time, changed the practice of public health.

The outbreak of the Korean War in 1950 was the impetus for creating CDC's EIS. The threat of biological warfare loomed, and Dr. Langmuir, the most knowledgeable person in PHS about this arcane subject, saw an opportunity to train epidemiologists who would guard against ordinary threats to public health while watching out for alien germs. The first class of EIS officers arrived in Atlanta for training in 1951 and pledged to go wherever they were called for the next 2 years. These "disease detectives" quickly gained fame for "shoe-leather epidemiology" through which they ferreted out the cause of disease outbreaks.

The survival of CDC as an institution was not at all certain in the 1950s. In 1947, Emory University gave land on Clifton Road for a headquarters, but construction did not begin for more than a decade. PHS was so intent on research and the rapid growth of the NIH that it showed little interest in what happened in Atlanta. Congress, despite the long delay in appropriating money for new buildings, was much more receptive to CDC's pleas for support than either PHS or the Bureau of the Budget.

Two major health crises in the mid-1950s established CDC's credibility and ensured its survival. In 1955, when poliomyelitis appeared in children who had received the recently approved Salk vaccine, the national inoculation program was stopped. The cases were traced to contaminated vaccine from a laboratory in California; the problem was corrected, and the inoculation program, at least for first and second graders, was resumed. The resistance of these 6- and 7-year-olds to polio, compared with that of older children, proved the effectiveness of the vaccine. Two years later, surveillance was used again to trace the course of a massive influenza epidemic. From the data gathered in 1957 and subsequent years, the national guidelines for influenza vaccine were developed.

CDC grew by acquisition.... When CDC joined the international malaria-eradication program and accepted responsibility for protecting the earth from moon germs and vice versa, CDC's mission stretched overseas and into space.

CDC played a key role in one of the greatest triumphs of public health, the eradication of smallpox. In 1962 it established a smallpox surveillance unit, and a year later tested a newly developed jet gun and vaccine in the Pacific island nation of Tonga.... CDC also achieved notable success at home tracking new and mysterious disease outbreaks. In the mid-1970s and early 1980s, it found the cause of Legionnaires disease and toxic-shock syndrome. A fatal disease, subsequently named acquired immunodeficiency syndrome (AIDS), was first mentioned in the June 5, 1981, issue of MMWR.

Although CDC succeeded more often than it failed, it did not escape criticism. For example, television and press reports about the Tuskegee study on long-term effects of untreated syphilis in black men created a storm of protest in 1972. This study had been initiated by PHS and other organizations in 1932 and was transferred to CDC in 1957. Although the effectiveness of penicillin as a therapy for syphilis had been established during the late 1940s, participants in this study remained untreated until the study was brought to public attention. CDC was also criticized because of the 1976 effort to vaccinate the U.S. population against swine flu, the infamous killer of 1918–1919. When some recipients of the vaccines developed Guillain-Barre syndrome, the campaign was stopped immediately; the epidemic never occurred.

As the scope of CDC's activities expanded far beyond communicable diseases, its name had to be changed. In 1970 it became the Center for Disease Control, and in 1981, after extensive reorganization, Center became Centers. The words "and Prevention" were added in 1992, but, by law, the well-known three-letter acronym was retained. In health emergencies, CDC means an answer to SOS calls from anywhere in the world....

Reproduced from Centers for Disease Control and Prevention. History of CDC. *Morbidity and Mortality Weekly Report*. 1996;45:526–528.

constitutional limitations on the authority of public health and other government agencies to impose actions on individuals. These may limit public health agencies' abilities to address issues ranging from tuberculosis and HIV control to responses to emergencies.

The social attitudes of Americans may also limit the authority and resources provided to public health agencies. Americans often favor individual or private efforts over governmental interventions when they believe that individuals and private organizations are capable of success. For instance, some Americans resist active efforts in schools to provide information and access to contraceptives, while others resist the type of case-finding efforts for HIV/AIDS that have

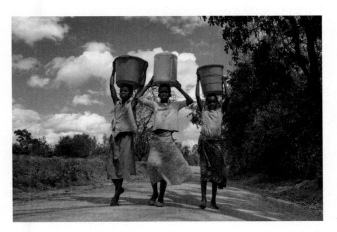

© Guido Dingemans, De Eindredactie/Moment/Getty

been used successfully in investigating and controlling other communicable diseases.

Today, governmental public health is a global enterprise. Let us take a look at the roles of global health organizations and agencies.

## ▶ What Are the Roles of Global Health Organizations and Agencies?

Public health is increasingly becoming a global enterprise. Global governmental efforts have grown dramatically in recent years. The World Health Organization (WHO) was created in 1948. Its impact has become more prominent in the 21st century with the increasing importance of global health issues. The WHO is a part of the United Nations organizations, which also include the United Nations Children's Fund and the Joint United Nations Programme on AIDS/HIV (UNAIDS).[11]

Today, the World Bank and other multilateral financial institutions are the largest funding source for global health efforts.[12] National governmental aid programs, including the United States Agency for International Development (USAID), also play an important role in public health. **TABLE 12.3** outlines the structure/governance, roles, and limitations of global public health agencies.

**TABLE 12.3** Global Public Health Organizations

| Type of agency | Structure/governance | Role(s) | Limitations |
|---|---|---|---|
| WHO | United Nations Organization<br>  Seven "regional" semi-independent components (e.g., Pan American Health Organization covers North and South America) | Policy development (e.g., tobacco treaty, epidemic control policies)<br>  Coordination of services (e.g., Severe Acute Respiratory Syndrome (SARS) control, vaccine development)<br>  Data collection and standardization (e.g., measures of healthcare quality, measures of health status).<br>  Director has authority to declare "public health emergency of global concern" | Limited ability to enforce global recommendations, limited funding, and complex international administration |
| Other U.N. agencies with focused agenda | UNICEF<br>UNAIDS | Focus on childhood vaccinations<br>  Focus on AIDS | Limited agendas and limited financing |
| International financing organizations | The World Bank<br>  Other multilateral regional banks (e.g., InterAmerican and Asian Development Banks) | World Bank is largest international funder. Increasingly supports "human capital" projects and reform of healthcare delivery systems and population and nutrition efforts<br>  Provides funding and technical assistance, primarily as loans | Criticized for standardized approach with few local modifications |

*(continues)*

**TABLE 12.3** Global Public Health Organizations                                                                 *(continued)*

| Type of agency | Structure/governance | Role(s) | Limitations |
|---|---|---|---|
| Bilateral governmental aid organizations | USAID<br>   Many other developed countries have their own organizations and contribute a higher percentage of their gross domestic product to those agencies than does the United States | Often focused on specific countries and specific types of programs, such as the United States' focus on HIV/AIDS, and maternal and child health | May be tied to domestic politics and global economic, political, or military agendas |

As we have seen, global health collaboration has increased in recent years as the world has faced new "public health emergencies of global concern." The Ebola epidemic of 2014–2016 and the ongoing spread of Zika have put increased pressure on national and international public health agencies to work together.

The complexity of local, state, federal, and global public health agencies has made collaboration difficult. It should not surprise you that close collaboration, while the goal, is often difficult to achieve with so many organizations involved. Thus, it is important to ask: How can public health agencies work together?

## ▶ How Can Public Health Agencies Work Together?

Coordination among public health agencies has been a major challenge that is built into our local, state, and federal systems of governance. Increasingly, coordination also requires a global aspect as well. Efforts on all levels have a long way to go. There are signs of

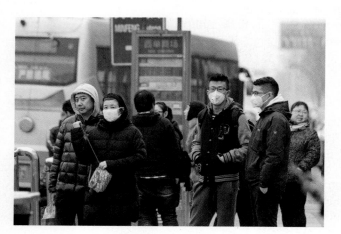

© testing/Shutterstock

hope with progress in such fields as tobacco control, food safety, as well as the responses to SARS, Ebola, and Zika.

**BOX 12.4** discusses the dramatic events of the 2003 SARS epidemic, providing an example of what can be done and what needs to be done to address future public health emergencies.[13]

Collaboration needs to be an everyday effort, and not just a requirement for emergencies or epidemics. Let us look at the relationships and needed collaboration among governmental public health and other governmental agencies, nongovernmental organizations, and the healthcare delivery system.

## ▶ What Other Government Agencies Are Involved in Health Issues?

To address health issues, it is important to recognize the important roles that government agencies not designated as health agencies play in public health. Such agencies exist at the local/state, federal, and global levels. To illustrate the involvement of these agencies in health issues, let us begin with the roles of nonhealth agencies at the federal level.

A number of federal agencies serve public health functions even though they are not defined as health agencies. The roles they play are important, especially when we take the population health perspective, which includes the totality of efforts throughout the life cycle to promote and protect health and prevent disease, disability, and death.

Environmental health issues are an important part of the role of the EPA. Reducing injury and hazardous exposures in the workplace are key goals of the Occupational Safety and Health Administration (OSHA), which is part of the Department of Labor.

**BOX 12.4** SARS and the Public Health Response

The SARS epidemic of 2003 began with little notice, most likely somewhere in the heartland of China, and then spread to other areas of Asia. The world took notice after television screens filled with reports of public health researchers sent to Asia to investigate the illness subsequently contracting and dying from the disease.

Not an easily transmissible disease except for between those in very close contact, such as investigators, family members, and healthcare providers, the disease spread slowly but steadily through areas of China. Among those infected, the case-fatality rate was very high, especially without the benefits of modern intensive care facilities.

The disease did not respond to antibiotics and was thought to be a viral disease by its epidemiological pattern of spread and transmission, but at first, no cause was known. The outside world soon felt the impact of the brewing epidemic when cases appeared in Hong Kong that could be traced to a traveler from mainland China. Fear spread when cases were recognized that could not be explained by close personal contact with a SARS victim.

The epidemic continued to spread, jumping thousands of miles to Toronto, Canada, where the second greatest concentration of disease appeared. Soon, the whole world was on high alert, if not quite on the verge of panic. At least 8000 people worldwide became sick and almost 10% of them died. Fortunately, progress came quite quickly.

Researchers coordinated by the WHO were able to put together the epidemiological information and laboratory data and establish a presumed cause, a new form of the coronavirus never before seen in humans, leading to the rapid introduction of testing.

The WHO and the CDC put forth recommendations for isolation, travel restrictions, and intensive monitoring that rapidly controlled the disease even in the absence of an effective treatment aimed at a cure. SARS disappeared as rapidly as it emerged, especially after systematic efforts to control spread were put in place in China. Not eliminated, but no longer a worldwide threat, SARS left a lasting global impact. The WHO established new approaches for reporting and responding to epidemics—these now have the widespread formal acceptance of most governments.

Once the world could step back and evaluate what happened, it was recognized that the potential burden of disease posed by the SARS epidemic had worldwide implications and raised the threat of interruption of travel and trade. Local, national, and global public health agencies collaborated quickly and effectively. Infection control recommendations made at the global level were rapidly translated into efforts to identify disease at the local level and manage individual patients in hospitals throughout the world. It is a model of communicable disease control that will continue to be needed.

Protecting health as part of preparation and response to disasters and terrorism is central to the role of the Department of Homeland Security. The Department of Agriculture shares with the FDA the role of protecting the nation's food supply. The Department of Housing and Urban Development influences the built environment and its impacts on health. The Department of Energy plays important roles in setting radiation safety standards for nuclear power plants and other sources of energy.

The multiple federal agencies involved in health-related matters often means that coordination and collaboration are required across agencies. This is certainly the case with food safety and disaster planning and response. It is true as well for efforts to address problems that cut across agencies, such as lead exposure or efforts to reduce the environmental causes of asthma.

The collaboration needed to address complex public health issues lends itself to a health in all policies approach, which acknowledges that the variety of influences impacting population health are outside the control of the health sector. Collaborative efforts are not restricted to governmental agencies. We will now explore the roles of NGOs in public health.

## What Roles Do Nongovernmental Organizations Play in Public Health?

NGOs play increasingly important roles in public health in the United States and around the world. The United States has a long tradition of private groups, often called nonprofits, organizing to advocate for public health causes, delivering public health services, and providing funding to support public health efforts. In recent years, these efforts have been expanding globally as well.

The American Red Cross and its network of international affiliates represent a major international effort to provide public health services. The organization plays a central role in obtaining volunteers for blood donations and ensuring the safety and effectiveness of the U.S. and world supply of blood products in collaboration with the U.S. Food and Drug Administration. The ability of the Red Cross to obtain donations, mobilize volunteers, and publicize the need for disaster assistance has allowed it to play a central role in providing lifesaving public health services.

Many private organizations provide public health education, support research, develop evidence-based recommendations, and provide other public health services. Many of these are organized around specific diseases or types of disease, such as the American Cancer Association, the American Heart Association, the American Lung Association, and the March of Dimes, which today focuses on birth defects. Other private organizations focus primarily on advocacy for individuals with specific diseases, but these organizations also may advocate for specific public health interventions. For instance, Mothers Against Drunk Driving (MADD) has had a major impact on the passage and enforcement of drunk driving laws. HIV/AIDS advocacy groups have influenced policies on confidentiality, funding, and public education.

Globally, NGOs increasingly play a key role in providing services and advocating for public health policies. CARE and Oxfam International are examples of the types of organizations involved in global health-related crises. Physician groups, including Physicians for Social Responsibility and Doctors without Borders, have been active in advocating for public health efforts, seeking funding for public health needs, and addressing the ethical implementation of public health programs.

New combinations of governmental and NGOs are increasingly developing to fill in the gaps. At the global level, the Global Fund to Fight AIDS, Tuberculosis, and Malaria, a public–private effort, provides funding for evidence-based interventions to address these diseases. It is funded not only by governments, but also by private foundations, such as the Bill and Melinda Gates Foundation.

Private foundations have long played major roles in funding public health efforts and also stimulating governmental funding. The Rockefeller Foundation's efforts were instrumental in developing local health departments and initiating schools of public health in the United States during the early 20th century. The Kellogg Foundation, the Robert Wood Johnson Foundation, and most recently the Gates Foundation have all played key roles in advancing public health efforts in areas ranging from nutrition to tobacco control to advancing new public health technologies.

Foundation funding has been the catalyst in initiating new funding efforts and sustaining those that are not adequately funded by governments. They cannot be expected, however, to provide long-term support for basic public health services. Thus, additional strategies are required. One key strategy is to link public health efforts with the efforts of healthcare professionals and the healthcare system.

## How Can Public Health Agencies Partner with Health Care to Improve the Response to Health Problems?

We have already seen a number of traditional connections between public health and health care. Clinicians and public health professionals increasingly share a common commitment to evidence-based thinking, cost-effective delivery of services, and computerized and confidential data systems. They also increasingly share a commitment to provide quality services to the entire population and eliminate health disparities. The potential for successful collaboration between public health and health care is illustrated by the National Vaccine Plan, which is discussed in **BOX 12.5**.[14]

In the mid-1990s, the Medicine-Public Health Initiative attempted to investigate better ways to connect public health with medicine, in particular, and health care, in general. Connecting these two fields has not always had easy or successful results. Additional structures are needed to formalize effective and efficient bonds. Models do exist, and new ideas are being put forth to connect clinical care and public health. **BOX 12.6** discusses one such model, called **community-oriented primary care (COPC)**.[16]

In the United States, community health centers have great potential to utilize the COPC approach to connect health care and public health. Despite efforts in the healthcare system to reach out to the community and address public health issues (such as COPC), it remains the primary responsibility of governmental public health to organize and mobilize community-based efforts. Working with NGOs and healthcare professionals and organizations is imperative to effectively and efficiently accomplish the goals of public health. But how exactly can public health agencies accomplish these goals?

## How Can Public Health Take the Lead in Mobilizing Community Partnerships to Identify and Solve Health Problems?

An essential service of public health is the mobilization of community partnerships and action to identify and solve health problems. These efforts by public health agencies are critical to putting the pieces of the

**BOX 12.5** National Vaccine Plan

In 1994, the first National Vaccine Plan was developed as part of a coordinated effort to accomplish the following goals:

1. "Develop new and improved vaccines".
2. "Ensure the optimal safety and effectiveness of vaccines and immunizations".
3. "Better educate the public and members of the health profession on the benefits and risks of immunizations".

A recent Institute of Medicine (IOM) evaluated progress since 1994 on achieving these goals and made recommendations for the development of a revised National Vaccine Plan.[15] The IOM highlighted a number of successes since 1994 in achieving each of the goals of the plan. These successes illustrate the potential for improved collaboration between public health systems and healthcare systems.

In terms of the development of new and improved vaccines since 1994, "more than 20 new vaccine products resulting from the collaborative efforts of the National Institutes of Health (NIH), academic, and industry researchers were approved by the Food and Drug Administration (FDA). Novel vaccines introduced include vaccines against pediatric pneumococcal disease, meningococcal disease, and the human papillomavirus (HPV)"—a cause of cervical cancer.

In terms of safety, vaccines and vaccination approaches with improved safety have been developed since 1994, including those directed against rotavirus, pertussis (whooping cough), and polio. "The FDA Center for Biologics Evaluation and Research (CBER),

which regulates vaccines, has had an expanding array of regulatory tools and legislative requirements that facilitate the review and approval of safe and efficacious vaccines… [The] FDA and CDC have collaborated on surveillance for and evaluation of adverse events… Efforts have also been made to increase collaboration with CMS, the Department of Defense, and the Department of Veterans Affairs to improve surveillance and reporting of adverse events following immunization in the adult populations these agencies serve."

In terms of better education of health professionals and the public, progress has also been made. The American Academy of Pediatrics (AAP) collaborates with the CDC for its childhood immunization support. The American Medical Association (AMA) cosponsors the annual National Influenza Vaccine Summit, a group that represents 100 public and private organizations interested in preventing influenza.

Despite the growing collaboration and success in vaccine development and use, new issues have appeared in recent years. Vaccines are now correctly viewed by the health professionals and the public as having both benefits and harms. In recent years, the public has grown more concerned about the safety of vaccines, including the issue of the use of large numbers of vaccines in children. The limitations of vaccines to address problems, such as HIV/AIDS, have also been increasingly recognized. Hopefully, the continued efforts to develop and implement national vaccine plans will build upon these recent successes and address the new realities and opportunities.

health system together to protect and promote health and prevent disability and death.

Increasingly, community members themselves are becoming active participants in addressing health and disease in their communities. One approach to engage community members in the process is through **community-based participatory research (CBPR)**. Through CBPR, community members are involved in all phases of the research process; contributing their expertise while sharing ownership and responsibility over the research; and assisting to build trust, knowledge, and skill to facilitate the research and development and implementation of interventions.

Examples of successful collaboration include state tobacco control programs that have been led by public health agencies, but rely heavily on nongovernmental organizations, healthcare professionals, and other governmental agencies. These efforts have been able to substantially reduce statewide cigarette smoking rates.

Efforts to organize coordinated programs for lead control have also been met with success. Collaborative efforts between public health and health care have identified and treated children with elevated lead levels. Cooperation with other agencies has provided for the removal of lead paint from homes and testing and control of lead in playgrounds, water, and, most recently, toys.

It is possible to view the coordinated mobilization of public and private efforts as **community-oriented public health (COPH)**. We can see this as a parallel to COPC. In COPC, healthcare efforts are expanded to take on additional public health roles. In COPH, public health efforts are expanded to collaborate with healthcare delivery institutions, as well as other community and other governmental efforts. Child oral health, an example of COPH, is illustrated in **BOX 12.7**.[17]

Developing community partnerships is a time-consuming and highly political process that

## BOX 12.6 Community-Oriented Primary Care (COPC)

COPC is a structured effort to expand the delivery of health services from a focus on the individual to also include an additional focus on the needs of communities. Serving the needs of communities brings healthcare and public health efforts together. COPC can be seen as an effort on the part of healthcare delivery sites, such as community health centers, to reach out to their community and to governmental public health institutions.

TABLE 12.4 outlines the six steps in the COPC process and presents a question to ask when addressing each of these steps. Notice the parallels between COPC and the evidence-based approach. In both cases, the process is actually circular because evaluation efforts often lead to recycling to move the process ahead.

A series of principles underlies COPC, including:

- Healthcare needs are defined by examining the community as a whole, not just those who seek care.
- Needed healthcare services are provided to everyone within a defined population or community.
- Preventive, curative, and rehabilitative care are integrated within a coordinated delivery system.
- Members of the community directly participate in all stages of the COPC process.

The concept of COPC, if not the specific structure, has been widely accepted as an approach for connecting the organized delivery of primary health care with public health. It implies that public health issues can and should be addressed when possible at the level of the community with the involvement of healthcare providers and the community members themselves.

**TABLE 12.4** The Six Sequential Steps of Community-Oriented Primary Care (COPC)

| Steps in the COPC process | Questions to ask |
| --- | --- |
| Community definition | How is the community defined based upon geography, institutional affiliation, or other common characteristics (e.g., use of an Internet site)? |
| Community characterization | What are the demographic and health characteristics of the community and what are its health issues? |
| Prioritization | What are the most important health issues facing the community and how should they be prioritized based upon objective data and perceived need? |
| Detailed assessment of the selected health problem | What are the most effective and efficient interventions for addressing the selected health problem based upon an evidence-based assessment? |
| Intervention | What strategies will be used to implement the intervention? |
| Evaluation | How can the success of the intervention be evaluated? |

Data from Gofin J, Gofin R. *Essentials of Global Community Health*. Sudbury, MA: Jones & Bartlett Learning; 2011.

## BOX 12.7 Child Oral Health and Community-Oriented Public Health (COPH)

The problem of childhood dental disease illustrates the potential for community-oriented public health (COPH). A lack of regular dental care remains a major problem for children in developed, as well as developing, countries. The need for this type of care is often high on the agenda of parents, teachers, and even the children themselves.

Public health efforts to improve oral health go back to the late 1800s and early 1900s, when tooth brushing and toothpaste were new and improved technologies. The public health campaigns of the early 1900s were

very instrumental in making tooth brushing a routine part of U.S. life.

The history of public health interventions in childhood oral health is a story of great hope and partial success. The benefits of the fluoridation of drinking water were well grounded in evidence. The American Dental Association and the AMA have supported this intervention for over half a century. Resistance from those who view it as an intrusion of governmental authority, however, has prevented universal use of fluoridation in the United States. After over a half century of effort, fluoridation has reached less than 66% of Americans through the water supply.

Today, new technologies from dental sealants to more cost-effective methods for treating cavities have again made oral health a public health priority. However, the number of dentists has not grown in recent years to keep up with the growing population. In addition, dental care for those without the resources to pay for it is often inadequate and inaccessible. Thus, a new approach is needed to bring dental care to those in need. Perhaps a new strategy using a COPH approach can make this happen.

Community-oriented public health can reach beyond the institutional and geographical constraints that COPC faces when based in a community health center or other institutions serving a geographically defined population or community. COPH as a governmentally led effort allows a greater range of options for intervention, including those that require changes in laws, incentives, and governmental procedures. These may include authorizing new types of clinicians, providing services in nontraditional settings such as schools, funding innovations to put new technologies into practice, and addressing the regulatory barriers to rapid and cost-effective delivery of services.

requires great leadership and diplomatic skills. Central authority and command-and-control approaches are generally not effective in the complex organizational structures of the United States. New approaches and new strategies are needed to bring together the organizations and individuals who can get the job done.

We have now looked at the organization of the public health system and the challenges it faces in accomplishing its core functions and providing its essential services. The role of public health will continue to evolve as current and emerging issues impact the health of the population.

## Key Words

Assessment
Assurance
Community-based participatory research (CBPR)
Community-oriented primary care (COPC)

Community-oriented public health (COPH)
Core public health functions
Essential public health services
Foundational areas
Foundational capabilities

Foundational Public Health Services
Healthcare safety net
Home rule
Nongovernmental organizations
Policy development

## Discussion Questions

Take a look at the questions posed in the following scenarios, which were presented at the beginning of this chapter. See now whether you can answer them.

1. A young man in your dormitory is diagnosed with tuberculosis (TB). The health department works with the student health service to test everyone in the dorm, as well as in his classes, with a TB skin test. Those who are positive for the first time are advised to take a course of a medicine called Isoniazid (INH). You ask: Is this standard operating procedure?

2. You go to a public health meeting and learn that many of the speakers are not from public health agencies, but from the Departments of Labor, Commerce, Housing, and Education. You ask: What do these departments have to do with health?

3. You hear that a new childhood vaccine was developed by the National Institutes of Health (NIH), approved by the Food and Drug Administration (FDA), endorsed for federal payment by the Centers for Disease Control and Prevention (CDC), and recommended for use by the American Academy of Pediatrics. You ask: Do all these agencies and organizations always work so well together?

4. A major flood in Asia leads to disease and starvation. Some say it is due to global warming, others to bad luck. Coordinated efforts by global health agencies, assisted by nongovernmental organizations (NGOs) and individual donors, help get the country back on its feet. You ask: What types of cooperation are needed to make all of this happen?

5. A local community health center identifies childhood obesity as a problem in the community. They collect data demonstrating that the problem begins as early as elementary school. They develop a plan that includes clinical interventions at the health center and also at the elementary school. They ask the health department to help them organize an educational campaign and assist in evaluating the results. Working together, they are able to reduce the obesity rate

among elementary school children by 50%. This seems like a new way to practice public health. What type of approach is this?

## References

1. The Public Health System and the 10 Essential Public Health Services. https://www.cdc.gov/nphpsp/essentialservices.html. Accessed July 25, 2017.

2. Institute of Medicine. *The Future of Public Health*. Washington, DC: National Academies Press; 1988.

3. Turnock BJ. *Public Health: What It Is and How It Works*. 4th ed. Burlington, MA: Jones & Bartlett Learning; 2016.

4. Turnock BJ. *Essentials of Public Health*. 3rd ed. Burlington, MA: Jones & Bartlett Learning; 2016.

5. Institute of Medicine. The future of the public's health in the 21st century. https://www.nap.edu/catalog/10548/the-future-of-the-publics-health-in-the-21st-century. Accessed July 25, 2017.

6. Public Health Accreditation Board. Accreditation overview. http://www.phaboard.org/accreditation-overview/. Accessed July 25, 2017.

7. Public Health Accreditation Board. Accreditation activity. http://www.phaboard.org/news-room/accreditation-activity/. Accessed July 25, 2017.

8. Public Health Leadership Forum. Defining and constituting foundational "Capacities" and "Areas." http://www.resolv.org /site-healthleadershipforum/files/2014/03/Articulation-of -Foundational-Capabilities-and-Foundational-Areas-v1.pdf. Accessed July 25, 2017.

9. U.S. Department of Health and Human Services. Organizational chart. http://www.hhs.gov/about/orgchart. Accessed July 25, 2017.

10. Centers for Disease Control and Prevention. History of CDC. *Morbidity and Mortality Weekly Report*. 1996;45:526–528.

11. World Health Organization. About WHO. http://www.who .int/about/en/. Accessed July 25, 2017.

12. The World Bank. Health. Who We Are. http://www.worldbank .org/en/who-we-are. Accessed July 25, 201712.

13. Duffin J, Sweetman A. *SARS in Context: Memory, History, Policy*. Montreal, Canada: McGill-Queen's University Press; 2006.

14. HHS.gov. U.S. National Vaccine Plan. https://www.hhs.gov /nvpo/national-vaccine-plan/index.html. Accessed July 25, 2017.

15. Institute of Medicine. Initial guidance for an update of the National Vaccine Plan: a letter report to the national vaccine program office. http://www.nap.edu/catalog/12257.html. Accessed July 25, 2017.

16. Gofin J, Gofin R. *Essentials of Global Community Health*. Sudbury, MA: Jones & Bartlett Learning; 2011.

17. Pfizer Global Pharmaceuticals. *Milestones in Public Health: Accomplishments in Public Health over the Last 100 Years*. New York, NY: Pfizer Global Pharmaceuticals; 2006.

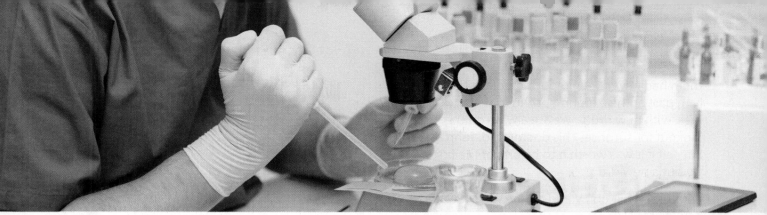

# CHAPTER 13

# Food and Drugs As Public Health Issues

## LEARNING OBJECTIVES

By the end of this chapter, the student will be able to:

- describe six ways that food affects health and disease.
- identify the steps in a foodborne outbreak investigation.
- identify the roles played by the Food and Drug Administration (FDA), Centers for Disease Control and Prevention (CDC), and U.S. Department of Agriculture (USDA) in food safety.
- describe the phases of drug approval by the FDA.
- explain the safety limitations of traditional approaches to drug approval.
- describe the role of postmarket surveillance in drug safety.
- describe recent changes in the FDA laws for food and also for drugs.
- identify other categories of products besides food and drugs regulated by the FDA.

"We are what we eat," you hear said again and again. "Sure," you say, "too little is bad, too much is bad, but what other ways can food affect our health?"

An outbreak of hepatitis A occurs among employees eating in your cafeteria. To your surprise, the local health department and the CDC quickly investigate the outbreak and trace its source to seafood grown and harvested in an Asian country and to the factory that handled the food in the United States far from your home. How is food being traced, you wonder, to allow outbreaks to be so rapidly and efficiently investigated?

Jessica wondered why she needed a pregnancy test each month to refill her prescription for acne medication. She was not even currently sexually active. The pharmacist told her that she needed to come in with proof of a recent pregnancy test because serious birth defects are so common with this medication. What a pain and what an embarrassment, she thought to herself. Why is all this bureaucracy needed anyway?

John's cancer was in remission, but he was still taking chemotherapy, and he often felt very sleepy. His doctor asked whether he wanted to try a new drug that was just approved by the FDA and showed evidence of reducing fatigue. John knew he was taking a chance, but he readily agreed. The side effects were worse than expected, and John's doctor told him some of them had never been reported before. "I guess I am part of the experiment," he told his doctor. "Yes, with new drugs, we are always on the lookout for surprises," his doctor said. John asked himself if it was worth it to be one of the first to try out a new drug.

Veronica saw it on TV and on the Web. It was a new dietary supplement that showed promise for reducing blood pressure, and that was just what Veronica needed. The fine print on the bottle said that it was not for the treatment or prevention of any disease. A low dose seemed to have some effect and a higher dose was even better. When Veronica started feeling a little dizzy, she went to the emergency room, where they found that she was losing blood in her stools. The dietary supplement was thought to be the cause of her bleeding and her reduced blood pressure. Veronica asked, "Do I need to treat dietary supplements as if they are drugs?"

Carlos's doctor told him he wanted to try him on a new treatment for his headaches because the standard treatment was not working. He told Carlos that the drug had been on the market for several years but was not officially recommended for headaches by the FDA. "I have been hearing that it works for headaches, and I would like to try it out, if you agree," the doctor said. Carlos wondered, Is that the way medicine is practiced?

Issues of food and drugs are central to public health. In this chapter, we will take a look at where we are in addressing the ongoing public health issues related to food and drugs. To understand where we are today, we need to take a look at the history of food and drugs and public health issues.

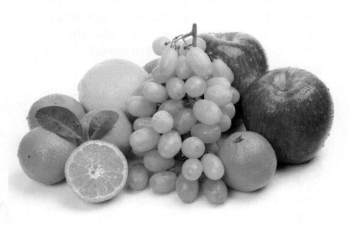

© Elena Itsenko/Shutterstock

## ▶ What Are Important Milestones in the History of Food and Drugs As Public Health Issues in the United States?[1]

Until the early 20th century, narcotics, cocaine, and other addictive substances were widely sold in the United States totally within the law. Drugs were falsely advertised to produce miraculous cures, and labeling of ingredients was not required. There were few limitations on what could be advertised or what substances the miracle cures of the day could contain. Abuses in the food industry included use of poisonous preservatives and dyes in food. Unsanitary conditions in the meatpacking industry were vividly portrayed in Upton Sinclair's classic novel *The Jungle*.

The aggressive journalists of the early 1900s, known as "muckrakers," brought to public attention many dangers from food and drugs. In 1906, these efforts resulted in the passage of federal legislation establishing what later became the FDA as part of the USDA. The Federal Food and Drugs Act of 1906 is often considered a key accomplishment of what has been called the Progressive Era of U.S. politics.

Though this legislation creating the FDA provided the foundation for modern food and drug regulation, the original law only required that products include accurate labeling indicating their ingredients. The burden was on the FDA to demonstrate safety problems before a drug could be removed from the market. It was not until the late 1930s that the authority of the FDA was expanded. This expansion was justified by use of the interstate commerce clause because most drugs are part of commerce between two or more states.

In 1937, a Tennessee drug company producing a pediatric liquid form of sulfa, the first antibiotic, precipitated the changes in FDA law. The solvent in this untested product was a highly toxic chemical related to antifreeze. Over 100 people died from kidney disease, mostly children. The public outcry brought Congress to action with the passage of the 1938 Federal Food, Drug, and Cosmetic Act. These amendments required safety testing prior to making a new drug available to the market. The process of safety regulation soon resulted in an additional requirement that certain drugs be prescribed only by a physician, while others were available as nonprescription drugs, or over-the-counter drugs. In addition, Congress expanded the authority and created a separate entity now called the Food and Drug Administration.

Congress gave the FDA authority to regulate cosmetics, authorized factory inspections, and gave the FDA increased authority to regulate both foods and drugs.

Over the years, the FDA's authority has been repeatedly increased in the wake of highly publicized tragedies. The production and distribution of a batch of polio vaccine that itself caused polio led to the regulation of vaccines in the 1950s. The Dalkon Shield, an intrauterine device (IUD) that produced thousands of cases of infection and subsequent infertility, brought about increased regulation of medical devices in the mid-1970s.

Perhaps the most famous U.S. drug disaster was the one that did not happen. In the early 1960s, FDA safety regulations resulted in a delay in approving a new, very effective sleeping pill called thalidomide. In Europe, the drug produced thousands of grossly deformed newborns with greatly shortened arms and legs, an event that did not occur in the United States. Ironically, the thalidomide case resulted in the Kefauver-Harris Drug Amendments, which focused on efficacy, not safety, and mandated efficacy testing before a drug could be approved and marketed. This landmark legislation laid the groundwork for today's process of drug approval and for the evolution of evidence-based medicine and public health.

The authority of the FDA, however, did not continue to expand. The 1980s and 1990s produced a social movement that sought smaller government and less authority over the lives of individuals. In addition, in the early 1990s, a U.S. Supreme Court decision allowed advertising of prescription drugs. The enormous expansion of prescription drug promotion encouraged a flood of direct advertisement to consumers and a rapid expansion of the quantity of prescription drugs marketed and prescribed. The greatly increased use of drugs in recent years has been associated with a large increase in drug side effects. As we will see, the FDA is now trying to address this 21st century-issue based on new federal legislation.

On the food front, the 21st century brought globalization of our food supply. The United States now obtains food products from well over 100 countries. Food increasingly originates in distant places, across the country, or from abroad and is processed in multiple locations. These foods are far more likely than locally grown and unprocessed foods to produce disease. The complexity of our food sources and food processing has magnified the potential for food-related disease, including outbreaks of disease. As we will see, several federal agencies are also now addressing this issue using tools provided by new federal food legislation as well as new technology.[2] Thus, the early years of the 21st century have brought new challenges and new approaches to both food and drug safety.

## ▶ Food and Food Safety

"We are what we eat" is a now familiar expression that suggests a wide range of ways that food can affect our health and lead to disease. Let us begin by taking a look at possible ways that food can affect our health.

### What Ways Can Food Affect Health and Disease?

There are a large number of ways that food can affect our health and can produce disease. Among the most important are:

- Too little food
- Too much food
- Deficiencies of vitamins and minerals
- Contaminants
- Individual susceptibilities
- Foodborne communicable diseases

Let us take a look at each of these:

*Too little food*: Undernutrition consisting of inadequate intake of calories and protein was among the most common causes of disease in the 20th century and earlier centuries, and it still is a common cause of disease, especially in today's developing world. Today, undernutrition remains an issue in a number of areas of the world, including some poor and remote areas of the United States. The world's food supply today is adequate to prevent undernutrition. Undernutrition today represents a society's failure to ensure basic services.

*Too much food*: Obesity is rapidly approaching tobacco use as the number one cause of death and disability in the United States. Over 30% of the adult

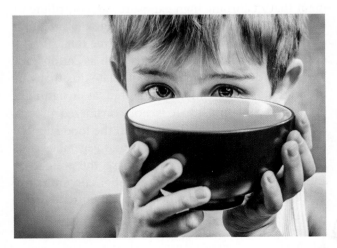

© Suzanne Tucker/Shutterstock

population is now considered obese, having a body mass index (BMI) of over 30. An even larger percentage of the adult population is considered overweight, having a BMI of over 25. The epidemic of obesity is rapidly expanding to include children. The rapid increase in type 2 diabetes and the potential for longer term complications have put obesity at or near the top of the U.S. public health agenda.

*Deficiencies of vitamins and minerals*: A growing list of vitamins and minerals, often called **micronutrients**, are now recognized as essential in small quantities to good health. These include vitamins A, B, C, D, E, and K, as well as the B-complex vitamins. The need for minerals—including iron, which is needed to prevent anemia, and iodine, which is needed to prevent thyroid enlargement or goiter—has been known for many years. A long list of minerals is being recognized as important to optimal health, including magnesium, selenium, copper, and zinc. A classic case of the importance of vitamins to public health is illustrated in **BOX 13.1** which takes a look at the history of pellagra.

Supplementation of foods with vitamins and minerals has been an important public health intervention for many years. Supplementation of foods with vitamin D has been used for decades to prevent bone disease. Other vitamins and minerals are increasingly being added to food products. For instance, folic acid, or vitamin B9, has been recognized as a key to the closure of the fetus's spinal column and skull during the first month of pregnancy. Supplementation of food with folic acid is now being used as an important intervention to prevent what are called neural tube defects, especially spina bifida, which is failure of the spinal column to close.[a]

*Contaminants*: Contamination of food comes in many varieties, both naturally occurring as well as introduced by humans either intentionally or unintentionally. Aflatoxins are a naturally occurring contaminant that in chronic high exposure can contribute to hepatoma or primary liver cancer. Aflatoxins are fungi or mold that may grow on peanuts, tree nuts such as pecans, corn, wheat, and oilseeds such as cottonseed. The FDA restricts the quantity of aflatoxins that can be present in susceptible foods, but as a naturally occurring contaminant, it is not considered practical to totally remove aflatoxins from the food supply.[5] Residual pesticides used on fruits and vegetables and residual antibiotics used to increase the weight of animals represent important potential contaminants introduced as part of commercial agriculture.

Humans may intentionally introduce contaminants to food as a form of terrorism. Alternatively, contaminants such as glass or metal products or food products such as nut or seafood shells may be included in food products unintentionally as part of harvesting or processing.

*Individual susceptibilities*: An increasing range of individual susceptibilities to diseases related to food are being recognized. Many of these are genetic or what has been called inborn errors of metabolism. For instance, phenylketonuria, or PKU, is a genetic inability to metabolize the amino acid phenylalanine, leading to mental deterioration and death at an early age. Genetic testing and avoidance of phenylalanine have allowed many of those with PKU to live normal lives.

Individual susceptibility may be a form of allergic reaction, producing symptoms ranging from a skin reaction to life-threatening anaphylaxis. Peanut allergy, for instance, is being recognized as a relatively common form of allergy that has the potential to cause anaphylaxis.

*Foodborne communicable diseases*: Last but by no means least is the potential for food to serve as a vehicle for transmission of disease-producing organisms, or pathogens. Food can be a vehicle for transmission of disease pathogens, including bacteria such as *Salmonella*, *Campylobacter*, and toxin-producing *E. coli*. Virus-related foodborne illnesses include hepatitis A and noroviruses. Noroviruses are highly contagious viruses and are increasingly recognized as the leading cause of foodborne outbreaks, especially in crowded environments ranging from nursing homes, to dormitories, to cruise ships.

Let us take a closer look at foodborne outbreaks of disease whose control has long been a part of public health efforts. In fact, when we speak of food safety, we are often referring to control of communicable diseases transmitted by food.

## How Important Is Foodborne Communicable Disease As a Cause of Morbidity and Mortality?

The CDC estimates that each year, roughly 1 in 6 Americans gets sick, over 100,000 are hospitalized, and over 3,000 die of foodborne diseases. As with many communicable diseases, the very young, the very old, and those who are immunologically compromised due to disease are the most vulnerable. Most foodborne diseases are not related to outbreaks. Nonetheless, outbreak investigations are an important means to understand the sources of food contamination and the methods for its control.[6]

---

a In recent years, food supplementation has also included adding physiologically active substances such as caffeine to other foods. Power drinks that have caffeine supplements have been an important and potentially dangerous form of food supplementation.

## BOX 13.1  Vitamin Deficiency Disease—Pellagra

The concept that food deficiencies could produce disease did not become fully accepted until the early 20th century. In 1905, Englishmen William Fletcher, researching the disease beriberi, found that eating unpolished, or brown, rice prevented beriberi and eating polished, or white, rice did not. Dr. Fletcher concluded that there were special nutrients contained in the husk of the rice. These nutrients were soon called "vitamins," after "vita," meaning "life" and "amine," which were compounds found in rice husks.[3]

Pellagra is the most deadly vitamin deficiency disease in the history of the United States. Between 1900 and 1940, approximately 3 million Americans developed pellagra, and over 100,000 died. In the rural southeastern United States in the early 20th century, physicians frequently began reporting this previously rare disease. Pellagra produces some or all of the features that came to be called the "four Ds": diarrhea, dermatitis (skin outbreaks, especially after sun exposure), dementia, and death. Initially, it was thought that pellagra was a communicable disease.

In 1914, the United States Public Health Service sent a public health physician named Joseph Goldberger to directly observe patients with pellagra and their living environment. He noted the following:

- Pellagra was almost exclusively present in poor rural areas, suggesting a socioeconomic relationship.
- Pellagra did not occur among nurses, attendants, or employees in hospitals or orphanages that took care of individuals with the disease, challenging the conclusion that pellagra was a communicable disease.
- Pellagra was present in association with cheap and filling diets, suggesting a dietary cause.

Goldberger and his U.S. Public Health Service colleagues conducted extensive cohort and case–control studies of mill towns in rural South Carolina where pellagra was common. They found a clear socioeconomic gradient, with far more disease among those with lower socioeconomic status. They looked for evidence of communicability through crowding and also a link with poor sanitation but found no evidence for either. They did find a lower incidence among men, especially those who worked in the mills and were often served a hearty and varied lunch. Regular consumption of food products low in nutrients and high in calories were strongly associated with pellagra.

After the occurrence of this epidemiological field investigation, Goldberger continued using epidemiological methods acceptable at the time to investigate a nutritional cause of pellagra.

- He identified 172 children with pellagra and 168 children without pellagra in the same orphanage. Both groups were given a new, more varied diet. Within weeks, almost all children were cured of symptoms of pellagra. After a year, no new cases of pellagra had occurred.
- In a prison where pellagra had never been reported, he identified a dozen volunteers who were offered pardons for participation. They were given an experimental diet consistent with the diet Goldberger had initially observed. Evidence of pellagra occurred in 6 of the 11 inmates within 9 months. When the initial diet was resumed, all 6 inmates recovered.
- In an effort to refute the theory that pellagra was infectious, Goldberger injected himself, his wife, and 16 healthy volunteers with blood from patients with pellagra. He also collected extracts from the nose, urine, and feces and mixed them with food consumed by volunteers. Despite episodes of diarrhea and nausea, no evidence of pellagra was ever noted.

Goldberger's studies demonstrate the strengths and limitations of traditional public health and clinical approaches to studying the cause of disease. Goldberger was able to successfully challenge the communicable disease theory of pellagra and strongly suggested the existence of a nutritional deficiency. However, convincing proof of the vitamin deficiency theory of pellagra required laboratory research as well. The definitive proof that pellagra was a vitamin deficiency had to wait until the late 1930s, when Conrad Elvehjem and his colleagues showed that nicotinic acid or vitamin B3 cured pellagra-like illness in dogs. Nicotinic acid was rapidly tried in humans and had a dramatic effect on the prevention and treatment of pellagra, demonstrating effectiveness even in the absence of a control group.[4]

Data from Elmore JG, Feinstein AR. Joseph Goldberger: an unsung hero of American clinical epidemiology. *Annals of Internal Medicine*. 1994;121:372–375.

## What Are the Steps in Foodborne Outbreak Investigation?

According to the CDC, the following steps should be followed in an outbreak investigation.[7]

1. *Detecting a possible outbreak*: Detecting an outbreak is the first step. An outbreak with hundreds of ill persons can be missed if the people are located over a wide geographic area. Public health officials may detect outbreaks through public health surveillance. By continuously gathering reports of illnesses, they know how many illnesses to expect in a given time period in a given area. If a larger number of people than expected appear to have the same illness in a given

time period and area, it is called a **cluster**. When ill persons in a cluster are found to have something in common to explain why they have the same illness, the group of illnesses is called an **outbreak**.

2. *Defining and finding cases*: Often, the initial illnesses that are recognized are only a part of the total outbreak. Finding more persons who are ill with the same condition is important to help public health officials understand the size, timing, severity, and possible sources of the outbreak. To determine who has the same disease, public health officials utilize or at times develop what is called a **case definition** to spell out which persons will be defined as having the disease as part of the outbreak.[b]

3. *Generating hypotheses about likely sources*: When exposure to a food is suspected, the investigators need to narrow the list to the foods that the ill persons remember eating before they got sick. Health officials interview persons who are or were ill to find out where and what they ate in the days or weeks before they got sick.

4. *Testing the hypothesis*: Case–control studies are the most common type of study conducted so investigators can analyze information collected from ill persons and comparable well persons to see whether ill persons are more likely than people who did not get sick to have eaten a certain food or to report a particular exposure. Food testing can also provide useful information and help to support a hypothesis. For instance, finding bacteria with the same DNA fingerprint in an unopened package of food and in the stool samples of people in the outbreak can be convincing evidence of a source of illness.

5. *Finding the point of contamination and the source of the outbreak*: If a likely source is identified, investigators may try to determine how the food was contaminated. If the people who got sick ate food prepared in only one kitchen, it is likely the contamination occurred in that kitchen. If an outbreak is linked to a food prepared in a number of different kitchens, such as food from many stores of the same chain, or to a food that was bought from many stores and eaten without further preparation, it is likely that contamination happened somewhere in the food production chain before the final kitchen. In that case, investigators do what is called a **source traceback** to find out where contamination occurred.

6. *Controlling the outbreak*: Once a food is found to be the source of illness, control measures are often needed immediately. If contaminated food stays on store shelves, in restaurant kitchens, or in home pantries, more people may get sick. Outbreak control measures may include cleaning and disinfecting food facilities, temporarily closing a restaurant or processing plant, recalling food items, and/or informing the public how to make the food safe or how to avoid it completely. Public health officials may decide on control measures based on strong epidemiological evidence on the disease's etiology. They do not need to wait for proof of contamination from the laboratory.

7. *Deciding that an outbreak is over*: An outbreak is considered over when the number of new illnesses reported drops back to the number normally expected in a particular geographic area. Even when new illnesses from the outbreak appear to have stopped, public health officials still continue active public health surveillance for a few weeks to be sure cases do not start to increase again. If that happens, they continue or restart their investigation because the source may not have been completely controlled, or a second contamination may have occurred.

**FIGURE 13.1** displays the seven steps in a food outbreak investigation as defined by the CDC.

Most foodborne outbreak investigations are handled by local or state health departments. However, the CDC may be called in by state health departments to help with an outbreak investigation. The CDC's Epidemic Intelligence Service can provide comprehensive outbreak investigation resources for a wide range of

---

b  A case definition is a set of criteria used to define which persons will be considered to have a disease as part of an outbreak. There may be more than one definition, such as definite, probable, or suspect. Alternatively, case definitions may be laboratory confirmed or not laboratory confirmed. Use of multiple definitions can be useful to epidemiologists who are investigating an outbreak or large-scale epidemic. Note that an epidemic like an outbreak represents a greater than usual occurrence of disease over a defined period of time. An epidemic implies a much greater number of cases, usually over a larger geographic area. For some diseases, such as influenza, the CDC defines the difference between an epidemic and an outbreak based on the percentage of the deaths that are due to influenza.

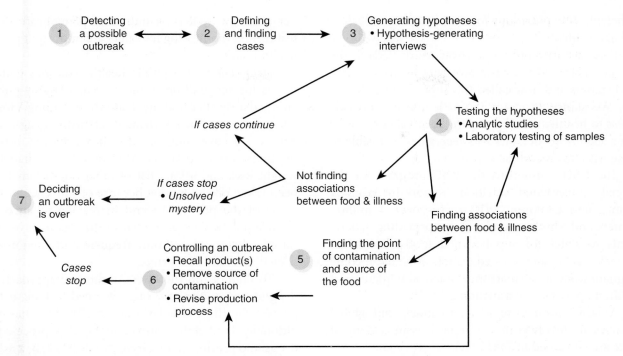

**FIGURE 13.1** Steps in a Foodborne Outbreak Investigation

types of outbreaks, including but not limited to food-borne outbreaks.

Investigation of foodborne diseases remains an important public health effort, but prevention of foodborne disease is the goal. Let us see what is being done to prevent foodborne diseases.

## What Is Being Done to Prevent Foodborne Diseases?

The FDA has a key regulatory role in food safety, including setting safety standards for food processing and distribution. The FDA shares this authority and responsibility with the USDA, which regulates meat, poultry, and eggs. The CDC has a lead role in collecting data on disease related to food along with its role in investigating possible foodborne outbreaks.

The successful implementation of food safety requires collaboration between the CDC, FDA, and USDA. This type of interagency collaboration is frequently needed in public health but often not easy to achieve. One example of successful collaborative efforts has been the FoodNet program. The FoodNet program aims to identify and investigate foodborne disease not only from outbreaks but also from routine exposures.

The Foodborne Diseases Active Surveillance Network, or FoodNet, has been tracking trends for infections commonly transmitted through food since 1996. FoodNet provides data for food safety policy and prevention efforts. It estimates the number of foodborne illnesses, monitors trends in incidence of specific foodborne illnesses over time, attributes illnesses to specific foods and settings, and disseminates this information.[8]

In 2010, the Food Safety Modernization Act was passed, giving the FDA and the USDA increased authority to ensure the safety of foods. Key to the law was the ability to track foods, including their origin, date of production, and other data that could be useful in locating the source of the food if a disease outbreak occurred and investigating the outbreak's cause. The law requires:[9]

- Farmers and food processors to maintain distribution records so that the FDA can more quickly trace an outbreak to its source
- Foreign food suppliers to meet the same safety standards as domestic suppliers
- Regular inspection of all food processing facilities, with more frequent inspections in higher risk facilities

## In the United States, What Other Programs Aim to Prevent Food-Related Disease and Disability?

In addition to its regulatory role, the USDA administers a series of **food security** programs. Food security as defined by the World Health Organization (WHO) requires that "all people at all times have access to sufficient, safe, nutritious food to maintain a healthy and active life."[10]

Food security programs cover nearly 15% of the U.S. population. The largest program, formerly called food stamps and now called the Supplemental Nutrition Assistance Program (SNAP), aims to provide access to healthy diets by making relatively expensive items such as fresh fruits and vegetables accessible to those with low incomes.

The USDA also runs the WIC program, or the Special Supplemental Nutrition Program for Women, Infants, and Children. WIC serves over 4 million women and children under 5 by providing federal grants to states for supplemental foods, healthcare referrals, and nutrition education for low-income pregnant women, postpartum women, and infants and children up to age 5 at nutritional risk.[11]

A large number of local, national, and global agencies are involved in food-related issues. Many of these are described in **TABLE 13.1**.

Food safety and food benefits have been long-standing issues in public health. The 21st century has brought new threats and new approaches for dealing with these threats. This century has also brought new possibilities for providing safe and nutritious food to everyone. As we have seen, food has multiple impacts on health and disease. Reducing the harms while maximizing the benefits is a continuing challenge to public health at all levels. Now let us turn our attention to drugs and drug safety.

# ▶ Drugs and Drug Safety

## Why Is Drug Safety Considered an Important 21st Century Public Health Issue?

The National Academy of Medicine has concluded that nearly 100,000 Americans die each year as a result of adverse effects of drugs.[12] Thus, from the population

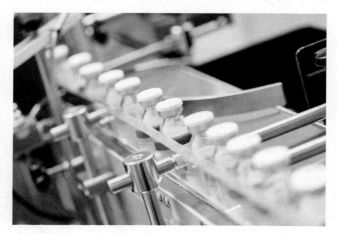

perspective as well as for individual patient care, drug testing and monitoring for safety are important public health issues.

Drug safety as a public health issue has gained increasing recognition in recent years. Highly publicized adverse effects of medications, including Vioxx® and other chemically related arthritis drugs, are believed to have contributed to heart disease in tens of thousands of patients. Medications for diabetes, weight loss, and a long list of other conditions have been taken off the market because of side effects. The aging of the population and increasing reliance on medications widely promoted in the media have also raised concerns about more frequent and often unexpected side effects of drugs.

To understand the FDA's traditional approach to drug testing and monitoring, we need to look at the phases of testing as used by the FDA. The FDA has traditionally divided the testing and approval process for drugs into preclinical research, **phases 1, 2, 3, and 4**. Phase 4 is also called postmarket surveillance.[13] Let us take a look at each of these phases.

## What Do We Mean by "Preclinical Research" on Drugs?

Drug testing begins before any human beings have received the drug. Prior to studying a drug on humans, the FDA requires animal safety studies. Animal testing is usually administered to two different species at levels well above the equivalent dosage expected to be used in humans. Studies are done primarily to detect cancer, teratogenicity (fetal malformations), and effects on fertility. In addition, toxic effects on drug-sensitive organs such as the liver, kidneys, and bone marrow are also investigated.

Unfortunately, the effects on animals may either fail to detect subsequent effects in humans or demonstrate high-dose effects that are difficult to interpret. For instance, thalidomide, the sleeping pill that caused severe limb shortening in newborns, did not demonstrate these effects in animal testing.

Humans may absorb, metabolize (alter its chemistry), and excrete (remove from the body) drugs differently than animal species. High-dose effects on one animal species alert us to the possibility of similar effects in humans but by no means guarantee their occurrence. In addition, humans have an enormous range of reactions to drugs even when given by the same route with the dose adjusted for body weight. Thus, it should not be surprising that animal testing can easily miss the rare but serious side effects occasionally experienced by humans.

**TABLE 13.1** Agencies and Their Role in Food Issues

| Level | Organizations involved | Roles |
|---|---|---|
| Global | Food and Agriculture Organization of the United Nations (FAO) | The United Nations agency with overall responsibility for the food supply, with special emphasis on ensuring an adequate supply of food worldwide |
| | WHO | Not a regulatory agency, but establishes policy and makes recommendations regarding the safety of the world food supply through its Department of Food Safety and Zoonoses |
| | Codex Alimentarius Commission | Initiated as a joint program of FAO and WHO that develops food standards, guidelines, and codes of practice; these now form the basis for the rules of global trade under the jurisdiction of the World Trade Organization |
| Federal | United States FDA | Overall responsibility for food safety regulation in the United States |
| | USDA | Regulatory responsibilities for meat, poultry, and eggs in the United States |
| | United States Environmental Protection Agency | Regulation of pesticide usage and the establishment of water quality standards |
| | CDC | Not a regulatory agency, but responsible for ongoing surveillance, as well as acute investigations in collaboration with state and local health departments |
| State/local | State and local health departments | Restaurant inspections, outbreak investigations |
| Consumer | Consumer protection agencies | Education in safe food purchasing, preparation, and storage |

## What Is Phase 1?

The initial administration of a drug to human beings is called phase 1. A phase 1 study focuses on the pharmacology of the drug—that is, its absorption, metabolism, and excretion. It aims to establish the dosage range and route of administration to be used in subsequent studies. It also looks at safety issues.

Phase 1 studies are capable of identifying common and serious side effects—even those that are not initially suspected. Thus, it is a critical component of the drug safety testing process. Phase 1 focuses on effects on organs that are known to be especially sensitive to the actions of drugs. These include the liver, kidney, bone marrow, and testicles. The liver may be especially prone to drug effects because it often concentrates drugs as it participates in their metabolism

and excretion. The kidneys likewise may be exposed to high doses as part of the excretion process. The rapid rate of cell division in the bone marrow and testicles may make them especially vulnerable to the effects of drugs.

Phase 1 may also focus on effects that may be expected based on the known actions of a particular class of drugs or a particular drug, perhaps based on animal studies. A new antidepressant may be subjected to examination of the electrical conduction system of the heart because antidepressants are known to produce heart rhythm changes, or arrhythmias. A new diuretic that removes salt and water from the body would be thoroughly examined for a range of electrolyte and metabolic effects because this class of medication is known to have a range of effects on the chemistry of the blood.

The duration of the exposure to the drug as part of phase 1 may be quite short—usually days to weeks. The length of exposure may be governed by the length of time needed to determine issues of absorption, metabolism, and excretion. Thus, phase 1 testing cannot be expected to detect longer term or chronic effects.

A phase 1 study is usually quite small, perhaps including only a few dozen individuals. The type of patients who are asked to participate in phase 1 studies is quite variable. Depending on the intended use of the drug, the patients may be severely ill with little or no chance of benefiting from the drug. Alternatively, they may be healthy volunteers who do not have a need for the drug. As a rule, patients at highest risk, such as pregnant women and young children, will not be part of a phase 1 study, even if they are the intended eventual recipients of the drug. Phase 1 studies by their very nature are designed to be short term. They intend to detect effects that occur in the short term and are predictable or produce clinical symptoms. Thus, it is expected that additional attention to safety will be needed.[c]

One of the major limitations of phase 1 in particular, and safety assessment in general, is the wide range of special sensitivities to drug actions that occur among a small number of people. These sensitivities may occur for a variety of reasons. These individuals may be unusual in the way they metabolize drugs, the way their other drugs interact with the new drug, or the way the presence of other diseases complicates the reactions to the new drug.

## What Are Phases 2 and 3?

Phase 2 and 3 studies are primarily designed to establish efficacy of a drug for a particular use or indication. That is, they aim to establish that on average, the drug improves outcomes under research conditions. Phase 2 consists of small, sometimes uncontrolled, trials designed to determine whether there is a suggestion of efficacy. Phase 2 trials are important because they serve as a precondition for moving ahead with the expense, time, and potential harm of conducting large randomized controlled trials, which are at the heart of phase 3.

Side effects identified in phase 1 trials are given special attention, but phase 2 trials are not primarily focused on safety. Phase 2 trials often aim to establish what is called **proof of concept** or provide suggestive evidence that the drug has efficacy (i.e., improves outcome). Phase 2 may also provide information that helps in the design of phase 3 randomized controlled trials as well as assist in the decision whether to pursue phase 3 randomized controlled trials.

Randomized controlled trials are the gold standard for establishing efficacy for one particular indication. Their key role in establishing efficacy often means that they are designed around the specific requirements for determining efficacy for a particular disease on a particular type of patient. Randomized controlled trials, even those that are well designed for establishing efficacy, have limitations in establishing safety. The key limitations of randomized controlled trials for evaluating safety can be summarized as follows:

- Too small—The sample size for randomized controlled trials is determined by the requirements of establishing efficacy. Thus, the number of patients generally ranges from several hundred to several thousand. Identifying rare but serious side effects often requires tens or even hundreds of thousands of users.[d]

- Too short—The duration of randomized controlled trials is geared to the length of time necessary to establish efficacy for the particular indication that is being investigated. Thus, an antibiotic for acute infections may be tested for 10–14 days, while a new drug for acute depression may be tested for 1–2 months. Long-term follow-up for safety is not an inherent part of randomized controlled trials.

- Too simple—The individuals eligible for inclusion in a randomized controlled trial are carefully defined by inclusion and exclusion criteria. These criteria make it easier to establish efficacy. Thus, patients with other complicating diseases or those on a variety of other drugs that make them

---

c  The process of phase 1 testing, like the overall process of safety assessment of drugs, is undergoing revision and hopefully improvement. For instance, advances in our understanding of the mechanism of drug action on a molecular basis may in the future allow us to do a better job of understanding what, where, and how a drug is acting, allowing researchers to focus on the impacts on the molecular as well as the clinical level.

d  An important statistical principle for establishing safety is known as the rule of three. The rule of three tells us that in order to be 95% confident that we will observe at least one case of a rare but serious side effect—for example, one with a true probability of once per 20,000 uses—we are required to observe 60,000 individuals. A sample size of this magnitude is generally only possible once the treatment is used in clinical practice.

especially susceptible to adverse effects of treatment are rarely included in randomized controlled trials.[e]

New drugs are approved on the basis of data collected in preclinical testing and phases 1, 2, and 3. These phases provide a great deal of assurance that the drug works or has efficacy to improve outcome for the average person in the groups that have been investigated. In recent years there have been efforts to speed up or expedite the approval of new drugs especially for conditions where currently approved drugs are of limited or no benefit. **BOX 13.2** describes recent efforts by the FDA to expedite review of new drugs.[14]

Phases 1, 2, and 3 do not, in-and-of-themselves, establish that the drug has effectiveness—that is, that it works under the conditions of clinical practice. Furthermore, while safety is considered throughout the approval process, the limitations of safety assessment leave open the possibility that new and more frequent side effects will be seen when the drug is widely used in clinical practice.

## What Are the Implications of FDA Approval of a Drug?

Understanding the process of assessing safety requires that we first understand what the FDA is indicating when it approves a drug. In general, FDA approval implies:

- The drug may be advertised and marketed for a particular indication, the one for which it was studied and approved.
- Once the drug is approved, it may be used by prescribing clinicians for any patient. That is, the prescribing clinician has the authority to use the treatment for indications or at dosages not specifically approved by the FDA. Use of FDA-approved drugs for indications not approved by the FDA is called **off-label prescribing**.

Thus, once approved, a drug may be prescribed for other conditions, at alternative doses, and for longer durations than those recommended for the particular indication for which the drug was approved. Frequently, clinicians will find that a drug works well in patients with more or alternatively less severe disease than those studied in the randomized controlled trial and will use the drug for these patients. A drug may be studied only for those who have failed other treatments, but clinicians in practice may use the drug as an initial treatment. Occasionally, there will

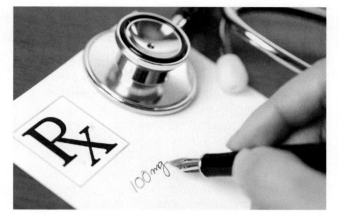

© bluestocking/E+/Getty Images

be suggestive evidence that the drug works for other conditions not previously approved, and clinicians will utilize the drug for these indications as well as the approved indications. A full evaluation of safety needs to take into account the actual uses of the drug in clinical practice. We can think of large-scale and long-term use in clinical practice as providing the gold standard for drug safety.

Many drugs are taken by individuals without a prescription. **BOX 13.3** looks at how nonprescription drugs differ from prescription drugs.

## How Are Adverse Effects of a Drug Monitored in Phase 4, After FDA Approval[16]

For many years, the system for detection of adverse side effects of drugs was limited to what is known as the **spontaneous reporting system**. In this system, those who prescribe the drug, and increasingly, patients themselves, are encouraged to report side effects to the FDA. However, they are not required to do so.

When a drug or vaccine produces a rare and dramatic side effect following soon after treatment is begun, spontaneous reporting systems may be useful in detecting their occurrence. For instance, a small number of cases of a rare and acute life-threatening condition called intussusception of the colon were seen in children within a few weeks of receiving a new rotavirus vaccine for the prevention of gastroenteritis. The unusual nature of the side effect, its dramatic presentation, and its clear time relationship to the vaccination provided convincing evidence that the side effect was due to the vaccine.

---

e  In addition to limitations due to the focus on efficacy, for many years, phases 2 and 3 testing routinely excluded those felt to be at the highest risk of complications—usually pregnant women and children. Recent changes have now made inclusion of children routine in phases 2 and 3 if the intention is to include children among those recommended to receive the drug if it is approved. Pregnant women are still generally omitted from phase 2 and 3 trials except in the unusual circumstance that a treatment is intended for women known to be pregnant.

## BOX 13.2 FDA Efforts to Expedite Approval of Drugs for Serious Conditions

The standard FDA criteria for drug approval include two independently conducted randomized controlled trials that demonstrate efficacy and adequate safety. One very large randomized controlled trial has long been acceptable when additional studies are not feasible. Beginning with the AIDS epidemic and the need for treatments that altered the course of the disease the FDA has been allowed to develop new procedures that speed-up or expedite the drug approval process.

These expedited review procedures have generally retained the same standards of evidence for efficacy and safety, at times requiring continued data collection after initial approval. However, these expedited review options use **surrogate endpoints**. Surrogate endpoints may not be a direct measurement of how a patient feels, functions, or survives, but they are considered likely to predict a desirable outcome. For example, a surrogate endpoint could be short-term lowering of HIV viral load. The FDA often requires ongoing studies of drugs approved using surrogate outcomes. If studies do not confirm the initial results, the FDA can withdraw the approval.

Recently the FDA, with pharmaceutical company support, has established a new category of expedited review called **breakthrough drugs**. According to the FDA a breakthrough drug is intended to treat a serious condition and preliminary clinical evidence indicates that the drug may demonstrate substantial improvement on a clinically significant endpoint(s) over available therapy.

Drugs with breakthrough drug designation may treat previously untreatable disease, produce substantially better results in short-term studies compared to existing treatments, or demonstrate improvement in situations where deterioration is expected.

New drugs for rare genetic diseases and new cancer therapies are increasingly receiving breakthrough drug approval. Breakthrough drug approval allows the FDA to approve drugs on the basis of studies that include smaller numbers of participants, studies that do not include randomized comparison group, and other types of studies called adoptive design that allow the investigators to alter the study design on the basis of blind analysis of preliminary data.

Other types of studies are also permitted under the breakthrough drug approval process. Cross-over studies in which participants' outcomes are assessed on and off the treatment may be allowed. In addition, studies called **N-of-1 trials** may be considered. N-of-1 trials may be conducted on one or a small group of patients who are observed off the treatment, on the treatment, and subsequently off the treatment again to determine whether they clearly benefit from the drug.

Expedited review procedures are more rapidly bringing new treatments to the drug approval stage. The reduced evidence for efficacy and safety at the time of approval, however, means that the effectiveness and safety-in-practice requires continuing collection of data post approval.

Data from U.S. Food and Drug Administration. Guidance for industry expedited programs for serious conditions – drugs and biologics. https://www.fda.gov/downloads/drugs/guidancecomplianceregulatoryinformation/guidances/ucm358301.pdf. Accessed July 25, 2017.

## BOX 13.3 Nonprescription Drugs[15]

Nonprescription drugs, often called over-the-counter drugs, are designed to be used without a clinician's prescription. Their sale is not limited to pharmacies. Nonprescription drugs are not necessarily designed to be used by one particular individual, as is the case with prescription drugs. While the FDA regulates the advertising of prescription drugs, the Federal Trade Commission regulates the advertisement of nonprescription drugs.[a]

There are over 300,000 nonprescription drug products available in the United States. Many of them contain the same ingredients. The FDA reviews the active ingredients and the labeling of over 80 therapeutic classes of drugs, such as pain-killers and

antacids, instead of reviewing individual drug products. For each category, a monograph is published, which the FDA describes as a "recipe book" covering acceptable ingredients, doses, formulations, and labeling. These monographs define the safety, effectiveness, and labeling of all nonprescription active ingredients. Companies can follow the recipe book and produce and market a nonprescription drug without the need for FDA preapproval.

New nonprescription drugs that utilize new active therapeutic agents need to satisfy the FDA requirement for a new drug or be converted from a prescription drug to a nonprescription drug. Conversion from a prescription

---

a The term "over the counter" will not be used here because it implies an interaction with an informed individual. Today, many nonprescription products can be purchased through vending machines, automated checkout counters, and the Internet without any human contact. In addition, a new option is being used by the FDA that may be called "behind the counter." Behind-the-counter drugs require identification of the purchaser and limitations on the quantity of drugs that can be purchased. Pseudoephedrine, often purchased as the brand name Sudafed®, is a nonprescription decongestant that was placed behind the counter after it was recognized that it could be used to make methamphetamine.

to a nonprescription drug is becoming an increasingly common action. In general, conversion requires that the drug is able to be safely used without the supervision of a prescribing clinician. In addition, the drug labeling must be tested to ensure that it can be generally understood by the groups of individuals for whom it is intended.

Nonprescription drugs such as aspirin and acetaminophen can have strong impacts on their own and can interact with prescription and nonprescription drugs.

Some nonprescription drugs can have life-threatening side effects at levels only modestly greater than those recommended on the label. Acetaminophen, for instance, can cause life-threatening liver disease with long-term use at levels only modestly above those recommended for short-term pain relief. Thus, the increased use of nonprescription drugs on their own and along with prescription drugs poses a potential public health hazard that needs continuing monitoring and ongoing education.

Data from U.S. Food and Drug Administration. Drug applications for over-the-counter (OTC) drugs. https://www.fda.gov/drugs/developmentapprovalprocess/howdrugsaredevelopedandapproved/approvalapplications/over-the-counterdrugs/default.htm. Accessed July 25, 2017

This example can be viewed as the exception rather than the rule. Spontaneous reporting systems often do not work this well because they have a number of limitations, including the following:

- Even with serious side effects, only a small percentage may be reported, especially when the effect is not dramatic or closely linked in time to the treatment.
- Side effects that result from a variety of causes or are similar to the consequences of the disease being treated may be difficult to recognize and attribute to the treatment.
- Unsuspected side effects may escape detection or not be attributed to the treatment.

The spontaneous reporting system cannot be expected to rapidly or completely detect rare but serious side effects. Patients who receive a new treatment over the first few months to the first few years

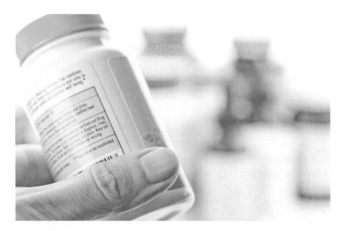

© Elena Elisseeva/Shutterstock

after initial marketing approval need to be regarded as part of the experiment. **TABLE 13.2** summarizes the roles that preclinical testing and phases 1, 2, 3, and 4 have traditionally played in the drug effectiveness and safety assessment process.

**TABLE 13.2** FDA Process of Assessing Safety and Effectiveness of Drugs

| | Definition | Objectives | Limitations |
|---|---|---|---|
| **Preclinical testing** | Safety assessment on at least two species at high dosages prior to initial use on humans. | Assess carcinogenic, teratogenicity, and fertility effects. | High-dose effects may not correlate with effects on humans. Species differences may result in missing effects that later appear in human testing or after widespread clinical use. |
| **Phase 1** | Initial testing of drug on humans may include healthy volunteers or terminally ill patients, but not necessarily those on whom drug will be used. | Designed to assess pharmacology, including metabolism and excretion, in an effort to establish dosage, timing, and route of administration. Safety assessed especially on vulnerable organs, including liver, kidney, testicles, and bone marrow. | Small numbers and short-term studies mean many effects may be missed. May not help predict side effects when patients are not representative of those the drug will be used on in practice. |

*(continues)*

| **TABLE 13.2** FDA Process of Assessing Safety and Effectiveness of Drugs | | | *(continued)* |
|---|---|---|---|
| | **Definition** | **Objectives** | **Limitations** |
| **Phase 2** | Initial small-scale, controlled or uncontrolled, trial of efficacy with secondary assessment of safety. | Establishes that there is enough evidence of efficacy to warrant phase 3 randomized controlled trials. | Primary intent is often "proof of concept" and information to help design and decide whether to pursue randomized controlled trials. |
| **Phase 3** | Two independently performed randomized controlled trials unless not practical or ethical. | Establish efficacy for one indication among a homogeneous group of patients compared to conventional treatment.    Investigate short-term safety relative to conventional treatment. | Randomized controlled trials may be too small, their duration too short, and their participants' conditions too simple or uncomplicated in terms of their disease(s) or their treatment(s) to observe side effects that will be seen in clinical practice. |
| **Phase 4 Postmarket surveillance** | Assessment of safety based on the use of the drug in clinical practice.    Spontaneous reporting system traditionally the basis for phase 4.    Databases from clinical practice and formal studies of safety increasingly used to assess safety in clinical practice. | Designed to detect rare but serious side effects as well as increased frequency of known side effects.    Once a drug is approved by the FDA for one particular indication, it may be used at different dosages, for different types of patients, and for other indications at the discretion of the prescribing clinician. | Spontaneous reporting system results may not detect side effects, especially if they simulate commonly occurring effects such as liver or kidney impairment.    Interactions between drugs or between drugs and diseases are common, making it difficult to assess and attribute causation. |

## What Else Can Be Done?

Until recently, the FDA did not have authority to require follow-up studies of drugs once they were approved for clinical practice. In addition, as opposed to the preapproval process, the burden of proof was on the FDA to establish a safety hazard before an approved drug could be removed from the market. In addition, the FDA had limited authority over drug advertisements as long as they did not contradict FDA language. Other than including warning labels, or what have been called black box warnings, in the drug use instructions, the FDA had limited authority over the process of prescribing or monitoring drug use.

The Food and Drug Administration Amendment Act of 2007 provided a wide variety of new authorities for the FDA. These new authorities were designed as a response to a range of safety issues that have

developed over several decades.[16] Congress provided the FDA with authority and a great deal of discretion over what should be done, how it should be done, and when it should be done. Many of the provisions of this law and other FDA laws take years or even a decade or more to be fully implemented.

The 2007 amendments to the FDA law provided the FDA with a wide range of new authority that it can use to monitor safety and act to reduce or eliminate side effects of drugs.[17] The use of this authority to protect against side effects while gaining the benefits of the drug use continues to be a difficult and controversial issue. Among the new authority granted to the FDA in the 2007 legislation are the following:

- The FDA was provided authority to require that more representative patients be included in randomized controlled trials with the aim to have randomized controlled trials more closely reflect the populations on whom the drug will be used.

- The FDA was given authority to require follow-up studies of drugs to monitor their performance in clinical practice.
- The FDA was given authority to develop large database systems to link pharmacy records with electronic medical records to assess side effects on an ongoing basis.
- The FDA was given authority to place increased restrictions on who can prescribe a particular drug and what conditions need to be fulfilled before it can be prescribed, including required testing prior to filling a prescription.
- The FDA was given increased authority to approve and monitor drug advertising to clinicians and directly to patients to ensure that they conform with FDA-approved language and accurately communicate risks.
- The FDA was given greater authority to withdraw drugs from the market when serious issues of safety are raised.

Today, a coordinated process of postmarket investigation of adverse effects of drugs has begun. The process relies not only on the spontaneous reporting system but also on follow-up of patients previously enrolled in randomized controlled trials. It also includes selective use of case–control studies and cohort studies, which take advantage of the greatly increased ability to link clinical and pharmacy records to investigate the relationship between drugs and adverse events.

## Do All FDA-Regulated Products Receive the Same Effectiveness and Safety Assessment As Prescription and Nonprescription Drugs?

Vaccines undergo many of the same phases of testing and monitoring that are required for drug approval. Because vaccines are often given to millions of healthy people, additional monitoring for safety is often expected prior to and after approval. A "no fault" system of financial compensation exists for adverse side effects related to vaccines. This has resulted in more complete and more comprehensive reporting of side effects of vaccines.

Many substances taken regularly by millions of people are not subject to the types of evaluation that we have discussed for drugs and vaccines. The FDA regulates what are called **dietary supplements**

under a different set of regulations than those covering "conventional" drug products (prescription and nonprescription).[18] Dietary substances include vitamins, minerals, and herbal treatments. The legal implication of dietary supplements that distinguishes them from drugs is that dietary supplements cannot be promoted as treatment for, or prevention of, a disease. Thus, when you hear about a dietary supplement, you will often see the disclaimer: "This product is not intended to diagnose, treat, cure, or prevent any disease."

As opposed to the makers of drugs and vaccines, the dietary supplement manufacturer is solely responsible for ensuring that a dietary supplement is safe before it is marketed. The FDA indicates that it is responsible for taking action against any unsafe dietary supplement product after it reaches the market. However, the burden of proof is on the FDA, making it very difficult to remove dietary supplements from the market.

Generally, manufacturers of dietary supplements need to register their products with the FDA. However, the FDA does not provide approval before the manufacturer may produce or sell dietary supplements. Manufacturers are responsible for making sure that product label information, including ingredients, is truthful and not misleading. The FDA describes its postmarketing responsibilities for dietary supplements as monitoring safety through voluntary adverse event reporting similar to the spontaneous reporting system for drugs. As opposed to its authority over advertising for drugs and vaccines, the FDA does not have any authority over dietary supplement advertising. The Federal Trade Commission regulates dietary supplement advertising.

Thus today, drugs and vaccines are subject to careful premarket review and to increasingly active postmarket surveillance. Dietary supplements, on the other hand, undergo very limited premarket or postmarket evaluation.

## What Other Products Does the FDA Regulate?

In addition to products classified as foods and drugs, the FDA has authority over a wide range of products. About 25% of every dollar spent by Americans is spent on products regulated by the FDA. The FDA regulates cosmetics, medical devices, biological products including the blood supply, and most recently tobacco products.

The FDA regulates the safety, labeling, and manufacture of cosmetics. Medical devices are a broad category with their own set of regulations, which are currently under active review.

The FDA promulgates and enforces standards for blood collection and for the production of blood products. The FDA also inspects blood banks and monitors reports of errors, accidents, and adverse clinical events. Authority over tobacco products is relatively new, and the FDA is beginning to utilize its authority in this area, including the regulation of nicotine and e-cigarettes.

Food and drugs, as well as other health and cosmetic products, play an important role in modern society. The United States has developed a complex public health system designed to maximize the benefits of these products, while identifying potential harms and minimizing their impact. The system is by no means perfect, but it continues to evolve and face new challenges. Do not expect these issues to go away. They have been a part of public health from the beginning and will continue to be key public health issues well into the future.

## Key Words

| | | |
|---|---|---|
| Breakthrough drugs | Micronutrients | Proof of concept |
| Case definition | N-of-1 trial | Source traceback |
| Cluster | Off-label prescribing | Spontaneous reporting system |
| Dietary supplements | Outbreak | Surrogate endpoint |
| Food security | Phases 1, 2, 3, and 4 | |

## Discussion Questions

Take a look at the questions posed in the following scenarios, which were presented at the beginning of this chapter. See now whether you can answer them.

1. "We are what we eat," you hear said again and again. "Sure," you say, "too little is bad, too much is bad, but what other ways can food affect our health?"

2. An outbreak of hepatitis A occurs among employees eating in your cafeteria. To your surprise, the local health department and the CDC quickly investigate the outbreak and trace its source to seafood grown and harvested in an Asian country and to the factory that handled the food in the United States far from your home. How is food being traced, you wonder, to allow outbreaks to be so rapidly and efficiently investigated?

3. Jessica wondered why she needed a pregnancy test each month to refill her prescription for acne medication. She was not even currently sexually active. The pharmacist told her that she needed to come in with proof of a recent pregnancy test because serious birth defects are so common with this medication. What a pain and what an embarrassment she thought to herself. Why is all this bureaucracy needed anyway?

4. John's cancer was in remission, but he was still taking chemotherapy, and he often felt very sleepy. His doctor asked whether he wanted to try a new drug that was just approved by the FDA and showed evidence of reducing fatigue. John knew he was taking a chance but he readily agreed. The side effects were worse than expected, and John's doctor told him some of them had never been reported before. "I guess I am part of the experiment," he told his doctor. "Yes, with new drugs, we are always on the lookout for surprises," his doctor said. John asked himself if it was worth it to be one of the first to try out a new drug.

5. Veronica saw it on TV and on the Web. It was a new dietary supplement that showed promise for reducing blood pressure, and that was just what Veronica needed. The fine print on the bottle said that it was not for the treatment or prevention of any disease. A low dose seemed to have some effect and a higher dose was even better. When Veronica started feeling a little dizzy, she went to the emergency room, where they found that she was losing blood in her stools. The dietary supplement was thought to be the cause of her bleeding and her reduced blood pressure. Veronica asked, "Do I need to treat dietary supplements as if they are drugs?"

6. Carlos's doctor told him he wanted to try him on a new treatment for his headaches because the standard treatment was not working. He told Carlos that the drug had been on the market for several years but was not officially recommended for headaches by the FDA. "I have been hearing that it works for headaches and I would like to try it out, if you agree," the doctor said. Carlos wondered, Is that the way medicine is practiced?

# References

1. U.S. Food and Drug Administration. Significant dates in U.S. food and drug law history. http://www.fda.gov/AboutFDA /WhatWeDo/History/Milestones/ucm128305.htm. Accessed July 25, 2017.

2. U.S. Food and Drug Administration. Food. http://www.fda .gov/Food/GuidanceRegulation/FSMA/ucm247559.htm. Accessed July 25, 2017.

3. About.com. The history of vitamins. http://inventors.about. com/library/inventors/bl_vitamins.htm. Accessed July 25, 2017.

4. Elmore JG, Feinstein AR. Joseph Goldberger: An unsung hero of American clinical epidemiology. *Annals of Internal Medicine*. 1994;121:372–375.

5. MedlinePlus. Aflatoxin. http://www.nlm.nih.gov/medlineplus /ency/article/002429.htm. Accessed July 25, 2017.

6. Centers for Disease Control and Prevention. Estimates of foodborne illness in the United States. http://www.cdc.gov /foodborneburden. Accessed July 25, 2017.

7. Centers for Disease Control and Prevention. Foodborne outbreak investigations. https://www.cdc.gov/foodsafety /outbreaks/investigating-outbreaks/investigations/figure _outbreak_process.html. Accessed July 25, 2017.

8. Centers for Disease Control and Prevention. Foodborne Diseases Active Surveillance Network (FoodNet). http://www .cdc.gov/foodnet. Accessed July 25, 2017.

9. U.S. Food and Drug Administration. FDA Food Safety Modernization Act (FSMA). http://www.fda.gov/food /guidanceregulation/fsma/default.htm. Accessed July 25, 2017.

10. World Health Organization. Nutrition and Food Security. http://www.who.int/foodsafety/areas_work/nutrition/en/. Accessed July 25, 2017.

11. U.S. Department of Agriculture. Women, Infants, and Children (WIC). https://www.fns.usda.gov/wic/women-infants-and -children-wic. Accessed July 25, 2017.

12. Institute of Medicine. *Preventing Medication Errors: Quality Chasm Series*. Washington, DC: National Academics Press; 2006.

13. U.S. Food and Drug Administration. Resources for You (Drugs). https://www.fda.gov/Drugs/ResourcesForYou/. Accessed July 25, 2017.

14. U.S. Food and Drug Administration. Guidance for industry expedited programs for serious conditions— drugs and biologics. https://www.fda.gov/downloads/drugs /guidancecomplianceregulatoryinformation/guidances /ucm358301.pdf. Accessed July 25, 2017.

15. U.S. Food and Drug Administration. Drug Applications for Over-the-Counter (OTC) drugs. http://www.fda .gov/drugs/developmentapprovalprocess/howdrugs aredevelopedandapproved/approvalapplications/over-the -counterdrugs/default.htm. Accessed July 25, 2017.

16. U.S. Food and Drug Administration. Postmarket drug safety information for patients and providers. http:// www.fda.gov/Drugs/DrugSafety/PostmarketDrugSafety InformationforPatientsandProviders/default.htm. Accessed July 25, 2017.

17. U.S. Food and Drug Administration. Food and Drug Administration Amendments Act (FDAAA) of 2007. https:// www.fda.gov/RegulatoryInformation/LawsEnforcedbyFDA /SignificantAmendmentstotheFDCAct/Foodand DrugAdministrationAmendmentsActof2007/default.htm. Accessed July 25, 2017.

18. U.S. Food and Drug Administration. Dietary supplements. http://www.fda.gov/food/DietarySupplements/default.htm. Accessed July 25, 2017.

# CHAPTER 14

# Systems Thinking: From Single Solutions to One Health

## LEARNING OBJECTIVES

By the end of this chapter, the student will be able to:

- explain how systems thinking differs from reductionist thinking.
- identify characteristics of a system.
- identify the steps in systems analysis using systems diagrams.
- explain the meaning of interactions between factors.
- explain the meaning of bottlenecks and leverage points.
- identify and explain uses of systems thinking in public health.
- discuss One Health as an example of systems thinking.

You are pregnant and have a 10-year history of cigarette smoking. You are surprised that at your first prenatal visit, there is a big sticker on your chart saying "Smoker." Everyone in the doctor's office asks you what they can do to help, and they quickly enroll you in special services for smoking cessation for which you were not eligible before you got pregnant. When you ask why so much time, attention, and money is now coming your way, they tell you pregnancy is a leverage point for stopping smoking. You ask: What do they mean by "leverage point"?

A patient with active tuberculosis (TB) is reported by the local hospital laboratory to the health department. The health department quickly connects with the patient to determine his close personal contacts. They also ask him if they can test him for HIV (the human immunodeficiency

virus). He turns out to be HIV positive, and permission is then requested to get in touch with his sexual contacts. You consider how you would describe the relationship between TB and HIV, and wonder how knowledge of this relationship can be used to reduce the risks of both TB and HIV.

You hear that motor vehicle injuries, especially those due to automobile collisions, have been dramatically reduced in recent years. Was there a magic bullet that accomplished this, you wonder, or was this reduction accomplished through a more complicated process?

You love rare hamburgers. "Just wave them over the flame," you like to say. Recently, you have heard that ground beef is a high-risk food—even a health hazard. You ask: What does that mean, and what is being done about it?

You hear that a new RNA (ribonucleic acid) virus is rapidly spreading and will likely soon reach the United States. Public health officials are rapidly mobilizing efforts to control the disease and respond to an outbreak but see little chance of stopping the disease from reaching the United States. Is this a common event you wonder or an emergency?

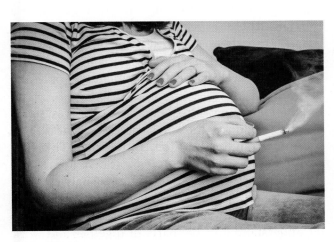

© andriano.cz/Shutterstock

Over the last 100 years, public health has evolved from having primarily a science focus to incorporating a problem focus and, most recently, a systems focus.

—Commission on Education of Health Professionals for the 21st Century[1]

Let us take a look at how population health thinking is changing in the 21st century and increasingly incorporating what we will call **systems thinking**. The focus on systems is so important that along with the population perspective, it is coming to define 21st century-population health.

We begin by taking a look at what makes systems thinking different.

## ▶ What Makes Systems Thinking Different?

Traditional thinking in public health, like most science-based disciplines, has used what is called **reductionist thinking**. Reductionist thinking looks at one factor or variable at a time.[2] That is, it reduces the problem to one potential "cause" and one potential "effect."[a]

Reductionist thinking has often been used in public health and medicine to search for the one-and-only answer to the why, or etiology, and the one-and-only answer to what should be done to improve outcome. This approach may be called the magic bullet or miracle cure approach.

Reductionist thinking has been very useful for establishing specific factors as contributory causes of disease, such as cigarettes and lung cancer, high blood pressure and vascular disease, as well as aspirin and Reye's syndrome. However, it is increasingly important that we look at the impacts of multiple factors and see how they work together as parts of systems. Systems thinking, or a systems approach, often utilizes data derived from reductionist thinking but goes beyond reductionist thinking to look at multiple factors that cause disease and disease outcomes. Thus, it is the focus on multiple factors and how they fit together that distinguishes reductionist thinking from systems thinking.[3,b]

---

a When using reductionist thinking, other factors are traditionally included in public health studies in order to take them into account or control for them. These factors are called confounding variables when they are related to both the cause and the effect. Confounding variables may confound or confuse the investigation of the relationship between a single cause and a single effect. Confounding variables may be differences between groups in age, severity, or disease, or other risk factors that affect the chances of developing disease or experiencing a poor outcome. It is important to remember that in reductionist thinking confounding variables are not being included in the research in order to investigate their relationship to the disease or other outcome being investigated. In addition systems thinking often differs from reductionist thinking since systems thinking aims to predict outcome, while reductionist thinking aims to explain outcome. Prediction and explanation are two quite different approaches that require different statistical methods. For instance, when predicting outcome statistical significance is less important than when explaining outcome.

b The terminology can be confusing. We will use the term "systems thinking" to describe the thinking process of the systems approach. We will use the term "systems analysis" as a broad term describing a range of methods for operationalizing systems thinking. Systems diagrams illustrated in this chapter are one such method for operationalizing systems thinking. The translational research model can be seen as another type of systems analysis. At times, the term "integrative" is used to describe systems thinking. "Integrative" describes the intention of systems thinking or the systems approach to bring together disparate influences into a coherent whole. Integrative thinking is at times used to distinguish systems thinking from reductionist thinking. Here we will use the term "systems thinking" as the broadest term, and "systems analysis" will be used as a term to describe a variety of methods to operationalize systems thinking. The definition chosen for the term "system," as indicated in the text, is an interacting group of items forming a unified whole. This definition was drawn and modified from a long list of potential definitions because it emphasizes the need to identify items or factors, their interactions, and how they fit together as a whole. We believe that these are the core elements of systems thinking.[5]

## ▶ What Is a System?

There are a large number of definitions of a system. We will define a **system** as an interacting group of items forming a unified whole.[4] According to O'Connor and McDermott, the key to identifying a system is that a system maintains its existence and functions as a whole through the interaction of its parts. They write:

> Your body is the perfect example. Your body consists of many different parts and organs, each acting separately, yet all working together and each affecting the others. Your thoughts affect your digestion and heart beat, the state of your digestion affects your thoughts—especially after a large lunch. The eye cannot see, nor the legs move without a blood supply, and the blood supply has to be oxygenated through the lungs. The movement of the legs helps pump the blood back to the heart. The body is a complex system.[5]

It is important to appreciate the features of a system and the implications of a system. O'Connor and McDermott go on to distinguish a system from what they call a heap or collection of pieces as follows:

- A system is a series of interconnected parts which function as a whole. A heap is merely a collection of parts.
- A system changes if you take away or add pieces; if you cut a system in half, you do not get two smaller systems: you get a system that will not function. A heap can be divided into pieces, each of which can function on their own.
- In a system, the arrangement of the pieces is crucial, while in a heap, the arrangement is irrelevant.
- In a system, the parts are connected to each other and work together, while in a heap, the arrangement of the pieces is irrelevant.
- The behavior of a system depends on its overall structure, while in a heap, size rather than structure determines behavior.

As we have seen, the term "system" may be used to describe complex biological relationships. "System" may also be used to describe organizations' relationships or processes, such as a healthcare system, a public health system, or a research system. Alternatively, "system" may be used to describe the working of factors or influences that bring about disease and the outcome of disease. Each of these uses of the term "system" shares the goal of understanding how the pieces or items fit together in a coherent whole. In recent years, population health has increasingly turned to systems thinking to better understand the operation of organizations and processes, as well as the development and outcome of disease.[c]

Implementing or operationalizing systems thinking requires tools for analyzing the pieces and understanding how they fit together. This process is called **systems analysis**. There are a wide range of these tools. Often, systems analysis relies on diagrams or graphics that visually display the relationships between the parts and allow us to better understand how the parts fit together and work together.

Let us look at the process of systems analysis and how it is being used in population health.

## ▶ What Are the Initial Steps in Systems Analysis?

When using systems analysis to understand disease and its outcomes, we need to start by identifying the most important **influences** on the outcome(s) of interest. Influences are factors or determinants that interact with each other to bring about outcomes, such as disease or the results of disease.[d]

Let us see how we might identify influences on smoking cessation. Using one-at-a-time reductionist studies, the following interventions have been shown to be effective: smoking cessation programs, prohibitions on smoking in public places, social marketing, and cigarette taxes. In addition, measures of the strength of a relationship such as relative risk obtained from reductionist studies often help us measure the

---

c  It may be argued that the U.S. healthcare and public health systems include many of the features of a heap rather than a system. While this is probably an overstatement, it points out the importance of thinking in systems and the potential contributions that thinking in systems can have on the development of healthcare and public health organizations.

d  The term "influences," like the term "risk factors," does not imply that all the criteria for a contributory cause have been established. We need to be careful with the use of the term "determinant" because it is often used as a synonym for "influences," even though it sounds like its presence carries an inevitability of developing a condition or disease.

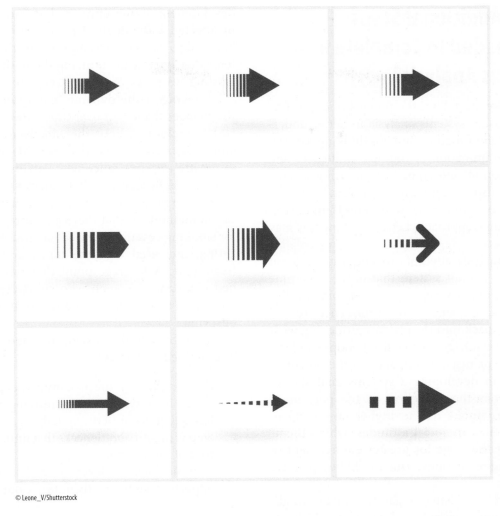

© Leone_V/Shutterstock

magnitude of the influence that a factor has on an outcome. Thus, the first two steps in systems thinking are often built on data derived using one factor at a time, or reductionist thinking.

Rather than looking at one intervention at a time, however, systems thinking asks about the best combination of interventions and how they can be used together. Let us assume that smoking cessation programs, prohibition on smoking in public, social marketing, and higher taxes have been identified as the four most important interventions or influences on the rate of cigarette smoking. The question then becomes how they can be effectively and efficiently combined.

Reductionist thinking usually assumes a straight-line or linear relationship between influences, implying that increased levels of an intervention, such as increasing taxes on tobacco, will produce a straight-line decrease in the levels of tobacco use. However, it is possible that small increases in taxes have little effect, while somewhat larger increases have dramatic effects. In addition, reductionist thinking does not look at

how the impact of one intervention may be affected by connecting it with other interventions, whereas systems thinking looks at these interactions. Thus, systems thinking would ask questions about how to most effectively utilize cigarette taxes by combining them with other approaches, such as using the taxes to support tobacco education programs, or reduce exposure to other causes of lung cancer, such as radon and asbestos.

The following summarizes the initial steps in a systems analysis:[6,7]

- Step 1: Identify the key influences or interventions on an outcome such as disease or the outcome of disease.
- Step 2: Indicate the relative strength of the impact of each of the influences or interventions.
- Step 3: Identify how these influences or interventions interact—that is, how they work together or, alternatively, interfere with each other.

These three steps in systems analysis are basic to understanding the structure of a system.

# ▶ What Additional Steps Are Needed to Complete a Systems Analysis?

Increasingly, we are taking the process one step further. We are using systems analysis to better understand how systems function. Systems thinking requires not only an examination of multiple influences and their interaction at one point in time using a static approach, but also encourages us to look at how these factors change over time. That is, systems thinking can lead to a dynamic approach. Let us see how this may be accomplished.

Systems analysis attempts to take into account changes in the overall system that occur over time due to changes in one or more of the factors or influences. These changes in a factor or influence are said to provide feedback into the process producing what are called **feedback loops**. Feedback loops can have either positive or negative impacts on the outcome. For instance, in developing a systems analysis, we might ask: Does the reduction in the percentage of people who smoke due to higher taxes lead to changes over time in social attitudes, which themselves may set the stage for greater enforcement of public smoking regulations? This would be a positive feedback loop.

Alternatively, raising cigarette taxes might reduce the money available to low income individuals to pay for smoking cessation programs if these services are not paid for by health insurance. This would be a negative feedback loop. Systems thinking does not view the impact of interventions as static. Rather, it tries to develop dynamic models, incorporating the feedback processes that reinforce or accelerate the impacts or alternatively dampen or reduce the impact.

Systems analyses encourage us to identify feedback loops, including positive feedback loops that reinforce or accentuate the process and negative feedback loops that dampen or slow down the process. Feedback loops are key to understanding how a system operates or functions. Complex systems, such as the human body, rely heavily on feedback loops in order to maintain stability. When one component gets out of control, such as body temperature or hydration, other components of the system respond to maintain the body within a tolerable range. This requires positive and negative feedback loops. Similarly, communicable disease in a population is controlled to a certain extent by responses or feedback, including voluntary isolation of sick individuals, development of immunity, and, unfortunately, death of affected individuals. Understanding these feedback loops can help us improve on the natural systems that exist, while utilizing the positive aspects of existing systems.

Looking at the dynamic nature of systems and the changes that occur over time allows us to identify **bottlenecks** that limit the effectiveness of systems and **leverage points** that provide opportunities to greatly improve outcomes. For instance, systems analysis might identify a bottleneck such as the need to train large numbers of clinicians in smoking cessation methods so that they can address the demand for smoking cessation services created by social marketing, increased cigarette taxes, and better drug treatments. A leverage point that might be identified is pregnant women who smoke but are highly motivated to quit due to the severe impact on their offspring.

Thus, the additional steps in systems analysis can be described as follows:[6,7]

- Step 4: Identify the dynamic changes that may occur in a system by identifying the feedback loops that occur in the system.
- Step 5: Identify bottlenecks that limit the effectiveness of the system.
- Step 6: Identify leverage points that provide opportunities to greatly improve outcomes.

# ▶ How Can We Use a Systems Analysis to Better Understand a Problem Such As Coronary Artery Disease?

Let us use each of the six steps we have identified in a systems analysis to better understand the problem of coronary artery disease.

*Step 1: Identify influences*—We know from reductionist research that there are multiple factors that increase the risk of coronary artery disease, including high blood pressure, high LDL (low-density lipoprotein) cholesterol, low HDL (high-density lipoprotein) cholesterol, abdominal obesity, diabetes, cigarette smoking, physical inactivity, family history, etc. Recognizing each of these factors has been an important part of addressing the problem of coronary artery disease. Further progress, however, requires us to think about how interventions to address these factors connect to each other.

*Step 2: Estimate the relative strength of the influences*—We need to estimate the relative strength or magnitude of the impact of each of the influences. We might estimate the relative risk for each of these factors, or we might classify their impacts as weak, moderate, or strong. In the case of coronary artery disease, each of these factors is generally considered of moderate strength with relative risks in the range of 2–4.

*Step 3: Examine the interactions between factors*— Examining the interaction between factors helps us understand what happens when two or more of the factors are present. Risk factors for disease may add together to increase the risk of disease, such as high blood pressure plus high LDL cholesterol and low HDL cholesterol. Alternatively, one factor, such as physical activity, may have a protective effect against coronary artery disease in and of itself. Interactions between factors may multiply the risk rather than resulting in an additive impact.

Risk factors for coronary artery disease are usually assumed to add together rather than to multiply the impact. However, a combination of risk factors known as the metabolic syndrome has been shown to interact and greatly increase the risk. Metabolic syndrome includes increased waist circumference, low HDL cholesterol, elevated triglycerides, hypertension, and elevated fasting blood sugar. When all or a number of these risk factors occur together, they greatly magnify the probability of coronary artery disease as well as other large blood vessel diseases such as strokes.

*Step 4: Identify feedback loops that lead to dynamic changes in the functioning of the system*— Understanding how systems operate over time requires us to identify feedback mechanisms, or feedback loops, that alter the likelihood of disease or impact its outcome. For instance, increased weight, especially increased abdominal girth, may lead to increased LDL cholesterol, diabetes, reduced exercise, reduced HDL cholesterol, and increased blood pressure. Alternatively, multiple interventions focused on weight, exercise, blood sugar control, and treatment of hypertension

may work together to have a surprisingly positive impact on the probability of coronary artery disease.[e]

*Step 5: Identify bottlenecks*—Bottlenecks imply that there are points in the system that need to be addressed in order for the other factors or influences to have their potential impacts. For instance, in coronary artery disease, if severe narrowing of the coronary arteries already exists, it is unlikely that interventions such as reducing blood sugar, reducing LDL cholesterol, increasing exercise, or stopping cigarette smoking are going to have a dramatic impact. If the bottleneck, the narrowed artery, can be addressed using angioplasty or surgery, attention to the other risk factors may have a much greater impact.

*Step 6: Identify leverage points*—The systems analysis that we have done so far suggests some leverage points where interventions may have greater than expected impacts. For instance, increasing exercise post angioplasty or surgery may be safer than when severe disease is present. Patients may also be highly motivated to exercise after having angioplasty or surgery. Exercise then might be effective in helping patients stop smoking cigarettes and reducing abdominal girth, as well as having an impact on HDL cholesterol and blood sugar.

**TABLE 14.1** summarizes the steps in the process, the meaning of each step, and the examples from cigarette smoking and coronary artery disease.

At times, we may be able to use the results of a systems analysis to display the structure and function of a system using what is called a **systems diagram**. A systems diagram is a graphic means of displaying the way we understand systems to be structured and/or to function. Let us see how we can use a systems diagram to display the functioning of a system.

# ▶ How Can We Use Systems Diagrams to Display the Workings of a System?[6,7]

Let us use an example to illustrate the development and use of systems diagrams. We will take a look at the

---

e   These dynamic effects may produce what are called stocks and flows. Stocks and flows can be thought of much like that of a dammed river system. The stocks are the reservoirs, or reserves, that we see. The flows represent the water coming into and out of the reservoir. Stocks and flows are especially important in systems analyses that address issues of the speed of events that occur when systems thinking is applied to organizational issues.

**TABLE 14.1** Steps and Their Meaning in Systems Analysis

| Step # | Meaning | Examples |
|---|---|---|
| 1. Identify influences | Identify factors or determinants that are thought to affect or influence the probability of occurrence of a disease or the outcome of a disease. | Coronary artery disease—High LDL cholesterol, cigarette smoking, increased abdominal obesity, etc., increase occurrence.<br><br>Cigarettes—Taxation of cigarettes, smoking cessation programs, prohibitions on public smoking, etc., improve outcome. |
| 2. Estimate the relative strength of the influences | Estimate the relative risks of each of the influences or at least the relative strength, such as weak, moderate, or strong. | Coronary artery disease—Most important factors are of moderate strength with relative risks between 2 and 4.<br><br>Cigarettes—Degree of addiction is a strong factor in determining outcome. Radon and asbestos each have relative risk of approximately 5. |
| 3. Examine the interactions between factors | How is the occurrence of disease or the outcome of disease affected when two or more influences are present? Do the impacts of the influences add together, does one influence protect against another influence, does the presence of two influences multiply the impact? | Coronary artery disease—The metabolic syndrome is an example of interactions between factors in which the presence of multiple factors has more than an additive impact.<br><br>Cigarettes—The impacts of radon and asbestos on lung cancer are multiplied in the presence of cigarette smoking. |
| 4. Identify feedback loops | Identify ways that an influence increases or decreases the impact of other factor(s) over time. | Coronary artery disease—Exercise can reduce weight, blood sugar, and blood pressure as well as having a protective impact in and of itself.<br><br>Cigarettes—Reduction in the percentage of the population who smoke may encourage greater use of other interventions such a laws against indoor public smoking to further reduce the percentage who smoke. |
| 5. Identify bottlenecks | Identify points in the system or constraints that need to be addressed in order for the other factors or influences to have their potential impacts. | Coronary artery disease—Severe constriction of major artery often needs to be addressed by angioplasty or surgery to enable other interventions to work effectively.<br><br>Cigarettes—Addiction often needs to be addressed directly in order for other intervention to be effective. |
| 6. Identify leverage points | Identify points in the system that presents opportunities for interventions to have greater than otherwise expected impacts. | Coronary artery disease—Exercise may have greater than expected impacts if used post angiography or surgery when exercise is safer and patients are motivated.<br><br>Cigarettes—Interventions aimed at pregnant women may have greater than expected impacts short term and longer term because women are highly motivated to stop cigarette smoking during pregnancy. |

etiology and outcomes of motor vehicle injuries, especially automobile injuries. **BOX 14.1** presents the "facts" that we will use in developing our systems diagrams.

The development of systems diagrams begins with identifying the key factors that will be included in the systems. For each factor, we need to:

▪ Indicate the direction in which it operates; in other words, which way the arrow points

▪ Indicate whether the factor operates to reinforce or increase another factor or outcome, which

is indicated by a (+), or operates to dampen or decrease another factor or outcome, which is indicated by a (−)

**FIGURE 14.1** looks at the direction of two factors, emergency response system and injury, as well as their type of impacts on death and disability. Note that both emergency response system and injury point toward death and disability because they presumably impact the frequency of occurrence of death and disability. However, emergency response has a negative sign

---

**BOX 14.1**  Background on Motor Vehicle Injuries As a Systems Issue

### Overview

In the United States, motor vehicle injuries, and automobile injuries in particular, have been the leading cause of death for children and young adults for at least the last half century. Today, they remain a critical problem; however, the death rates from motor vehicle collisions, especially when measured as death per miles driven, have fallen so dramatically that the Centers for Disease Control and Prevention (CDC) classified highway safety as one of the 10 great public health achievements of the 20th century. This progress has not been due to any one intervention or magic bullet—it is the combination of systems thinking and coordinated interventions that have made the difference.

We might regard the dramatic fall in automobile-related deaths as a systems thinking success story. However, change brings new issues and new challenges. The widespread practice of texting while driving poses new safety hazards that need to be addressed.

We will use motor vehicle injuries as an example that allows us to illustrate principles of systems thinking. We will aim to analyze the issue of motor vehicle injuries from both an etiology and an outcome perspective. That is, we will look at both the reason for motor vehicle injuries and consequences of motor vehicle injuries. We will see how we can impact one, the other, or both of these. In using a systems thinking approach, we need to incorporate the following information. For purposes of this example, you need to act as if the following represents important factual information.

### Etiology

In terms of etiology, motor vehicle collisions are greatly influenced by alcohol use, which has direct impacts on the risk of motor vehicle collisions but also leads to speeding, which itself strongly influences the chances of a motor vehicle collision. Speeding greatly increases the likelihood of a collision as well as reducing available response times. Efforts aimed at speeding as well as at

alcohol use have been especially effective in reducing motor vehicle injuries.

Motor vehicle collisions are also increased by texting, which greatly increases the response time when potential hazards occur. In addition, texting may directly produce motor vehicle collisions by the body movements or mechanical issues produced by texting, which disrupt safe driving.

Motor vehicle collisions can be reduced by road safety technology such as wider shoulders, barriers, and straighter roads. Vehicle collision prevention technology such as more visible brake lights, occupied blind spot notification systems, and out of lane notification systems may reduce the probability of collisions. Vehicle collision safety technology such as crumple zones, which absorb impacts, roll-over protections, and safety glass can reduce injuries when collisions do occur. Passenger restraint systems including safety belts and airbags can reduce the chance of injury from motor vehicle collisions.

### Outcome

In terms of outcome, an emergency response system can take advantage of the "golden hour," a period of time when emergency intervention can save many lives, which can reduce death and disability after injuries do occur. The emergency response system can be thought of as including first responders, emergency department preparedness, as well as a trauma triage system helping ensure that those injured get appropriate care as fast as possible. By eliminating the long delays in reaching care, the emergency response systems have been especially effective in reducing the rate of death and disability due to motor vehicle injuries.

A systems analysis of both etiology and outcome can diagram the approaches that have been used to address motor vehicle injuries. The collaborative efforts of public health and clinical medicine have been an essential ingredient in this success.

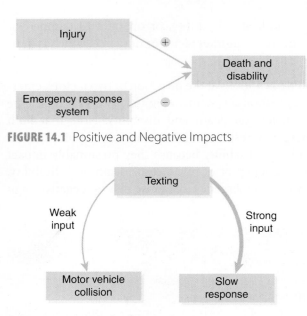

**FIGURE 14.1** Positive and Negative Impacts

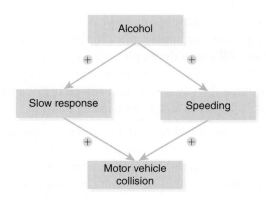

**FIGURE 14.3** Positive Feedback Loop

magnifies the effect of alcohol alone. A positive feedback loop can help us identify leverage points where extra efforts can have great benefits. Efforts to address both alcohol use and speeding, often together, have been especially effective in having a major impact on the reduction of motor vehicle collisions.

**FIGURE 14.4** demonstrates what is called a negative feedback loop. As shown in the figure, the occurrence of injuries leads to increased use of the emergency response system, which itself is intended to reduce the probability of death and disability. The increased use of the system may provide increased experience and increased competence for these health professions, so the increased use may actually improve outcome. A negative feedback loop can help us identify bottlenecks, which later prevent otherwise effective interventions from working. Efforts to eliminate long delays in reaching trauma care and taking advantage of the golden hour have largely removed this bottleneck. These interventions have been especially effective in reducing the deaths and disabilities due to motor vehicle injuries.[g]

**FIGURE 14.2** Strength of Response

because it hopefully reduces the frequency of death and disability. Injury itself increases the frequency of death and disability.[f]

In addition to indicating the direction of influence and whether the influence is positive or negative, systems diagrams often indicate the strength or magnitude of the impact. The strength or magnitude of the impact is indicated by the width of the arrow used; the thicker the arrow, the greater the impact. **FIGURE 14.2** illustrates the strength or magnitude of two relationships. The thicker arrow between texting and slow response indicates a stronger impact, while the thinner arrow between texting and motor vehicle collision indicates a weaker direct impact.

Texting has a strong impact on response time because those who are texting often fail to see and respond to hazards in a timely way. In addition, texting may in and of itself lead to collisions due to the body movements or mechanical issues produced by texting, which disrupt safe driving, such as having one or both hands off the steering wheel while writing a text, or inadvertently swerving when reaching for the phone.

**FIGURE 14.3** demonstrates what is called a positive feedback loop. In a positive feedback loop, one factor reinforces another to magnify the impact. Alcohol use reduces inhibitions and often leads to driving well beyond the speed limit. It also decreases response time, and together with the increased speed, greatly

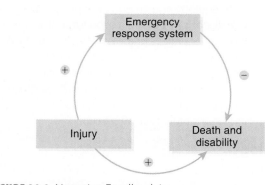

**FIGURE 14.4** Negative Feedback Loop

---

f   At times, arrows may point in both directions. Stoplights, for instance, may reduce the occurrence of injuries. The increased occurrence of injuries might also increase the frequency of placement of stoplights. When this occurs, expect there to be arrows in both directions. Each of these arrows may have a positive or a negative sign, and the magnitude or strength of the impacts may be different in the two directions.

g   In systems analysis, positive and negative feedback loops are distinguished by the product of the signs. Two negative signs or two positive signs therefore produce a positive feedback loop. Three negative signs or two positive signs and one negative sign produce a negative feedback loop. In general, when the product of the signs is positive, the loop is considered a positive feedback loop, and when the product of the signs is negative, the loop is considered a negative feedback loop.

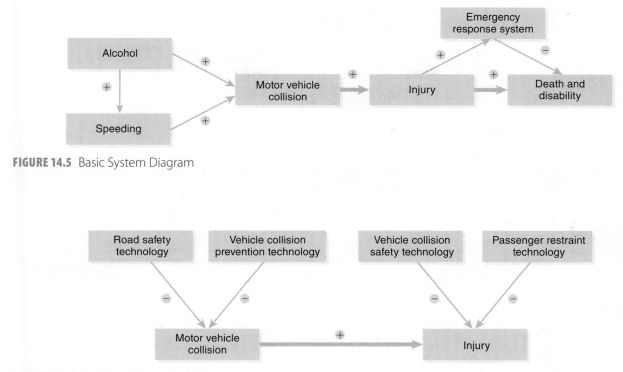

**FIGURE 14.5** Basic System Diagram

**FIGURE 14.6** Additional Negative Influences

**FIGURE 14.5** represents a basic systems diagram putting together the impact of the positive and the negative feedback loops and indicating the direction of influence and the strength or magnitude of the impacts. This is the simplest type of full systems diagram.

Often additional factors can be included in the systems diagram. **FIGURE 14.6** diagrams the dampening or negative impact of a series of factors on the probability of motor vehicle collisions and also on the occurrence of injury once motor vehicle collisions occur. These factors are road safety technology, vehicle collision prevention technology, vehicle collision safety technology, and passenger restraint technology.

**FIGURE 14.7** illustrates additional positive or accelerating/magnifying impacts of the combination of speeding and texting on motor vehicle collisions. It indicates how both speeding and texting have direct and indirect impacts that increase the probability of motor vehicle injury. Here it is assumed that texting has its major impact by slowing response time, while speeding has its greatest impact by directly increasing the chances of a collision.

Finally, **FIGURE 14.8** attempts to put all of these components together to develop a systems diagram incorporating all the factors or influences that we indicated have an impact on the occurrence of collision or the outcome of collisions.[h] Figure 14.8 may be used as the basis for developing potential interventions or future research on the expected impact of interventions.[i]

---

h Systems diagrams are designed to communicate the author's understanding or belief about the relationships that produce disease or impact the outcomes. Thus, there can be variations, with no single one serving as the correct version. Systems diagrams often do not include all the potential interactions that occur. Which interactions to include is often a judgment call. One consideration in drawing systems diagrams is to avoid having arrows cross each other, which makes the completed diagram more complicated and difficult to read and interpret. Because one of the aims of systems diagrams is to communicate efficiently, systems diagrams should not be any more complex than necessary to convey an appreciation of what the author believes are the key relationships.

i Systems diagrams at times can be converted into what is called a systems model if measureable variables are used to describe each factor. For instance, instead of using alcohol as a factor, a measure of alcohol consumption needs to be used, such as blood level of alcohol. Systems models aim to simulate the actual operation of a system. By developing a systems model, we may be able to use computerized methods to perform simulations of the operation of the model and quantitatively test the model to estimate how the outcome(s) may be altered by altering one or more of the factors. Simulations imply calculating quantitatively the outcome(s) of the model after making one or more changes in the model. The simulation may be "run" a large number of times based on chance selection of particular values from a possible distribution of values for each factor. The results of the simulation can then be presented as a range of values using the mean and standard deviations of each outcome. The process of running the model a large number of times is called sensitivity analysis and allows us to determine whether the outcome is sensitive to the level or value of a particular factor. This process can help us judge the potential impact of a number of possible interventions, or, at times, changes that occur over time.

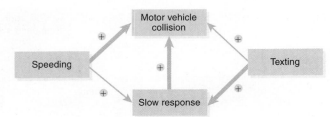

**FIGURE 14.7** Additional Positive Influences

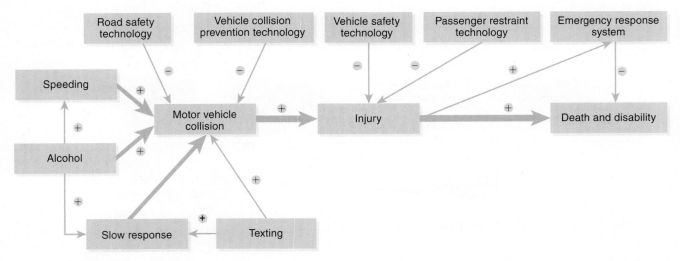

**FIGURE 14.8** Systems Diagram

## ▶ How Can We Apply Systems Thinking to Population Health Issues?

Even when we do not have enough data to do a full systems analysis or develop a systems diagram, specific components of systems thinking can be applied to population health issues. Let us take a look at the roles that systems thinking can play in population health. In doing this, we will look at five population health questions that systems thinking can help us answer:

- How can systems thinking help us incorporate interactions between factors to better understand the etiology of disease?
- How can systems thinking help take into account the interactions between diseases?
- How can systems thinking help identify bottlenecks and leverage points that can be used to improve population health?
- How can systems thinking help us develop strategies for multiple simultaneous interventions?
- How can systems thinking help us look at processes as a whole to plan short- and long-term intervention strategies?

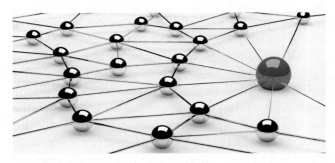

© 3DProfi/Shutterstock

## ▶ How Can Systems Thinking Help Us Incorporate Interactions Between Factors to Better Understand the Etiology of Disease?

Understanding the interactions between factors, influences, or determinants has become central to population health, as illustrated by new approaches such as the social determinants of health. Let us examine a specific interaction that has received a great deal of attention in public health in recent years: the interaction between radon and cigarette smoking in causing lung cancer.[8] As we have discussed, radon is a naturally occurring radioactive gas. It is colorless and odorless. Radon is produced by the decay of uranium in soil, rock, and groundwater. It emits ionizing radiation during its radioactive decay. Radon is found all over the country, though there are areas of the country with substantially higher levels than other areas. Radon gets into the indoor air primarily by entering via the soil under homes and other buildings at the basement or lowest level.

Today, it is recognized based on high-quality epidemiological studies that radon causes lung cancer. Radon is the second most important cause of lung cancer after cigarettes and the most common cause of lung cancer among nonsmokers. The Environmental Protection Agency (EPA) estimates that radon accounts for over 20,000 cases of lung cancer, as compared with the over 100,000 cases attributed to cigarettes. The average indoor level in the United States is about 1.3pCi/L. The EPA has set a level of 2pCi/L as an attainable level and a level of 4pCi/L as the maximum recommended level. Approximately 15% of homes in the United States have basement radon levels above 4pCi/L.

Cigarette smoking and radon exposure are multiplicative; that is, when both are present, the hazard is multiplied. For instance, using the EPA's figures, the relative risk of lung cancer for the average smoker is approximately nine times the risk compared to a nonsmoker. The relative risk from radon when the level is 10pCi/L compared to 2pCi/L is over 4.5. When both cigarette smoking and a level of radon exposure of 10pCi/L are present, the relative risk of lung cancer increases almost 40 times.[8]

The recognition that radon multiplies the impacts of cigarette smoking has had a key impact on the approaches used to address these potential hazards. For smokers with exposure to these hazards, the risk can be greatly reduced by reductions in radon as well as by stopping smoking. Because radon is a measurable and controllable environmental exposure, there has been a great deal of attention and effort given to control of this hazard. Thus, the recognition of interactions that multiply or greatly increase the risk have become an important tool for setting priorities and developing approaches to risk reduction.

## ▶ How Can Systems Thinking Help Take into Account the Interactions Between Diseases?

The classic connection between diseases was Edward Jenner's observation that children who develop cow pox were very unlikely to get smallpox even when exposed. This fundamental observation led to the concept and term "vaccination," from the Latin word "vacca," or cow. It also established that there can be a relationship between diseases.

In recent years, it has been increasingly recognized that some diseases predispose to other diseases. In addition, there are patterns of risk factors or symptoms that tend to occur together. These are often called **syndromes**. As we have seen, the components of the metabolic syndrome frequently occur together and greatly increase the probability of coronary artery and other large blood vessel diseases. The recognition of the frequent occurrence of the metabolic syndrome has led to concerted efforts to identify individuals with the syndrome and make a multi-intervention approach to reducing the risk.

HIV provides a good example of the complex interactions that occur between diseases. A number of sexually transmitted diseases, especially those that interrupt the mucosal membranes lining the genital organs, such as syphilis and herpes genitalis, increase the risk of being infected with HIV if exposed. In addition, diseases such as gonorrhea greatly increase the level of the HIV virus that appears in semen, thus increasing the communicability of HIV.

HIV itself predisposes to a large number of infections, the most important of which from the public health perspective is tuberculosis. Finally, HIV is found in association with other conditions, including drug abuse and intimate partner violence, which greatly increases the burden of disease. These types of interactions of HIV with other diseases and conditions have been described as a **syndemic**. A syndemic is the occurrence together of two or more diseases that interact to magnify the occurrence and/or burden of disease.[9]

Disease interactions are not always detrimental. At times, one disease may provide protection against other diseases. Early infection with bacteria and other pathogens in environments such as that which occurs on farms has been shown to be associated with reduced incidence of food and skin allergies.

Systems thinking can not only help us understand the relationship between diseases, but it can also help us understand the impact that a disease has over the life span.

## ▶ How Can Systems Thinking Help Identify Bottlenecks and Leverage Points That Can Be Used to Improve Population Health?

Looking at the dynamics of systems helps us to identify two types of points that benefit from special attention. The first of these is called a bottleneck or a constraint. A bottleneck is a point at which events are slowed down, presenting obstacles to success of an intervention. We have already identified some important bottlenecks. In the 1960s, it was recognized that after trauma, such as injuries from war or motor vehicle collisions, many victims are able to physiologically respond and temporarily tolerate blood loss and other injuries before rapidly deteriorating. This early period became known as the golden hour.

Few victims of motor vehicle injuries before the 1970s were reaching emergency care during the golden hour. To address this bottleneck, a sophisticated system of emergency response was put into place in the United States, which, as we have discussed, greatly reduced the response time and resulted in a large reduction in deaths and disabilities from motor vehicle collisions.

We identified another example of a bottleneck in the course of cigarette smoking. The vast majority of cigarette smokers start before age 18 and often many years earlier. These smokers often have a great deal of difficulty stopping smoking, even when they are intellectually committed to stopping in later years. Addiction to nicotine in cigarettes has been recognized as a key bottleneck to successful control of cigarette smoking. Recent interventions are addressing this bottleneck, including new authority for the Food and Drug Administration (FDA) to regulate the quantity of nicotine in cigarettes.

On the other hand, leverage points are points in systems in which successful interventions produce better than expected outcomes. We can see them as opportunities to make major improvements in outcomes. At leverage points, there is no bottleneck, but the conditions are right to take advantage of the interactions that exist between factors. For instance, with cigarette smoking, pregnant women who smoke are at greatly increased risk of delivering premature infants. In addition, they are highly motivated to stop smoking and often have encouragement to do so by family and friends. New efforts to put extra resources and extra efforts into smoking cessation for pregnant women are having a large payoff for their newborns and themselves.

In addition to helping us identify bottlenecks and leverage points, systems thinking can help us develop a coordinated approach or strategy for combining multiple simultaneous interventions.

## ▶ How Can Systems Thinking Help Us Develop Strategies for Multiple Simultaneous Interventions?

As we have seen, the approach to coronary artery disease has successfully utilized multiple simultaneous interventions for several decades. Today, we are moving to a coordinated strategy of utilizing primary, secondary, and tertiary interventions. Primary interventions include control of high blood pressure, cholesterol, cigarette smoking, obesity, diabetes, and a growing list of other contributory causes of coronary artery disease.

Secondary interventions designed to prevent heart damage and death—including interventions in the early hours of a myocardial infarction—have become an increasingly successful part of an overall strategy. Drug treatment and post myocardial exercise rehabilitation are now a standard part of medical care. Finally, tertiary interventions to prevent sudden death in public places have now become a population health intervention, with placement of automated defibrillators in places where people congregate, such as airports and sporting events.

New approaches to disease often combine primary, secondary, and tertiary interventions. For instance, efforts to address HIV may in the future include primary prevention through barrier protection, circumcision, precoital and intracoital treatment, and eventually vaccination. Postexposure treatments are being extensively investigated as well. Detection during the first few weeks, when transmissibility is greatest, is being investigated as an important new intervention. In addition, early and continuous drug treatment of HIV has been found not only to help the individual but also to reduce his or her infectivity.

The dramatic reduction in maternal to child transmission of HIV is an example of the potential for multiple intervention to improve outcome. **BOX 14.2** discusses the success of the multiple intervention approach to prevention of maternal–child transmission of HIV.

Prevention of maternal–child transmission of HIV in the United States has been highly successful. Today, infection with HIV by the maternal–child route should be considered a failure of public health and medicine. HIV can be transmitted across the placenta during pregnancy. The higher the level of virus in the mother's blood, the greater the probability of transmission. Thus, early testing and active treatment of pregnant women is fundamental to prevention of maternal–child transmission.

In addition, there is an increased risk during vaginal delivery. Selective use of cesarean delivery can reduce this risk. Early treatment of infants has been shown to reduce the risk still further. Finally, breastfeeding carries a small but important risk of transmission. Avoidance of breastfeeding or active maternal drug treatment during breastfeeding among women with HIV can greatly reduce this risk as well.

The strategy of coordinated use of multiple simultaneous complementary interventions has become a highly successful population health strategy. For many years, interventions were studied and applied one intervention at a time, with little thought to how they interact or how they could be used in combination to produce the best results. In recent years, systems thinking and systems analysis approaches have contributed to the development of increasingly effective strategies that combine multiple interventions.

Fully developed systems thinking approaches, when feasible, can also be used to help us see entire processes to help us plan short-term as well as long-term intervention strategies.

## How Can Systems Thinking Help Us Look at Processes As a Whole to Plan Short-Term and Long-Term Intervention Strategies?

Efforts to see the entire processes rather than pieces of the pie have become key to planning interventions and have been incorporated into the "health in all policies" approach.

Systems thinking approaches to food safety have taken this type of approach in recent years.[10] Initially, systems thinking has focused on identifying interventions for high-risk food one type of food at a time. This process has been called the Hazard Analysis and Critical Control Points (HACCP) system. **BOX 14.3** takes a look at the HACCP approach and the efforts to control the hazard of ground beef.

New approaches to food safety build on the HACCP system and its big picture look at the process as a whole. In an emerging systems thinking approach, most food's detailed location and time of production down to the level of the farm or factory are being identified on the label. This allows public health officials to trace the food back to where and when the problem occurred. Adding this approach to the HACCP provides a mechanism for quickly responding to early indications of foodborne outbreaks, regardless of the type of food involved. The combination of the HACCP system and food tracing provides the potential for a fully developed systems thinking approach to food safety.

We have now looked at the basic principles and applications of systems thinking to population health. Let us now take a detailed look at the concept of **One Health** which aims to develop a systems thinking approach to perhaps the most complex of all systems which affects us all; the system of humans, animals, and ecosystem health.

## What Is Meant by One Health?

One Health is about the larger system, the world we live in. The One Health movement asserts that human health is dependent on animal health and the health of the ecosystem. The One Health movement focuses on the connections between human, animal, and ecosystem health as illustrated in **FIGURE 14.9**.

The history of the One Health approach can be traced to Rudolph Virchow a 19th century German pathologist and public health leader who coined the term **zoonotic disease** or diseases that exist in animals but can be transmitted to humans. We now know that zoonotic diseases can be caused by viruses, bacteria, parasites, and fungi. Virchow's aphorism "between

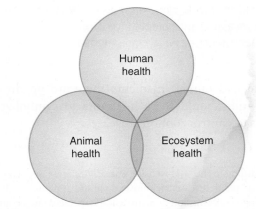

**FIGURE 14.9** One Health: From AIDS to Zika: The Relationships Between Human Health, Animal Health, and Ecosystem Health Are Central to One Health

---

**BOX 14.3** The HACCP System and Ground Beef

The HACCP is a systems approach that looks for key leverage or control points to manage food safety issues. It is built upon a series of prerequisite conditions designed to first ensure basic environmental and operating conditions. These prerequisite conditions might be viewed as efforts to remove the bottlenecks to an effectively functioning system. These include facilities that maintain sanitary conditions; proper equipment construction, installation, and maintenance; personal hygiene by employees; etc.

Once these basic conditions of food safety are accomplished, HACCP looks for options for interventions at multiple leverage or control points and institutes a series of safeguards at these specific points.

Meat safety issues reflect this approach. Ground beef, which often combines meat from leftover portions of multiple animals, has been identified as a high-risk product or hazard. Toxin-producing strains of *Escherichia coli* were previously widespread in ground beef products and have been responsible for a number of fatal outbreaks of foodborne illness in the past. The threats to health have led to a more coordinated systems thinking approach using the HACCP system. Let us take a look at the HACCP process and the ground beef example.

The systems thinking approach known as HACCP attempts to understand, monitor, and quickly respond to breakdowns in the food safety system. This methodology, originally developed for the U.S. space program, is based on the principle that risks to food safety exist from the field to the fork. HACCP is increasingly being adopted for such products as seafood, meat, poultry, and fruit juices. HACCP includes the following seven steps:

- *Analyze hazards.* Potential hazards associated with a food and potential interventions to control those hazards are identified. The hazard could be biological, such as a microbe; chemical, such as a toxin; or physical, such as ground glass or metal fragments.
- *Identify critical control points.* These are points in a food's production—from its raw state through processing and shipping to consumption by the consumer—at which the potential hazard can be

controlled or eliminated. Examples are cooking, cooling, packaging, and metal detection.

- *Establish preventive measures with critical limits for each control point.* For a cooked food, for example, this may include setting the minimum cooking temperature and time required to ensure the elimination of any harmful microbes.
- *Establish procedures to monitor the critical control points.* Such procedures may include determining how and by whom cooking time and temperature should be monitored.
- Establish corrective actions to be taken when monitoring shows that a critical limit has not been met. An example is reprocessing or disposing of food if the minimum cooking temperature is not met.
- *Establish procedures to verify that the system is working properly.* An example is testing time- and temperature-recording devices to verify that a cooking unit is working properly.
- *Establish effective recordkeeping to document the HACCP system.* This would include records of hazards and their control methods, the monitoring of safety requirements, and actions taken to correct potential problems.

Each of these principles must be backed by sound scientific knowledge—for example, published microbiological studies on time and temperature factors for controlling foodborne pathogens.

Key control points at which ground beef may be contaminated in the meatpacking process have been identified. Monitoring by testing now includes a random testing process on all batches of ground beef. The process uses rapid testing of a sample of the finished ground beef and holding up distribution until the results are available. Education of consumers about the danger of eating rare or raw ground beef is also a key component of this strategy. In addition, separating beef products from other food preparation, especially from food products eaten raw, is an important educational effort.

The HACCP process has already had a major impact on the incidence of disease associated with ground beef. It is not a cure-all, but looking at the process as a whole has helped us come up with effective interventions.[11]

---

animal and human medicine there are no dividing lines—nor should there be" came to symbolize the efforts to control zoonotic diseases.[12,j]

The control of zoonotic diseases was part of wider efforts to control infectious diseases in the first half of the 20th century. By the 1960s and 1970s, the medical

---

j   According to the NIH website, one of Virchow's important contributions was establishing the round worm *Trichinella* as the cause of the human disease trichinosis, a painful and potentially fatal disease of muscles caused by eating raw or undercooked pork as well through consumption of many wildlife species which contain the round worm larvae. Virchow was opposed to Otto von Bismarck, the Iron Chancellor's military budget, "…which angered Bismarck sufficiently to challenge Virchow to a duel. Virchow, being entitled to choose the weapons, chose 2 pork sausages: a cooked sausage for himself and an uncooked one, loaded with *Trichinella* larvae, for Bismarck. Bismarck, the Iron Chancellor, declined the proposition as too risky."[12]

and public health communities often felt that victory was in sight in the battle against infectious diseases. Antibiotics were curing most bacterial diseases including tuberculosis, vaccines were controlling many viral disease outbreaks, and smallpox eradication was on the horizon. Malaria and other mosquito borne disease had been reduced by widespread mosquito control often through use of DDT and other pesticides.

All that began to change in the 1980s with the emergence of HIV infection and the recognition that it likely had its origins in the African tropical forests. Mosquito borne diseases including dengue fever, West Nile Virus (WNV), Chikungunya, and most recently, Zika virus, began a relentless expansion. In addition, new life-threatening diseases including most notably severe acute respiratory syndrome (SARS) emerged and rapidly spread person-to-person posing the threat of international epidemics and disrupting the rapid growth of global trade as well as international travel.[13]

In the 21st century it has become evident that environmental change, population growth, and economic disparities have accelerated the pace of spread of existing diseases. It is now apparent that we need to take a new look at the relationship between humans, animals and the ecosystem and better understand their connections. That's what One Health is all about.

## ▶ What Is the One Health Initiative?

The One Health Initiative has been a response to these increasing threats. Initially developed by the veterinary medicine community it has been widely accepted by national and international organizations.[k]

The One Health Initiative defines One Health as "the collaborative effort of multiple health science professions, together with their related disciplines and institutions – working locally, nationally, and globally – to attain optimal health for people, domestic animals, wildlife, plants, and our environment."[14]

One Health is designed to serve as an umbrella under which collaboration is facilitated between the full range of disciplines and professions that connect human health, animal health, and health of the ecosystem as illustrated in the One Health "umbrella" displayed in **FIGURE 14.10**.

We examine the One Health initiative mostly from the perspective of human health. Ideally, however, these benefits flow both ways. Animals may also benefit from control of zoonotic diseases and from the human–animal bond. In addition, reducing the rate of human-mediated species loss and artificial introduction of nonnative species may help sustain ecosystems.

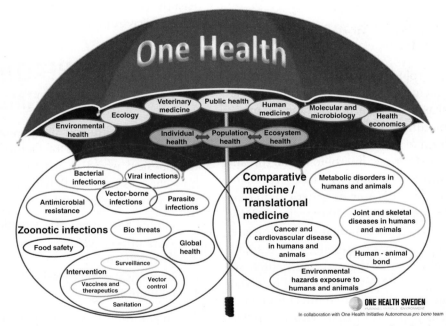

**FIGURE 14.10** The One Health Umbrella Indicating the Need for Broad Collaboration to Achieve the Goals of One Health

Reproduced from One Health Sweden. http://www.onehealthinitiative.com/about.php.

k The organizations include CDC, World Health Organization, World Organization for Animal Health (IOE), the European Union, and the World Bank. It is increasingly recognized by a range of health professions as a key component of the education of all health professionals.

## ▶ What Is the One Health Educational Framework?

The One Health educational framework was developed by the One Health Interprofessional Education Working Group made up of representatives of medicine, nursing, pharmacy, and veterinary medicine, as well as public health.[15] The framework includes the following three components:[1]

■ Microbiological influences on health and disease
■ Ecosystem health/physical environment
■ Human–animal interaction

We can view these components as important factors or influences that affect the system of human, animal, and ecosystem health. We have not reached the stage where we can draw complete systems diagrams or fully understand the relationships between the components of the system. Nonetheless looking at these three influences can get us to start to think about how we can improve the health of humans, animals, and the ecosystem. We will begin by taking a look at microbiological influences on health and disease.

## MICROBIOLOGICAL INFLUENCES ON HEALTH AND DISEASE

### What Are the Most Important Microbiological Threats to the Public's Health?

A wide range of microbiological entities can produce human disease including DNA (deoxyribonucleic acid) and RNA viruses, bacteria, a wide range of parasites, protozoa, and fungi, as well as prions which are a disease-causing form of a normal brain protein.

Many of the most serious microbiological threats to the public's health are due to RNA viruses. An **RNA virus** is a virus that has RNA as its genetic material. There are currently approximately 200 species of RNA viruses that are known to infect humans, and more are being added each year. This represents only a small fraction of the RNA viruses that exist in nature, so there is an abundance of RNA viruses which have the potential to mutate to enable them to infect humans.

RNA viruses, as opposed to DNA viruses, are far more likely to produce mutations during their frequent replications since they do not have the same protective mechanism against copying or coding errors. This high rate of mutation in RNA viruses is believed to enhance their ability to cross species lines and, once established in a new species, to continue to mutate. RNA viruses often have multiple animal species as hosts and are believed to easily cross species lines, creating new host species including human beings. Crossing of RNA viruses between similar species such as nonhuman primates and humans is believed to be more likely than crossing between less closely related species.[10]

RNA viruses that have "spilled over" or crossed the species line and included humans in their list of hosts often do not immediately or inevitably cause severe disease or produce epidemics. Most of the recently recognized epidemic diseases caused by RNA viruses existed in humans for years, decades, or longer before they became epidemic diseases.

Often, human populations exposed to RNA viruses as well as other pathogens gain immunity and do not experience frequent or severe illnesses. However, when previously unexposed populations encounter the same pathogen, they may experience severe and/or epidemic disease.

RNA viruses are so important to the relationship between human health, animal health and ecosystem health that is may be helpful to identify what we will call the "top 10" RNA viruses as discussed in **BOX 14.4**. Let us now turn to the second component of the One Health educational framework: ecosystem health/physical environment.

## ECOSYSTEM HEALTH/PHYSICAL ENVIRONMENT

Ecosystem health and its impact on human health involves a wide range of factors that directly affect the physical world in which we live.[26] We examine how changes in the following factors can have major impacts on human health:

■ Global movement of populations
■ Agriculture changes and changes in food distribution
■ Ecological changes in land and resource use
■ Climate change

In addition, as we use a systems analysis approach we need to keep in mind key underlying mechanisms

---

1   The One Health Inter-professional Education Working Group was convened by the Association of American Veterinary Medical Colleges with the collaboration of the Healthy People Curriculum Task Force of the Association for Prevention Teaching and Research.

**BOX 14.4**  The "Top 10" Emerging RNA Viruses

Let us take a look at what we will call the "Top 10" emerging RNA viruses. These have been chosen not just for their frequency of occurrence but also the impact they have had and the lessons which they can teach. Together they reflect the spectrum of emerging human infections caused by RNA viruses.

## AIDS/ HIV

Despite the fact that HIV, as the name implies, is currently exclusively transmitted from person to person, recent evidence strongly supports its origin in non-human primates in Africa.

## Chikungunya

Chikungunya is a classic example of an emerging infectious disease. In the 1950s it was first detected in humans in Sub-Saharan Africa. It was named Chikungunya from African languages meaning "to become contorted" or to "walk bent over" reflecting the severe joint pain it produced and the efforts of patients to find a comfortable position.

In 2004, a mutation of Chikungunya virus was documented which allowed spread of infection with a lower amount of the virus during mosquito feeding. This in turn allowed another mosquito species *Aedes albopictus* (commonly called the Asian tiger mosquito) which is now present in the southeastern United States to transmit the disease. The combination of the right mutation and the right mosquito most likely led to the major outbreaks of Chikungunya in the Caribbean and could lead to outbreaks in the United States as well.[16]

## Dengue

Dengue is an example of a long standing human disease that has increased in frequency and expanded into new territory in recent years. Known in the United States since colonial times, Dengue is transmitted by the *Aedes aegypti* mosquito.

Dengue is usually a relatively mild disease, but a severe disease known as dengue hemorrhagic fever can occur. An estimated 500,000 people with severe dengue require hospitalization each year, a large proportion of who are children. Approximately 2.5% of those affected die. In recent years, over 2 million cases of dengue per year have been reported in the Americas alone, of which over 10,000 cases were diagnosed as severe dengue.

In the 1960s, only nine countries had experienced severe dengue epidemics. The disease is now endemic in more than 100 countries with approximately half the world's population including Africa, the Americas, the Eastern Mediterranean, South-East Asia, and the Western Pacific including Hawaii where repeated outbreaks have occurred.[17]

## Ebola

Ebola, another RNA virus, was first identified in 1976 near the Ebola River in what is now the Democratic Republic of the Congo. Since then, over 25 outbreaks have appeared sporadically in Africa. Ebola, which causes Ebola hemorrhagic fever, is a tragic disease in which the victims experience internal and external bleeding and damage to almost every organ before succumbing to the infection. As the disease progresses, the virus is contained in blood or body fluids (including but not limited to urine, saliva, sweat, feces, vomit, breast milk, and semen) making it potentially contagious through close contact as well as through needlesticks. For those who recover, the virus can remain in the system for long periods of time.

The natural reservoir host of Ebola virus remains unconfirmed. However, researchers believe that bats are the most likely reservoir species and initial source of the infection in human and nonhuman primates. Nonhuman primates are susceptible to Ebola and have died in large numbers. There are four species of Ebola which can cause disease so it is possible for individuals to contract Ebola more than once.

Previous Ebola outbreaks occurred in sparsely populated rural areas where the potential to perpetuate the epidemic by person-to-person transmission was limited. The 2014–2016 epidemic of Ebola was different since it spread rapidly across three West African countries including their densely populated capital cities causing nearly 30,000 cases and 11,000 deaths, including over 500 among healthcare workers who experienced close personal contact with the disease.[18]

## Hantavirus

Though a rare disease in humans which cannot be transmitted person-to-person, Hantavirus is part of our top 10 RNA diseases because it reflects how humans can develop disease through routine exposures to nature and how they can be prevented. Hantavirus is carried by mice and other rodents in many parts of the United States, especially the Southwest and West.

Transmission usually occurs when humans breathe the virus contained in rodent urine or feces which has become airborne or aerosolized, and may go on to produce Hantavirus pulmonary syndrome which has a case-fatality rate of over one-third.

The most famous Hantavirus outbreak in recent years occurred in Yosemite National Park. A large number of cases and three deaths occurred there in 2012 in newly constructed cabins that were found to harbor rodent nests built with insulation from the new cabins. Hantavirus illustrates how new or previously unrecognized diseases from human–animal contact can appear in very unexpected places, including the most natural and beautiful of settings in the United States.[19]

## Influenza A

Influenza A has been an ongoing annual threat to health for many years as evidenced by the 1918–1919 pandemic which killed approximately 50 million people, many of whom were previously young and healthy. Influenza A remains a disease that infects humans by person-to-person respiratory transmission. Wild birds and pigs or swine serve as reservoirs and provide opportunities for the emergence of new strains. The mixing of the different subtypes of the virus is believed to allow genetic changes which may result in new subtypes capable of human-to-human respiratory transmission.

When a major change in the Influenza A virus occurs, previous immunity does not provide protection from the disease. In this situation entire populations may be susceptible, potentially leading to a worldwide pandemic. In 2009–2010, an Influenza A pandemic occurred with a new strain of Influenza A which is believed to have been transmitted to humans from swine in Mexico and rapidly spread to the United States and beyond. Fortunately, the 2009–2010 pandemic did not result in a high case-fatality rate, but the same might not be true in future pandemics.[20]

## Middle Eastern Respiratory Syndrome (MERS)

Middle Eastern Respiratory Syndrome, or MERS, is a newly recognized coronavirus (CoV) related to SARS. MERS affects the respiratory system. Most patients with MERS develop severe acute respiratory illness with symptoms of fever, cough, and shortness of breath. Three to four of every 10 patients diagnosed with MERS have died.

The CDC reports that the first cases of the disease were recognized in Saudi Arabia in 2012. MERS-CoV has been found in camels, and many MERS patients have reported contact with camels. The World Health Organization suggests general precautions for anyone visiting farms, markets, barns, or other places in affected countries where animals are present.

Approximately 2,000 people have developed the disease, and about 25% of those have died. So far, all cases of MERS around the world, including in the United States, have been linked to travel to or residence in countries in and near the Arabian Peninsula. MERS CoV has spread from ill people to others through close contact, such as caring for or living with an infected person.[21]

## Severe Acute Respiratory Syndrome (SARS)

The SARS CoV virus has been traced to a mutation of the RNA CoV carried by civets, a delicacy in China, which shed large numbers of the virus in their feces.

It is now well established that once the disease took hold in humans it could be transmitted by airborne aerosol droplets. The 2003 epidemic of SARS was able to quickly spread to 30 countries causing 8,000 cases and 800 deaths.

The documentation of a small number of "super spreaders" was shown to greatly enhance the potential for epidemic spread. Fortunately, with careful isolation and quarantine, person-to-person spread of SARS was interrupted, and there have not been any recent reports of its re-emergence. Given its animal reservoirs in bats and its ability to infect civets, a recurrence is always possible.[22]

## West Nile Virus (WNV)

West Nile Virus was first recognized in 1937 in the West Nile region of Uganda and was soon identified in parts of the Middle East. It usually caused mild disease. In the late 1990s it began to spread to other regions, perhaps due to a recently recognized mutation. It reached New York City in 1999 and spread throughout most of the continental United States over the next few years.

WNV is transmitted often in the late summer or early fall to humans and horses by the bite of the Culex mosquito, better known as the common house mosquito. The Culex mosquito typically obtains its blood meal from birds instead of humans but can then transmit the virus to humans when it bites humans, usually at dawn or dusk.

For approximately 80% of people who are exposed to WNV the disease does not produce symptoms. Most of the remaining 20% experience a brief period of fever and nonspecific symptoms such as headache, joint pain, and nausea. Less than 1% develops severe neurological disease that can include high fever, neck stiffness, disorientation, coma, tremors, seizures, or paralysis.[23]

## Zika Virus

In 1947 researchers identified a new virus in a rhesus monkey in the Zika forest of Uganda and named it Zika virus. The virus was soon isolated from mosquitos from the same forest suggesting mosquito-borne transmission.

From the 1960s through the 1980s, the spread of Zika virus was traced to Central and West Africa as well as tropical areas of Asia. Evidence of infection was found to be widespread, but there was little evidence of human symptoms or complications.

The world learned of Zika virus in 2015 after physicians in poverty stricken Northeast Brazil reported an enormous increase in the number of new cases of microcephaly in newborns whose mothers were found to have had Zika virus infection during pregnancy. Studies soon established that Zika virus can invade the brain of a fetus and cause direct injury to the developing brain.

In 2015, 2016, and 2017, Zika virus spread rapidly throughout South and Central America and the Caribbean, transmitted by *A. aegypti* mosquitos. Mosquito-borne transmission can be expected in the Americas, including the United States, wherever *A. aegypti* mosquitos thrive. In addition, sexual transmission was confirmed with the potential for transmission for extended periods after initial infection.[24,25]

Much still remains to be learned about Zika virus, but it is already all too clear that it is an emerging infectious disease that illustrates how rare emerging diseases that spillover from other species can suddenly and unexpectedly emerge as epidemic and even pandemic diseases.

Our "top ten" RNA viruses illustrate the diverse challenges humans face. Even though RNA viruses have been established as the causal pathogen, social and economic factors as well as individual behavior and local cultures all play a role in the system that determines where, when, and how many individuals will be affected by RNA viruses.

Data from One Health Initiative. About the One Health Initiative. Available at http://www.onehealthinitiative.com/about.php. Accessed July 25, 2017.

that often impact these factors. These mechanisms include poverty and social-economic conditions as well as population growth.

The factors that directly affect the ecosystem and human health can often be affected by poverty and the social and environmental conditions created by poverty. Therefore, it should not be surprising that changes in socioeconomic conditions can alter these factors for better or for worse. Because of the connection between socioeconomic factors and the health of the ecosystem, environmental health is increasingly being linked to the broader concept of social determinants of health.

Population growth also has a direct impact on ecosystem health through human presence in previously uninhabited areas as well as an indirect impact through increased demands for food and other resources that lead to potentially damaging impacts on the environment. The impacts of population growth continue in many areas of the developing world and have both subtle and not so subtle impacts on ecosystems.

## ▶ How Can Global Movements of Populations Affect Health?

Major migrations of human populations and exposure to new diseases have been accompanied by epidemic and pandemic spread of disease. Anthony Fauci, the Director of the National Institute of Allergy and Infectious Diseases, and his colleagues have described the two-way expansion of disease caused by the exploration and conquest of the Americas as follows:

"From the 15th through to the 19th century, a time when previously isolated continents were discovering each other and thereby exchanging microorganisms, re-emergence of epidemic diseases associated with geographic spread of microbes became common..."

Syphilis spread from the Americas to Europe causing widespread outbreaks. Smallpox spread from Europe to the Americas early in the 1500s. Fauci et al. write "Historians believe that about 3.5 million people in central Mexico died in the first year ..... By the end of the century some 18.5 (74%) of the 25 million population had died, presumably largely because of smallpox and additional imported diseases. Smallpox spread southward into South America, ultimately destroying two great civilizations, the Aztec and Inca empires, facilitating Spanish conquests that greatly altered history."[27,m]

Today's movement of populations dwarfs those of 500 years ago and 100 years ago. The ability to move around the globe in hours rather than days or months has created the potential for rapid spread of disease as we saw with the SARS epidemic and which we are now witnessing with the Zika virus. Today, large-scale movements of populations include those due to

---

m According to Fauci et al. "Francisco Pizarro, who continued Spanish conquests of South America in the 1530s, is alleged to have undertaken a bioterrorist attack on native peoples using smallpox contaminated blankets. Mexico became a regional geographic reservoir for smallpox and was the source of repeated exportations until the 1940s."[30]

humanitarian crises. In the not too distant future, they may be caused by climate change as well. These large-scale movements of people may complicate efforts to prevent the outbreak of a wide range of communicable diseases. The impact of population movements are likely to fall most heavily on countries and populations with the fewest resources to effectively respond to these threats.

# ▶ How Can Agricultural Practices and Changes in Food Distribution Influence the Occurrence of Infectious Diseases in Humans?

Zoonotic diseases such as anthrax and bovine TB have been exacerbated by agricultural changes since humans first developed agricultural practices over 10,000 years ago. Today we are developing new ways to produce and distribute food which pose new types of threats. The United States, which is a net exporter of food, actually imports food from more than 100 countries.

Concerns about agricultural practices affect not only human health but also animal health and the health of the ecosystem, and have enormous potential economic impacts. The use and misuse of pesticides, for instance, has raised concerns ranging from the health effects of human exposure to the destructive impacts on pollinating bees which are essential for food production.

An example of the impact of recent changes in agriculture is the way that livestock and poultry are

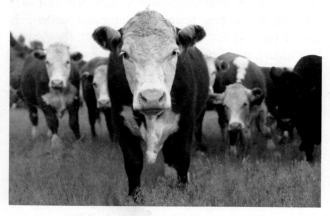

© John P Kelly/The Image Bank/Getty Images

raised. The increased affluence in many parts of the world as well as the continued growth in populations has led to a demand for more animals raised for food. A livestock revolution began in the 1980s with the rapid expansion of intensive pig and poultry production as well as the growth of milk production. This industrial food production system resulted in close confinement of animals which are often inbred to maximize growth. It was also accompanied by rapid expansion of the use of antibiotics designed to prevent disease as well as increase animal weight and contributed to the development of antibiotic resistance in animals and humans.

While this livestock revolution increased production it also increased the risk of emerging and re-emerging infectious diseases. Most dramatically it has been at the forefront of the emergence of new strains of Influenza A. The 2009–2010 influenza pandemic was first recognized among industrially raised pigs in Mexico and rapidly spread to the United States and beyond. In 2015, a highly pathogenic avian influenza strain spread rapidly through industrially raised U.S. poultry. Approximately 50 million chickens, ducks, and turkeys were infected with the virus requiring large-scale euthanasia of these bird species. Despite the fact that this particular strain of avian flu was not transmissible to humans, avian influenza in the United States cost farmers billions of dollars and more than doubled the price of eggs in the United States despite a large-scale increase in imports.[28]

# ▶ How Can Ecological Changes in Land and Resource Use Affect the Development of Infectious Diseases?

A wide range of types of ecological changes can increase or reduce the frequency of infectious diseases. For instance, the building of dams has been shown to increase the presence of schistosomiasis which affects approximately 200 million mostly poor people in the developing world. Schistosomiasis is caused by a flatworm which develops within freshwater snails that thrive in slow-moving, vegetation-heavy water bodies. Dam construction produces ideal conditions for the disease to proliferate, often affecting those who swim or wade in infected waters and spreading quite frequently to the bladder and other organs where it can produce severe disease.[29]

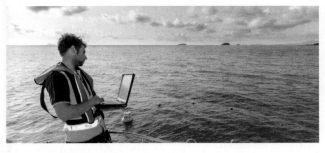

© MB Photography/Moment/Getty

Lyme disease is an example closer to home. Lyme disease, which is transmitted to humans by tick bites, has increased dramatically in the United States in the 21st century affecting as many as 300,000 people each year. Lyme disease has been associated with increases in forest land and increased human exposure to forests, especially in the eastern United States. The increase in Lyme disease has also been associated with an increase in the deer population and the white footed mice population, which serve as part of the life cycle of ticks and provide a reservoir for the bacteria which causes Lyme disease. A controversy exists about the ability to control Lyme disease though reduction in the deer population.[30]

Not all environmental changes are detrimental to health. Chagas disease, caused by a parasite, is transmitted to animals and people by insect vectors and can cause chronic heart and intestinal diseases. Over 8 million cases due to local disease transmission are estimated to be found in the Americas, mainly in rural areas of Mexico, Central America, and South America where poverty is widespread. The bugs are found in houses made from materials such as mud, adobe, straw, and palm thatch. Improvement in living standards and changes in the environment in which people live, especially better housing, is reducing the frequency of Chagas disease.[31]

## ▶ How Can Climate Change Affect Human Health?

*The Impacts of Climate Change on Human Health in the United States: A Scientific Assessment* (Health Impacts of Climate Change Report) was published in 2016 as part of the President's Climate Action Plan.[32] It assessed the scientific evidence for a wide range of potential climate impacts on human health over the next 15 to 35 years. These impacts are summarized in **TABLE 14.2**.

The table shows specific examples of how climate change can affect human health, now and in the future. These effects could occur at local, regional, or national scales. Moving from left to right along one health impact row, the three middle columns show how climate drivers affect an individual's or a community's exposure to a health threat and the resulting change in health outcome. The overall climate impact is summarized in the final column.

## HUMAN–ANIMAL INTERACTIONS

The final component of the One Health educational framework is human–animal interaction. Pet ownership is by far the most common way that most human beings come in contact with animals. There has been an estimated three-fold increase in the number of dogs and cats owned as pets in the United States in the last half century. Today nearly two-thirds of Americans own at least one pet. Over one-third of households have at least one dog and nearly one-third have at least one cat. In addition to the approximately 140 million pet dogs plus cats in the United States there are estimated to be approximately 5 million horses, 8 million birds as well as more than 5 million small mammals plus a similar number of reptiles kept as pets.[33]

## ▶ What Is the Human–Animal Bond and What Are Its Health Benefits?

According to the American Veterinary Medical Association, the **human–animal bond** is a mutually beneficial and dynamic relationship between people and animals that is influenced by behaviors that are essential to the health and well-being of both. This includes, but is not limited to, emotional, psychological, and physical interactions of people, animals, and the environment.[34]

The CDC recognizes the following benefits to human health from the interaction with pets:[35]

- Reduced blood pressure
- Reduced cholesterol and triglycerides
- Reduced feelings of loneliness
- Increased opportunities for exercise and outdoor activities
- Increased opportunities for socialization

**TABLE 14.2** Examples of Climate Impacts on Human Health

| | Climate Driver | Exposure | Health Outcome | Impact |
|---|---|---|---|---|
| **Extreme Heat** | More frequent, severe, prolonged heat events | Elevated temperatures | Heat-related death and illness | Rising temperatures will lead to an increase in heat-related deaths and illnesses. |
| **Outdoor Air Quality** | Increasing temperatures and changing precipitation patterns | Worsened air quality (ozone, particulate matter, and higher pollen counts) | Premature death, acute and chronic cardiovascular and respiratory illnesses | Rising temperatures and wildfires and decreasing precipitation will lead to increases in ozone and particulate matter, elevating the risks of cardiovascular and respiratory illnesses and death. |
| **Flooding** | Rising sea level and more frequent or intense extreme precipitation, hurricanes, and storm surge events | Contaminated water, debris, and disruptions to essential infrastructure | Drowning, injuries, mental health consequences, gastrointestinal and other illness | Increased coastal and inland flooding exposes populations to a range of negative health impacts before, during, and after events. |
| **Vector-Borne Infection** (Lyme Disease) | Changes in temperature extremes and seasonal weather patterns | Earlier and geographically expanded tick activity | Lyme disease | Ticks will show earlier seasonal activity and a generally northward range expansion, increasing risk of human exposure to Lyme disease-causing bacteria. |
| **Water-Related Infection** (*Vibrio vulnificus*) | Rising sea surface temperature, changes in precipitation and runoff affecting coastal salinity | Recreational water or shellfish contaminated with *Vibrio vulnificus* | *Vibrio vulnificus* induced diarrhea and intestinal illness, wound and bloodstream infections, death | Increases in water temperatures will alter timing and location of *Vibrio vulnificus* growth, increasing exposure and risk of waterborne illness. |
| **Food-Related Infection** (*Salmonella*) | Increases in temperature, humidity, and season length | Increased growth of pathogens, seasonal shifts in incidence of *Salmonella* exposure | *Salmonella* infection, gastrointestinal outbreaks | Rising temperatures increase *Salmonella* prevalence in food; longer seasons and warming winters increase risk of exposure and infection. |
| **Mental Health and Well-Being** | Climate change impacts, especially extreme weather | Level of exposure to traumatic events, like disasters | Distress, grief, behavioral health disorders, social impacts, resilience | Changes in exposure to climate- or weather-related disasters cause or exacerbate stress and mental health consequences, with greater risk for certain populations. |

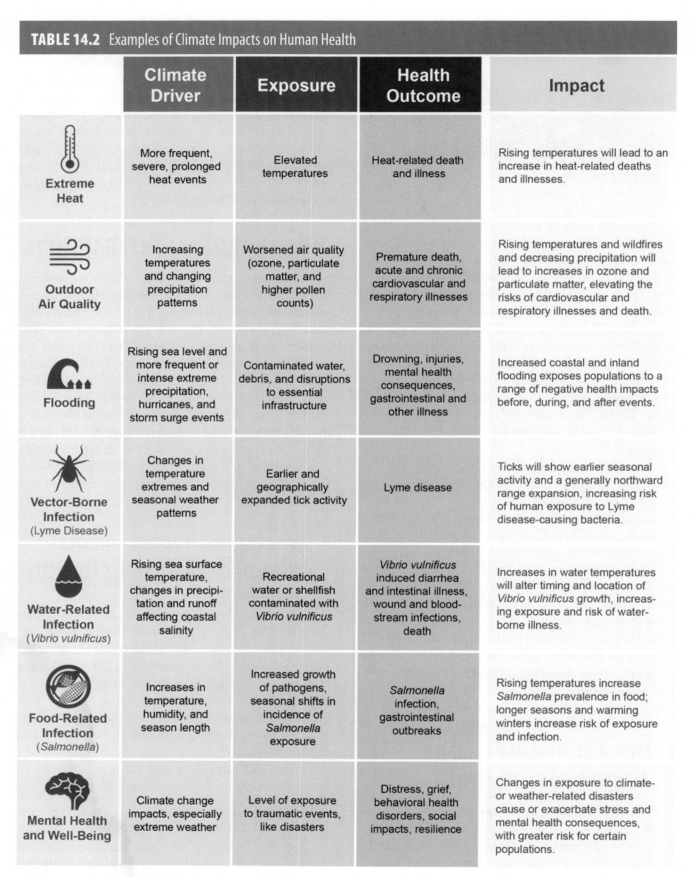

The NIH (National Institute of Health) News in Health provides some research evidence of the benefits of pet ownership. NIH indicates that:

> Some of the largest and most well-designed studies in this field suggest that four-legged friends can help to improve our cardiovascular health… The general belief is that there are health benefits to owning pets, both in terms of psychological growth and development, as well as physical health benefits.[36]

Evidence suggests additional benefits including reduced allergies and asthma among children exposed to pets during the first year of life and increased ability to communicate among children with autism. Perhaps the most well publicized benefit of pet ownership has been the use of service animals, usually dogs. Service animals are now recognized as helpful not only to those with blindness and seizure disorders but also to individuals with posttraumatic stress syndrome.[37]

While domesticated animals such as dogs and cats can provide considerable benefits to humans they are not free of risk from zoonotic diseases.

## ▶ What Are the Major Risks from Cats and Dogs and How Can They Be Minimized?

Dogs and, to a lesser extent, cats are a potential source of rabies. Fortunately, proper vaccinations effectively protect dogs and cats as well as humans. Today the transmission of rabies to humans from dogs and cats is very rare. The CDC recognizes a number of other preventable risks including:

- Toxoplasmosis is an infection caused by a microscopic parasite called *Toxoplasma gondii*. Toxoplasmosis can cause severe illness in infants, including vision loss and seizures, when infected from their mothers before birth. The most common way for a pregnant woman to become infected is through contact with a cat's litter box. According to the CDC, pregnant women ideally should avoid changing a cat's litter box and avoid adopting stray cats. Everyone should cover outdoor sandboxes to keep cats away.[38]
- Cat-scratch disease is a bacterial infection spread by cats. The disease spreads when an infected cat licks a person's open wound, or bites or scratches a person hard enough to break the surface of the skin often leading to spread of the infection to the lymph nodes. Washing cat bites and scratches well with soap and running water helps prevent human disease. People should not allow cats to lick human wounds. About 40% of cats carry the disease producing bacteria *Bartonella henselae* at some time in their lives, although most cats with this infection show no signs of illness.[39]

A wide range of bacterial diseases can be transmitted by cats and dogs and require caution especially when disposing of feces. Perhaps the most serious disease transmitted to humans by dogs (and far less frequently by cats) is toxocariasis which the CDC has identified as a "neglected parasitic infection in the United States" one of a group of diseases that results in significant illness among those who are infected and is often poorly understood by health care providers."[40]

Toxocariasis is a preventable parasitic infection caused by the larval form of the dog or cat roundworms *Toxocara canis* and *Toxocara cati*. *Toxocara* eggs are often found in dog feces and occasionally cat feces. People can acquire toxocariasis if they accidentally come in skin contact with or ingest dirt containing *Toxocara* eggs after gardening or playing in dirt or sand contaminated with infected feces. After skin contact with the *Toxocara* eggs, the larvae hatch and may travel under the skin (cutaneous larva migrans or creeping eruption). Toxocariasis can rarely invade the eyes and other organs including the brain where they can cause severe damage. Preventive measures greatly reduce the risk of toxocariasis. These measures include controlling *Toxocara* infection in dogs and cats through deworming by a veterinarian and reducing contact with the larvae by promptly disposing of dog and cat feces to a place away from people.[40]

The preventable diseases caused by cats and dogs are viewed by most Americans as far less of a threat than the many benefits of the human–animal bond. The same cannot be said of other types of pets that the CDC has called "exotic pets."

## ▶ What Is Meant by Exotic Pets and What Risks Do They Pose for Infectious Disease?

There are approximately 10 million animals imported into the United States each year including amphibians, birds, mammals, and reptiles. Check out the Internet and you will see that included in these numbers is a thriving trade in what has been called exotic species. Exotic species are nonnative species including many large and small animals not found in the United States. For most of these animals, except for nonhuman primates, there are no federal requirements for disease screening. Exotic pets also include native species of reptiles and amphibians. It is controversial whether domestic small mammals, many of which can carry diseases transmittable to humans, should be considered as exotic species.[41]

According to National Geographic,

> …in Americans' backyards and garages and living rooms, in their beds and basements and bathrooms, wild animals kept as pets live side by side with their human owners. It's believed that more exotic animals live in American homes than are cared for in American zoos… Privately owning exotic animals is currently permitted in a handful of states with essentially no restrictions: You must have a license to own a dog, but you are free to purchase a lion or baboon and keep it as a pet.[42]

The risks posed by exotic pet ownership illustrate the components of One Health including risks to humans, animals and the ecosystem. For example, Monkeypox, a less severe relative of smallpox, has been spread by imported pets. Pet pythons that have been released into wetlands have become unchecked predators. Lionfish, an invasive marine species common in the aquarium trade, are now threatening reefs throughout the Caribbean and Gulf of Mexico due to release by pet owners in Florida.

In summary, the One Health movement may be seen as the ultimate effort to view the health of the public as part of one large system in which we all live. Despite our growing attention to the interactions between humans, animals, and the ecosystem we are just beginning to understand how these factors influence health. The One Health movement is helping us understand that addressing microbiological threats, the impact of ecosystem change, and the impacts of close human–animal interactions is key to developing a healthy planet. We are "all in it together" is no longer just about the human race, it's about the health of all living things.

## Key Words

| | | |
|---|---|---|
| Bottlenecks | One Health | System |
| Feedback loops | Reductionist thinking | Systems analysis |
| Human–animal bond | RNA virus | Systems diagram |
| Influences | Syndemic | Systems thinking |
| Leverage points | Syndromes | Zoonotic disease |

## Discussion Questions

Take a look at the following discussion questions and see how well you can apply principles of systems thinking.

1. You are pregnant and have a 10-year history of cigarette smoking. You are surprised that at your first prenatal visit, there is a big sticker on your chart saying "Smoker." Everyone in the doctor's office asks you what they can do to help, and they quickly enroll you in special services for smoking cessation for which you were not eligible before you got pregnant. When you ask why so much time, attention, and money is now coming your way, they tell you pregnancy is a leverage point for stopping smoking. You ask: What do they mean by "leverage point"?

2. A patient with active tuberculosis (TB) is reported by the local hospital laboratory to the health department. The health department quickly connects with the patient to determine his close personal contacts. They also ask him if they can test him for HIV (the human immunodeficiency virus). He turns out to be HIV positive, and permission is then requested to get in touch with his sexual contacts. You consider how you would describe the relationship between TB and HIV, and wonder how knowledge of this relationship can be used to reduce the risks of both TB and HIV.

3. You hear that motor vehicle injuries, especially those due to automobile collisions, have been dramatically reduced in recent years. Was there a magic bullet that accomplished this, you wonder, or was this reduction accomplished through a more complicated process?

4. You love rare hamburgers. "Just wave them over the flame," you like to say. Recently, you have heard that ground beef is a high-risk food—even a health hazard. You ask: What does that mean, and what is being done about it?

5. You hear that a new RNA (ribonucleic acid) virus is rapidly spreading and will likely soon reach the United States. Public health officials are rapidly mobilizing efforts to control the disease and respond to an outbreak but see little

chance of stopping the disease from reaching the United States. Is this a common event you wonder or an emergency?

# References

1. Frenk J, Chen L, Bhutta ZA, et al. Health professionals for a new century: Transforming education to strengthen health systems in an interdependent world. *Lancet.* 2010;376: 1923–1958.
2. Meadows H. *Thinking in Systems: A Primer.* White River Junction, VT: Chelsea Green Publishing; 2008.
3. National Cancer Institute–U.S. Department of Health and Human Services. *Greater Than the Sum: Systems Thinking in Tobacco Control—Executive Summary.* Washington, DC: U.S. Department of Health and Human Services–National Institutes of Health; 2007.
4. Merriam-Webster. System. http://www.merriam-webster .com/dictionary/system. Accessed July 26, 2017.
5. O'Connor J, McDermott I. *The Art of Systems Thinking: Essential Skills for Creativity and Problem Solving.* Phoenix, AZ: Premium Source Publishing; 2006.
6. Kirkwood CW. System dynamic methods: A quick introduction. http://www.public.asu.edu/~kirkwood/sysdyn/SDIntro /SDIntro.htm. Accessed July 26, 2017.
7. The Open University. Systems thinking and practice: Diagramming. http://systems.open.ac.uk/materials/T552. Accessed July 26, 2017.
8. U.S. Environmental Protection Agency. Radon. http://www .epa.gov/radon. Accessed July 26, 2017.
9. Centers for Disease Control and Prevention. CDC grand rounds: The TB/HIV syndemic. http://www.cdc.gov /mmwr/preview/mmwrhtml/mm6126a3.htm. Accessed July 26, 2017.
10. Woolhouse MEJ, Adair K, and Brierley L. RNA viruses: A case study of the biology of emerging infectious diseases. *Microbiology Spectrum.* 2013;1(1):OH-0001-2012. doi:10 .1128/microbiolspec.OH-0001-2012.
11. U.S. Food and Drug Administration. Hazard analysis & critical control points (HACCP). http://www.fda.gov/Food /GuidanceRegulation/HACCP. Accessed July 25, 2017.
12. Schultz M. Photo quiz. Emerging infectious diseases. Rudolph Virchow. http://www.ncbi.nlm.nih.gov/pmc/articles /PMC2603088/. Accessed July 26, 2017.
13. Cardiff RD, Ward JM, and Barthold SW. 'One medicine—one pathology': are veterinary and human pathology prepared? *Laboratory Investigation.* 2008;88:18–26.
14. One Health Initiative. About the One Health Initiative. http://www.onehealthinitiative.com/about.php. Accessed July 25, 2017.
15. American Association of Veterinary Medical Colleges. One health educational framework for health professional students. http://www.aavmc.org/One-Health/Case-Studies.aspx. Accessed July 25, 2017.
16. Centers for Disease Control and Prevention. Chikungunya Virus. http://www.cdc.gov/chikungunya/. Accessed July 25, 2017.
17. World Health Organization. Dengue and severe dengue. http://www.who.int/mediacentre/factsheets/fs117/en/. Accessed July 25, 2017.
18. Centers for Disease Control and Prevention. Ebola. http:// www.cdc.gov/vhf/ebola/index.html. Accessed July 25, 2017.
19. Centers for Disease Control and Prevention. Hantavirus. http://www.cdc.gov/hantavirus/hps/transmission.html. Accessed July 25, 2017.
20. Centers for Disease Control and Prevention. Influenza (Flu). http://www.cdc.gov/flu/. Accessed July 25, 2017.
21. Centers for Disease Control and Prevention. Middle East respiratory syndrome (MERS). http://www.cdc.gov/coronavirus /mers/about/index.html. Accessed July 25, 2017.
22. Koplan JP, Butler-Jones D, Tsang T, et al. Public health lessons from severe acute respiratory syndrome a decade later. Emerging Infectious Disease [Internet]. June 2013. http://wwwnc.cdc .gov/eid/article/19/6/12-1426_article. Accessed July 26, 2017.
23. Centers for Disease Control and Prevention. West Nile Virus. http://www.cdc.gov/westnile/. Accessed July 26, 2017.
24. World Health Organization. The history of Zika virus. http:// www.who.int/emergencies/zika-virus/history/en/. Accessed July 26, 2017.
25. Centers for Disease Control and Prevention. Zika virus. http://www.cdc.gov/zika/symptoms/. Accessed July 26, 2017.
26. Morse SS. Factors in the emergence of infectious diseases. Emerging Infectious Diseases. January 1995. http://wwwnc .cdc.gov/eid/article/1/1/95-0102. Accessed July 26, 2017.
27. Morens DM, Folkers GK, and Fauci AS. Emerging infections: A perpetual challenge. *Lancet Infectious Diseases.* 2008;8: 712–213. doi: 10.1016/S1473-3099(08)70256-1.
28. Entis L. Will the worst bird flu outbreak in US history finally make us reconsider factory farming chicken? *The Guardian.* July 14, 2015. http://www.theguardian.com/vital-signs/2015 /jul/14/bird-flu-devastation-highlights-unsustainability -of-commercial-chicken-farming. Accessed July 26, 2017.
29. Goldsmith E and Hildyard N. Dams and disease. January 1, 1984. http://www.edwardgoldsmith.org/1018/dams-and -disease/. Accessed July 26, 2017.
30. Centers for Disease Control and Prevention. Lyme disease. https://www.cdc.gov/lyme/index.html. Accessed July 25, 2017.
31. Centers for Disease Control and Prevention. Parasites— American Trypanosomiasis (also known as Chagas Disease). http://www.cdc.gov/parasites/chagas/gen_info/detailed.html. Accessed July 26, 2017.
32. Crimmins A, Balbus J, Gamble JL, et al. 2016: Executive Summary. The Impacts of Climate Change on Human Health in the United States: A Scientific Assessment. U.S. Global Change Research Program, Washington, DC, 1–24. http:// dx.doi.org/10.7930/J00P0WXS.
33. American Veterinarian Medical Association. U.S. Pet Ownership Statistics. https://www.avma.org/KB/Resources/Statistics /Pages/Market-research-statistics-US-pet-ownership.aspx. Accessed July 26, 2017.
34. American Veterinary Medical Association. Human-animal bond. https://www.avma.org/kb/resources/reference/human -animal-bond/pages/human-animal-bond-avma.aspx. Accessed July 26, 2017.
35. Centers for Disease Control and Prevention. Healthy pets healthy people. http://www.cdc.gov/healthypets/. Accessed July 26, 2017.
36. National Institutes of Health. Can pets help keep you healthy? *NIH News in Health.* February 2009:1–2. https:// newsinhealth.nih.gov/2009/February/feature1.htm. Accessed July 26, 2017.
37. O'Haire ME, Guérin NA, and Kirkham AC. Animal-assisted intervention for trauma: A systematic literature review. *Frontiers in Psychology.* 2015;6:1121. doi: 10.3389 /fpsyg.2015.01121.

38. Centers for Disease Control and Prevention. Parasites—Toxoplasmosis (Taxoplasma infection). www.cdc.gov/parasites/toxoplasmosis. Accessed July 26, 2017.

39. Centers for Disease Control and Prevention. Cat-Scratch Disease. http://www.cdc.gov/healthypets/diseases/cat-scratch.html. Accessed July 26, 2017.

40. Centers for Disease Control and Prevention. Parasites—Toxocariasis (also known as Roundworm Infection). http://www.cdc.gov/parasites/toxocariasis/. Accessed July 26, 2017.

41. Marano N, Arguin PM, and Pappaioanou M. Impact of globalization and animal trade on infectious disease ecology. *Emerging Infectious Diseases* [serial online]. 2007;13(12): 1807–1809. doi: 10.3201/eid1312.071276.

42. Slater L. Exotic pets. *National Geographic*. April 2014. http://ngm.nationalgeographic.com/2014/04/exotic-pets/slater-text. Accessed July 26, 2016.

# SECTION V

# Cases and Discussion Questions

# ▶ Public Health Departments— Getting the Lead Out

A series of articles appears in your local newspaper investigating reports of elevated lead levels and reduced academic performance among students in a local grade school. The series ends with an editorial asking: "Where was the health department and what are they going to do now?"

The health department was aware of these reports and had sent a letter to each parent alerting them to the dangers of increased lead levels and letting them know of doctors and local clinics that could follow up and provide treatment through a health department-funded program. The mayor is not satisfied. He asks: "But isn't public health about prevention? How can we prevent this from happening again?" He asks the health department for a full report within a month.

The health department sets out to evaluate the range of potential sources of lead exposure in the community. They find the following possible factors: a local factory releases fumes that contain lead, local playgrounds are still contaminated by lead from gasoline despite the fact that lead was completely removed from gasoline well over a decade ago, lead paint in older homes, possible exposure from lead used in water pipes, and lead from painted toys and glazes on homemade pottery. The health department's report to the mayor concludes that prevention of lead exposure requires not just the health department's role, but also the cooperation of schools, parks, the environmental protection agency, the water system, the housing agency, as well as local industry and merchants. "We cannot do it alone," the report concludes.

"Okay," says the mayor, "it sounds like this is a job for the whole city. I am issuing an order requiring all city agencies to cooperate with the health department to find the sources of lead and develop a plan to reduce them." Then he turns to you, a new health department employee. "Work on this and write me a report by next month, but I want a press release out this afternoon."

## Discussion Questions

1. How would you recommend reducing or eliminating the hazard from each of the sources of lead identified by the health department? Explain.
2. How does this case reflect the role that the media and effective communications play in public health? Explain.
3. How does this case reflect the multiple collaborations that are needed to practice public health effectively? Explain.
4. How does this case reflect the relationship between public health agencies and clinicians? Explain.
5. How does this case illustrate the inherently political nature of public health? Explain.

# ▶ Community-Oriented Primary Care (COPC)

A community-oriented primary care team was developed in a large Hispanic/Latino community defined by census tracks. The vast majority of the community is employed, and over half of the working population receive minimum wage and have no health insurance. There are a large number of immigrants from Central America. Over 25% of the community is estimated to be undocumented aliens, most of who live in crowded conditions. A high percentage of those over 18 are married with an average family size of 5—considerably larger than other communities in the same city. The population of the community is generally younger than the surrounding more affluent communities. The vast majority of the community receives its health care at one community clinic.

The community's priority issues according to community residents include TB, HIV/AIDS, a lack of recreational facilities for children, a lack of dental services, and a lack of Spanish-speaking healthcare professionals. The COPC team, consisting of health professionals, public health experts, a clinical administrator, and members of the community, identified tuberculosis for further study. They found CDC evidence-based guidelines that recommend the following:

- Early and accurate detection, diagnosis, and reporting of TB cases leading to initiation and completion of treatment
- Identification of contacts of patients with infectious TB and treatment of those at risk with an effective drug regimen
- Identification of other persons with latent TB infection at risk for progression to TB disease and treatment of these persons with an effective drug regimen
- Identification of settings in which a high risk exists for transmission of Mycobacterium tuberculosis and application of effective infection-control measures

To implement these recommendations, risk factors for tuberculosis were identified in the community, including crowded conditions, HIV infections, high numbers of recent immigrants from endemic areas, and poor follow-up of treatment.

The COPC team found data on the estimated prevalence of a positive skin test for TB, the prevalence of active TB, the percentage of HIV-positive patients among those with active TB, and the percentage of active TB patients who completed a full course of treatment. The team recommended interventions for those factors that are most amenable to change, including intensive testing and follow-up of HIV-positive patients and special home health assistance to ensure completion of TB treatment.

The team recommended monitoring the percentage of HIV patients who were given tuberculosis skin tests and the percentage of TB patients who completed a full course of treatment. They also recommended measuring the prevalence of active TB before and after the interventions. Finally, they advised working closely with the local health department so that recommended TB follow-up practices are successfully performed. This included making sure that whenever active TB is diagnosed all those in contact with the individual are offered TB skin testing and preventive treatments if they convert to positive.

## Discussion Questions

1. Identify how the COPC team accomplished each of the six steps in the COPC process.
2. What factors would you consider in selecting a particular condition, such as tuberculosis, for special intervention efforts?
3. Identify one of the community's other priority issues and suggest interventions that you would use for addressing it and assessing, monitoring, and evaluating the impact of your intervention.
4. What are the strengths and limitations of the COPC approach?

## ▶ Hurricane Karl and the Public Health Success in Old Orleans

Hurricane Karl, a category 4 hurricane, made landfall last August 29th on the gold coast of the state of Good Fortune. The state is home to the town of Old Orleans, a historical community built below sea level and home to a large community from a range of socioeconomic backgrounds. Old Orleans has a model health department that seeks to provide the 10 essential public health services.

Before Hurricane Karl made its impact on the community, preparation for hurricanes had been an ongoing activity of the health department, which worked closely with first responders to ensure safe evacuation and protection from fire and looting. The department also worked with the local TV and radio stations to advise citizens on the purchasing and storing of essential food, water, and first aid supplies. It organized a community-wide emergency care network to ensure that 911 calls were responded to as quickly as possible in the event of a hurricane and worked with local hospitals to ensure that a triage system was in place to allocate patients to available emergency facilities, while not overwhelming any one healthcare institution.

When Hurricane Karl did strike, the damage was more extensive than expected. Leaks in the public sewer system led to water contamination. A local chemical plant experienced a major chemical discharge. Almost 200 residents were stranded in their homes without adequate food. Nearly half of the homes experienced water damage and rapid growth of mold. Many older residents did not have access to their daily medications.

The local health department had prepared for disasters like Hurricane Karl. After testing the water for contamination, supplies of stockpiled bottled water were distributed to homes in the contaminated areas by the National Guard. The police department had purchased specially equipped vehicles on the recommendation of the health department and was able, with the help of community organizations, to evacuate the stranded residents. The health department also sent out trained teams to diagnose the type and extent of hazards related to chemical contamination. With the help of the emergency radio system and cell phones, all individuals in the contaminated areas were notified and educated about methods for protecting themselves and their children.

Based on the emergency plan, the health department set up temporary healthcare sites and pharmacies staffed by nurses, physicians, and pharmacists who had been certified as emergency responders. The department also worked with representatives of the building industry to test water-exposed homes for mold and provided assistance to minimize the damage.

After the emergency, the health department joined with the local schools of public health and medicine to evaluate the response to Hurricane Karl and make recommendations for future emergencies. The data on infections, injuries, and deaths, as well as the use of services during the emergency, was collected and published. A national network was set up as a result to coordinate efforts for future disasters and learn from the experience in dealing with Hurricane Karl.

## Discussion Questions

1. Which of the 10 essential services did the health department of Old Orleans fulfill? Explain.
2. What efforts beyond those of the health department were needed to accomplish the 10 essential public health services? Explain.
3. In addition to providing the 10 essential public health services, to what extent are efforts required to deal with a disaster such as Hurricane Karl? Explain.
4. How does this case illustrate the complementary relationship between public health and medicine? What are the benefits of working together?

## ▶ Lung Cancer: Old Disease, New Approaches

Lung cancer in the United States today is the most commonly diagnosed life-threatening cancer among both men and women, with over 150,000 deaths per year. Cases of lung cancer increase with advancing age, with the disease rarely occurring before age 50. Lung cancer is usually diagnosed at a late stage. The duration of the disease after diagnosis is often measured in months, and the chance of death once the diagnosis is made is well above 90%.

Cigarette smoking has been recognized as the most important contributory cause of lung cancer since 1964, when the data was sufficient for the U.S. surgeon general to publish the first of a series of reports on smoking and health concluding that cigarette smoking is a cause of lung cancer and that interventions are needed to reduce the rate of cigarette smoking.

A large number of specific interventions have been studied and implemented, many with some success. Nearly 50% of men and 25% of women smoked cigarettes in the United States in the early 1960s. Initial efforts to reduce smoking included public service announcements and warning labels on cigarettes. The rate of smoking in the 1960s was modestly reduced among men, but little or no change occurred among women. In fact, over the subsequent decades, the rates of cigarettes smoking increased among young women. During these years tobacco companies advertised Virginia Slims and other products which associated smoking with weight loss and may have led to increased smoking among young women.

During the 1980s and early 1990s, efforts included increased taxes on cigarettes and restrictions of cigarette smoking in public places, including airplanes and increasingly in the workplace justified by evidence of the hazards of second-hand smoking. Evaluation efforts indicated a gradual reduction in smoking, with rates falling to less than 25% among both adult men and women.

The evaluation data indicated that the rates among adolescents were increasing to above 35% by the mid-1990s. In addition, it was recognized that nearly 90% of adult smokers began smoking before age 18 and most at a much earlier age. This led to a better understanding of the addictive nature of smoking and the need for interventions aimed at preventing addiction and addressing it through behavioral modification and drug treatments.

By the late 1990s, efforts were directed at reducing the rate of smoking among adolescents. A range of interventions was introduced. Peer education, even higher taxes on cigarettes, and laws preventing advertising of cigarettes and selling cigarettes to minors, such as the Joe Camel campaign, were among the interventions used. The subsequent rates of cigarette smoking among adolescents gradually fell to approximately the same rates as those of adults.

Data suggests that most of the approximately 20% of the population who continue to smoke are strongly addicted to nicotine and that education and even motivation are not likely to be effective. Recent efforts have turned to the regulation of nicotine in cigarettes, and the FDA has authority to regulate but not eliminate nicotine in cigarettes. Pregnant women have been recognized as a group who are highly motivated to stop smoking to prevent the adverse effects on their offspring. Efforts to stop smoking during pregnancy have the potential to carry over beyond delivery. Early detection, extra attention, and insurance coverage for cessation efforts have become widespread strategies for addressing smoking during pregnancy.

The declining rate of cigarette smoking in the United States has been coupled with a better recognition of other factors that today play roles in the development of lung cancer. A large number of Americans have been exposed to asbestos, a substance used as insulation in building, in brake linings, and in many other applications. It was widely used in the shipbuilding industry during World War II, where several million workers were heavily exposed. Restrictions on the use of asbestos and regulations of renovation and demolition of asbestos-containing buildings have greatly reduced exposures to asbestos.

Uranium miners in several countries have been found to have an increased risk of developing lung cancer even in the absence of cigarette smoking.

Radon, a naturally occurring invisible, odorless gas that is produced by the breakdown of uranium, was found to be widely present in homes in many geographic areas not just those with uranium mines. Public health investigators began to examine whether there was a connection between radon gas exposure and lung cancer. Approximately 20,000 cases of lung cancer per year are now attributed to radon exposure by the Environmental Protection Agency. About 1 in 15 homes currently have radon exposures above the levels at which the Environmental Protection Agency recommends action. The EPA recommends voluntary routine home testing. However, the major effort to successfully control radon exposure has been laws requiring testing prior to sale of a property and compulsory reductions in levels when high levels are detected.

The importance of asbestos and radon exposures have been apparent based on data indicating that these risk factors for lung cancer have multiplicative effects on the risk when combined with cigarette smoking. For instance, when the relative risk of asbestos is 5 and the relative risk of cigarette smoking is 10, the risk when there is exposure to both is nearly 50. Thus reductions in either of these risk factors can have dramatic impacts on the overall risk of lung cancer among those who also smoke cigarettes.

Early detection and treatment of lung cancer by chest X-rays have been shown to have little if any impact. Studies of routine chest X-rays for long-term smokers have been shown to produce a slightly earlier diagnosis, but to merely extend the time between diagnosis and death. Once evident on chest X-ray, the lung cancer is nearly always beyond the point of cure. Recent studies have confirmed that a newer type of X-ray test called a spiral computerized tomogram, or spiral CT, is capable of diagnosing lung cancer at an earlier stage. The test is expensive and has false positives as well as false negatives. However, it has been shown to reduce the deaths due to lung cancer by about 20%. Controversy continues over if and when to use spiral CT for screening for lung cancer.

An appreciation of the causes of lung cancer has led to multiple efforts to reduce exposure and to detect and treat it early. The rates of lung cancer in recent years have begun to fall, but the disease remains the most common cause of cancer deaths in both men and women. Increasingly, a systems thinking approach is being used to develop a coherent approach to reducing the incidence rate and the mortality rate due to lung cancer.

## Discussion Questions

1. Identify the interventions discussed for cigarette smoking in this case as primary, secondary, and tertiary, and discuss the advantages and disadvantages of using each of these types of interventions.
2. Identify the interventions discussed in this case for cigarette smoking as using education, motivation, or obligation, and discuss the advantages and disadvantages of using each of these types of interventions.
3. Discuss how the systems analysis approach of identifying multiple factors and investigating their interactions is illustrated in this case.
4. Discuss how systems analysis goals of identifying bottlenecks and leverage points are illustrated in this case.

## ▶ Restorital—How Do We Establish Safety?

The family wanted to know what went wrong. The FDA had approved the drug; her doctor had prescribed it; and her local pharmacy had filled the drug. Why had they been told in the ER that it looked like their mother, Noreen, had a bad drug reaction and may not survive?

The FDA had approved a new drug called Restorital to prevent fractures due to osteoporosis that did not respond to other available treatments. Restorital worked by blocking action of a newly recognized enzyme that was central to bone destruction. Animal studies showed no evidence of teratogenic, carcinogenic, or fertility problems except at doses well beyond the range that would be used for treating patients. Phase 1 studies on 30 healthy patients established dosage levels and did not detect side effects in vulnerable organs, including the liver, kidneys, and bone marrow. Phase 2 studies supported the efficacy of Restorital and suggested that randomized controlled trials with approximately 1000 patients, 500 each in the study and in the control groups, would be adequate for establishing the efficacy of Restorital.

The results of two randomized controlled trials conducted on approximately 1000 patients each demonstrated that the drug was able to modestly increase bone density for postmenopausal women with osteoporosis who had failed on other existing treatments. The drug was tested over a 1-year period on patients with severe osteoporosis who were taking no other prescription drugs. The only side effects observed more frequently in the study group were occasional nausea and diarrhea.

The drug was approved by the FDA and widely advertised for prevention of fractures due to osteoporosis. The advertisement noted in small print that Restorital had been approved for treatment of osteoporosis when all other available treatments had failed.

Physicians were impressed with Restorital's rapid improvement in bone density, its once-a-day dosage, its apparent lack of side effects, and its acceptance by patients. Patients found that most of the nausea and diarrhea could be avoided if they took their medicine with food. The success of the treatment encouraged many physicians to use Restorital as initial treatment for osteoporosis.

Noreen had begun Restorital 4 years ago, along with five other medications. She was pleased that Restorital did not seem to have any side effects and was successful in slowing down her bone loss, according to the follow-up tests ordered by her doctor.

Over the next few months, there seemed to be a subtle change in Noreen. She did not have her usual energy or enthusiasm and just wanted to stay home. When her family checked her medication, they found that she had been taking double the prescribed dose of Restorital. When they finally got her to her doctor, he ordered a series of blood tests. The next day, he called, saying, "Meet me in the ER. We need to look into this right away. Noreen's liver is not doing well."

Her doctor was worried about whether Restorital could have been the problem. He went so far as to file a report with the FDA's spontaneous reporting system, the first time he had ever done this in 20 years of practice. The FDA told him that they now had a series of 10 such reports suggesting that Restorital can cause life-threatening liver failure when used for 3 or more years at higher than recommended dosages, usually along with other drugs that can injure the liver. The FDA, he was told, was reviewing whether to put a black box warning label on Restorital, recommending liver function tests on patients taking it for more than a year.

It was too late to help Noreen, her doctor thought, but he was not going to prescribe Restorital again. "I guess even wonder drugs are not always so wonderful for every patient," he said to himself.

## Discussion Questions

1. What does this case study illustrate about the limitations of safety testing of drugs in animal studies?
2. What does this case study illustrate about the limitations of phase 1 and phase 2 drug testing?
3. What does this case study illustrate about the limitations of safety testing of drugs using randomized controlled trials?
4. What does this case study illustrate about the potential dangers of using approved drugs?
5. How could the FDA use its new authority provided in the 2007 amendments to prevent this type of problem from occurring?

## ▶ West Nile Virus: What Should We Do?

It is September 1, and Sean is beginning his infectious disease rotation in Regional Medical Center, a referral center for a large section of a Midwestern state. He hears that there are patients to see with suspected WNV in both the adult and child intensive care units. Sean's attending physician tells him this is becoming a late summer ritual at Regional Medical Center.

Sean learns that these patients have gone into coma after experiencing a short period of fever, headache, and fatigue. Clinicians usually diagnose the disease using the newest antibody tests, but occasionally the test results are negative until late in the course of the disease. Alpha interferon therapy, a type of immune therapy, shows some evidence of benefit in animal models but is not approved by the FDA for use in WNV. Because alpha interferon has been FDA approved for other uses, however, clinicians occasionally use it "off label" when patients are not doing well. Often, all that clinicians can do to help the patients is provide support, frequently in intensive care, while the body either heals or deteriorates.

Sean goes to the research literature available on the Internet to learn more about WNV. Sean learns that WNV is spread by mosquitos, which bite infected birds and then bite humans. Mosquitos are more likely to bite birds with high levels of WNV in the summer and early fall, explaining the high incidence of WNV in humans in the same time period. Sean learns in his reading that birds, especially jays and crows, are particularly susceptible to WNV. In fact, public health officials have used testing of these species as a way to anticipate increased disease in humans.

The vast majority of those infected with WNV show no symptoms. About 20% experience fever, headaches, fatigue, and, occasionally, a reddish raised rash on the back, legs, or stomach and/or swollen lymph nodes. A small percentage of those with symptoms progress to experience central nervous system symptoms, which can include meningitis, encephalitis, and/or paralysis, potentially progressing to coma and possibly death. Over 90% of those with severe WNV survive, but a small percentage is left with brain damage. Based on hospital reports of severe WNV from hospitals like Regional Medical Center and recognizing that these reports are just the tip of the iceberg, the CDC estimates that 100,000 or more individuals in the United States may be infected with WNV in high-incidence years.

Severe WNV especially affects the very young and old, whose immune systems are most vulnerable to progression of the disease. HIV/AIDS patients and others with reduced immunity are also vulnerable to severe WNV. Person-to-person transmission has only been observed through blood transfusions and organ transplantation. There is now a vaccine for WNV approved for use in horses, given that horses often experience severe consequences of WNV. The vaccine is a DNA vaccine, which has not been approved for human use because of the theoretical possibility of altering the human DNA and causing cancer. Other vaccines, including those with live attenuated viruses, are under investigation.

Sean's attending physician tells him that WNV was unknown in the United States before 1999. It may have mutated to be more easily transmitted to humans. The virus first appeared in New York and within 3 years had spread across the country. In epidemic years, associated with high volumes of mosquitos, thousands of patients have been hospitalized, and several hundred people have died from WNV.

Personal protection is provided by using mosquito repellant, avoiding dawn and dusk exposures (when mosquitos most often bite), and preventing stagnant pools of water in close proximity to humans. Community-wide mosquito spraying may have short-lived effects on the intensity of mosquito populations.

WNV drops dramatically after the first frost, which kills most of the disease-causing mosquitos. By extending the length of the frost-free period, global climate change has the potential to extend the West Nile "season" later into the fall.

We know a lot about WNV, Sean concludes, but there is a lot more we need to know, and a lot more we need to do.

## Discussion Questions

1. What is the role of individual prevention in WNV?
2. What is the role of medical treatment in addressing the issues of WNV?
3. If an effective and safe vaccine was approved for WNV, who should receive the vaccine?
4. What population health measures do you recommend to control the spread of the disease?
5. What One Health concepts are illustrated by this case study?

# ▶ Antibiotic Resistance: It's With Us for the Long Run

It was too good to be true: when penicillin was first introduced in clinical practice during World War II, it had dramatic impacts on a range of infectious diseases, from pneumococcal pneumonia, to gonorrhea, to staphylococcal wound infections. No randomized controlled trials were needed to demonstrate its efficacy or effectiveness compared with previous treatments. In short order, however, higher dosages of penicillin were required, and by the early 1950s, penicillin stopped working altogether for many infections.

In the 1950s, new classes of antibiotics were developed that headed off a crisis. However, it was already apparent that bacteria had the ability to develop resistance to antibiotics using a range of mechanisms. The more aggressively antibiotics were used, the more common resistance became, especially in hospitals where antibiotics had literally become standard operating procedure.

In addition to the use of antibiotics to treat bacterial infections, it became common clinical practice to try antibiotics as a first-line approach when the cause of the problem was not clear or was most likely due to a virus. In addition, it was found that antibiotics could modestly increase the growth rate of many animals raised for food. Widespread use of antibiotics in farm animals allowed the development of feedlots and whole industries devoted to raising animals together in close quarters.

By the late 20th century, animal use of antibiotics far exceeded human use. These antibiotics often ended up in public water systems, where the runoff from feedlots contaminates streams and groundwater. It has been called a "double hit": We got antibiotics in our food and in our drinking water, both of which promote bacterial resistance.

By the early years of this century, the problem of antibiotic resistance returned with a vengeance. Methicillin-resistant *Staphylococcus aureus* infections, or MRSA, became widespread not only in the hospital but in the community as well. Healthy athletes as well as those undergoing outpatient surgeries were now at risk for life-threatening diseases. Community-acquired MRSA skin infections are increasingly common in groups that share close quarters or experience more skin-to-skin contact, such as team athletes, military recruits, and prisoners. However, MRSA infections are being seen in the general community as well, including in individuals without known risk factors.

The problem is broader than staphylococcal infection; in fact, the vast majority of bacteria that causes infections in hospitals are resistant to at least one of the antibiotics previously used for their treatment. Recently, gram-negative infections, which are the most common causes of urinary tract infections and an increasingly frequent cause of pneumonia and postsurgical infections, have often become resistant to multiple antibiotics. The CDC estimates that over 20,000 people per year die in the United States alone from antibiotic-resistant bacterial infections.

Reducing the consequences of the existing antibiotic resistance is critical. Increased hand-washing and use of other sterilizing procedures is under way in healthcare institutions. Parallel precautions might be needed in athletic and fitness facilities. Early nonantibiotic treatments of wounds and other acute conditions may also become necessary.

Previously unrecognized impacts of overuse of antibiotics are increasingly being recognized. These are likely to include increases in childhood asthma and in juvenile idiopathic arthritis. There is even suggestive evidence of an increase in childhood obesity associated with early use of antibiotics. These previously unexpected impacts are all being linked to changes in the human microbiome that are due to overuse of antibiotics. The human microbiome consists of billions of bacteria and other microbes that live outside and inside all human beings, most commonly in the gastrointestinal tract.

In recent years, routine feeding of antibiotics to animals has been banned in much of the developed world and is now being curtailed in the United States. New approaches to reducing the development and spread of antibiotic-resistant bacteria are under way,

and new classes of antibiotics are under investigation. Before clinical approval, they will need FDA approval. Once approved, the FDA will need to decide whether they should be available for all licensed prescribers or restricted to specifically qualified prescribers and/or specific conditions/diseases.

Alternative or complementary approaches, such as greater reliance on vaccinations, may reduce the need for antibiotics. For instance, vaccines to prevent pneumococcal and meningococcal bacterial disease have been highly successful. Use of nonprescription probiotics, or "good bacteria," has been shown to improve the tolerance for, and at times the effectiveness of, existing antibiotics. They are increasingly being used as a routine adjunct to treatment and possibly for prevention.

New approaches to antibiotic resistance may come from the rapidly expanding understanding of the relationship between human health, animal health, and ecosystem health. The issue of antibiotic resistance to treatment is not new, and it is not going away.

## Discussion Questions

1. What are the positive and negative aspects of routine use of antibiotics on animals raised for food use? What types of restrictions, if any, do you favor?
2. If a new class of antibiotics is developed and approved by the FDA, what type of restrictions should be placed on its use, if any?
3. What interventions do you recommend for reducing the impact of bacteria that are already resistant to multiple antibiotics?
4. How should the recently recognized impacts of antibiotic overuse affect recommendations for use of antibiotics in primary care practice?

# Glossary

**Absolute risk** The actual chances or probability of developing the disease expressed as a probability, such as 0.01, or a percentage, such as 1%.

**Academic health center** An organization that includes a medical school, one or more other health profession schools, and an affiliated hospital.

**Accreditation** A process applied to educational institutions, healthcare institutions, and governmental health departments, to define and enforce required structures, processes, and outcomes.

**Activities of daily living** Routine activities that people tend to do every day without needing assistance. They include eating, bathing, dressing, toileting, transferring (walking), and continence.

**Actual causes** Modifiable factors that lead to major causes of mortality.

**Administrative regulations** In the United States, the type of law produced by executive agencies of federal, state, and local governments.

**Affordable Care Act** U.S. legislation passed in 2010 that made major changes to the U.S. health insurance system.

**Age adjustment** Taking into account age distribution of a population when comparing populations or when comparing the same population at two different points in time.

**Age distribution** The number of people in each age group in a population.

**All-hazards approach** An approach to public health preparedness that uses the same approach to preparing for many types of disasters, including use of surveillance systems, communications systems, evacuations, and an organized healthcare response.

**Altered environment** The impact of chemicals, radiation, and biological products that humans introduce into the environment.

**Ancillary criteria** Criteria that may be used to argue for a cause-and-effect relationship when the definitive requirements have not been fulfilled (synonym: supportive criteria).

**Antibody** A protein produced by the body in response to a foreign antigen that can bind to the antigen and facilitate its elimination.

**Artifactual** Differences between populations or changes in a population over time due to changes in interest in identifying the disease, change in ability to recognize the disease, or changes in the definition of the disease.

**Assessment** A core public health function that includes obtaining data that defines the health of the overall population and specific groups within the population, including defining the nature of new and persisting health problems.

**Association** The occurrence together of two factors, such as a risk factor and a disease, more often than expected by chance alone.

**Assurance** A core public health function that includes governmental public health's oversight responsibility for ensuring that key components of an effective health system, including health care and public health, are in place even though the implementation will often be performed by others.

**Asymptomatic** Without symptoms. When referring to screening for disease, it implies the absence of symptoms of the disease being sought.

**At-risk population** The group of people who have an increased chance or probability of developing a disease.

**Attributable risk percentage** The percentage of the disease or disability that can potentially be eliminated, among those with the factor being investigated, assuming a contributory cause and assuming the impact of the "cause" can be immediately and completely eliminated (synonym: percent efficacy).

**Authoritative decision** A decision made by an individual or a group that has the power to implement the decision.

**Bayes' theorem** A mathematical formula that can be used to calculate posttest probability of disease based on the pretest probability of the disease plus the test's sensitivity and specificity.

**Behavioral economics** A method of economic analysis that seeks to utilize new psychological insights into human behavior to explain and change patient and clinician decision making.

**Belmont Report** The commonly used name for a report of the National Commission for the Protection of Human Subjects of Biomedical and Behavioral Research that established key principles upon which the current approach to protection of human subjects is based.

**Beneficence** An ethics principle that states that persons are treated in an ethical manner not only by respecting their decisions and protecting them from harm, but also by making efforts to secure their well-being.

**BIG GEMS** A mnemonic that summarizes the determinants of disease, including behavior, infection, genetics, geography, environment, medical care, and socioeconomic-cultural status.

**Bioethics** Lies at the intersection of health law and policy and attempts to apply individual and group values and morals to controversial issues.

**Biological plausibility** An ancillary or supportive criteria for contributory cause in which the disease can be explained by what is currently known about the biology of the risk factor and the disease.

**Bottlenecks** Factors that limit the effectiveness of systems.

**Branding** A marketing concept for creating identification with a product or service that is also used in social marketing.

**Breakthrough drugs** An FDA category of drugs intended to treat a serious condition and preliminary clinical evidence indicates that the drug may demonstrate substantial improvement on a clinically significant endpoint(s) over available therapy.

**Built environment** The physical environment constructed by human beings.

**Burden of disease** Generically, an analysis of the morbidity and mortality produced by disease.

**Cap** A limit on the total amount that the insurance will pay for a service per year, per benefit period, or per lifetime.

**Capitation** A system of reimbursement for health care based upon a flat payment per time period for each person for whom a provider of care assumes responsibility for providing healthcare services, regardless of the services actually provided.

**Carrier test** A test to determine whether an individual has a genetic mutation for an autosomal recessive disorder.

**Case–control studies** A study that begins by identifying individuals with a disease and individuals without a disease. Those with and without the disease are identified without knowledge of an individual's exposure or nonexposure to the factors being investigated (synonym: retrospective study).

**Case definition** A set of criteria used to define which persons will be considered to have a disease as part of an outbreak.

**Case-fatality** The chances of dying from a condition once it is diagnosed.

**Case finding** As used in public health, an effort to identify and locate contacts of individuals diagnosed with a disease and evaluate them for possible treatment.

**Cell-mediated immunity** Immunological protection that is produced by t-lymphocytes and other white blood cells that combats intracellular pathogens and tumor cells.

**Certainty effect** A risk-taking attitude in which the decision maker favors the status quo rather than a probability of obtaining a better or a worse outcome.

**Certification** A nongovernmental process designed to ensure competence by individual health professionals based upon completion of educational requirements and performance on an examination or other evaluation procedure.

**Chance node** A circle in a decision tree that indicates that once a decision is made, outcomes occur with known probabilities indicated in the decision tree.

**Choice node** A square or rectangle in a decision tree that indicates that a selection needs to be made.

**Chronic carriers** Those individuals without symptoms of the disease but with the ability to chronically transmit the disease.

**Cluster** Occurrence of an increased number of cases of a disease over a defined time period.

**Cohort study** An investigation that begins by identifying a group that has a factor under investigation and a similar group that does not have the factor. The outcome in each group is then assessed (synonym: prospective study).

**Coinsurance** The percentage of the charges that the insured is responsible for paying.

**Communicable disease** A disease due to an organism such as bacteria or a virus that is transmitted person-to-person or from animals or the physical environment to humans by a variety of routes, including from air and water, contaminated articles or fomites, and insect bites and animal bites. Here considered a subset of infectious disease.

**Community-based participatory research (CBPR)** Research in which community members are involved in all phases of the research process, contributing their expertise while sharing ownership and responsibility over the research.

**Community-oriented primary care (COPC)** A structured six-step process designed to move the delivery of health services from a focus on the individual to an additional focus on the needs of communities.

**Community-oriented public health (COPH)** An effort on the part of governmental health agencies to reach out to the community and to the healthcare delivery system to address specific health issues.

**Community rating** Insurance rates set the same for all eligible individuals and families based on the previous expenses in a defined community.

**Concierge practice** A form of private practice of medicine that aims to provide personalized health care to those who can afford to pay for additional access and services out of pocket.

**Confounding variable** A difference in the groups being compared that makes a difference in the outcome being measured and which is not part of the chain of causation.

**Consistency** A supportive or ancillary criteria implying that the relationship has been observed in a wide range of populations and settings.

**Constitutional law** In the United States, a form of law based upon the U.S. Constitution or the constitution of a state.

**Contributory cause** A definition of causation that is established when all three of the following have been established: (1) the existence of an association between the "cause" and the "effect" at the individual level, (2) the "cause" precedes the "effect" in time, and (3) altering the "cause" alters the probability of the "effect."

**Copayment** An amount that the insured is responsible for paying even when the service is covered by the insurance.

**Core public health functions** Describes governmental public health functions that cannot be delegated and remain the responsibility of governmental public health. The Institute of Medicine has defined these functions as assessment, assurance, and policy development.

**Cost-effective** A measure of the cost of an intervention relative to its benefit. In interventions, implies that any additional benefit is considered worth the cost. The term can also imply that a large cost savings is worth a small reduction in net effectiveness.

**Cost sharing** An effort to reduce healthcare costs by shifting the costs of health care to individuals on the assumption that individuals will spend less when the costs are coming out of their pockets.

**Course of a disease** A description of a disease or other condition often using incidence, prevalence, and case-fatality.

**Covered service** A service for which health insurance will provide payment if the individual is otherwise eligible.

**Credentialing** A general term indicating a process of verifying that an individual has the desirable or required qualifications to practice a profession.

**Customary, prevailing, and reasonable** These standards are used by many insurance plans to determine the amount that will be paid to the provider of services.

**Data** Facts or the representation of facts as opposed to information.

**Database** A collection of data organized in such a way that a computer program can select and compile the desired pieces of data.

**Decision analysis** A process that compares the outcomes of two or more interventions based on principles of expected utility.

**Decision maker** A generic term that can be applied to a range of individuals and organizations that make health decisions, including individuals, health professionals, and organizations ranging from nonprofits to corporations to government agencies.

**Decision tree** A graphic method for displaying the benefits and harms of two or more options for intervention.

**Deductible** The amount that an individual or family is responsible for paying before being eligible for insurance payments.

**Demographic transition** Describes the impact of falling childhood death rates and extended life spans on the size of populations and the age distribution of populations.

**Determinants** Underlying factors that ultimately bring about disease; has been referred to as the causes of causes.

**Dietary supplements** A category within FDA law that includes vitamins, minerals, and many herbal remedies.

**Diffusion of innovation** A theory that identifies stages of dissemination and types of adopters of new technology and other changes, including behavioral change.

**Disability-adjusted life years (DALYs)** A population health status measure that incorporates measures of death and disability and allows for measurement of the impact of categories of diseases and risk factors.

**Discounting** A process in which we place greater importance on events that are expected to occur in the immediate future than on events that are expected to occur in the distant future.

**Dissemination** The widespread circulation of information often aimed at integration into public health and/or clinical practice.

**Distribution of disease** How a disease is spread out in a population, often using factors such as person, place, and time.

**Dose–response relationship** A relationship that is present if changes in levels of an exposure are associated with changes in frequency of the outcome in a consistent direction.

**Downstream factors** Factors affecting behavior that directly involve an individual and can potentially be altered by individual interventions, such as an addiction to nicotine.

**Dread effect** Perception of an increase in the probability of occurrence of an event due to its ease of being able to be visualized and its feared consequences.

**Ecological assessment** An assessment of the impact of an alteration of the physical environment on plants and animals.

**Effectiveness** An intervention has been shown to increase the positive outcomes or benefits in the population or setting in which it will be used.

**Efficacy** An intervention increased positive outcomes or benefits in the population on which it is investigated.

**Eligible** Used in the context of health insurance, an individual may need to meet certain criteria to be allowed to enroll in a health insurance plan.

**Endemic** A term that implies that a disease is present in a community at all times but at a relatively low rate.

**Epidemic** A term used when a disease has increased in frequency in a defined geographic area far above its usual rate.

**Epidemiological transition** A concept indicating the change that has been historically observed as part of social and economic development, from mortality and morbidity dominated by infections, to morbidity and mortality dominated by what has been called noncommunicable disease or degenerative and human-made diseases (synonym: public health transition).

**Epidemiological treatment** Treatment of contacts of an individual with a disease even in the absence of evidence of transmission of the disease.

**Epidemiologist** An investigator who studies the occurrence and control of disease or other health conditions or events in defined populations.

**Essential health benefits** Ten healthcare services defined by the Affordable Care Act that are required to be included as part of most health insurance policies.

**Essential public health services** The 10 services that have come to define the responsibilities of the combined local, state, and federal governmental public health system.

**Estimation** A statistical term implying a measurement of the strength of an association or the size of a difference.

**Etiology** The cause of a disease or health condition.

**Evidence** Reliable quantitative or qualitative information or data upon which a decision can be based.

**Expected utility** In decision analysis, the probability multiplied by the utility to produce a probability that takes into account the utility of the outcome.

**Experience rating** Health insurance rates set on the basis of a group's past history of healthcare expenses (synonym: medical underwriting).

**Exposure assessment** A step of risk assessment which assesses who has been exposed to a pollutant and the extent to which exposure took place.

**False negative** Individuals who have a negative result on a screening test but turn out to have the disease.

**False positive** Individuals who have a positive result on a screening test but turn out not to have the disease.

**Fee-for-service** A system of reimbursement for health services provided based on charges for health services actually provided to patients.

**Feedback loops** In systems analysis, the impact of changes in one influence or factor on other influences or factors in a positive or negative direction.

**Food desert** A geographic area that lacks grocery stores and other establishments in which low-income individuals are able to purchase nutritious food due to high prices or inaccessibility.

**Food security** As defined by the World Health Organization, requires that all people at all times have access to sufficient, safe, nutritious food to maintain a healthy and active life.

**Foundational Areas** Substantive areas of expertise or program-specific activities in all state and local health departments essential to protect the community's health.

**Foundational Capabilities** Cross-cutting skills that need to be present in state and local health departments everywhere for the health system to work anywhere.

**Foundational Public Health Services** Skills, programs, and activities that must be available system-wide in state and local health departments.

**Gini index** A measure of income distribution. The index, ranging from 0 to 1, measures the extent of deviation between an economy's distribution of income among individuals or households and that of perfectly equal distribution or an index of 0.

**Group association** Two factors, such as a characteristic and a disease, occur together more often than expected by chance alone in the same group or population. Does not require that the investigator have data on the characteristics of the individuals that make up the group or population (synonym: ecological association).

**Hazard** A measure of the inherent capability of a substance to produce harm.

**Hazard identification** A step in risk assessment that looks at the health effects caused by a pollutant.

**Health-adjusted life expectancy (HALE)** A population health status measure that combines life expectancy with a measure of the population's overall quality of health.

**Health belief model** A model of behavioral change that posits that personal beliefs influence health behavior and people will be more likely to take action if they believe they are susceptible to the condition; the condition has serious consequences; taking action would benefit them, with the benefits outweighing the harms; people are exposed to factors that prompt action; and people believe in their ability to successfully perform the action.

**Health communications** The full range of uses of information in health, from data collection to decision making.

**Health disparity** A type of difference in health that is closely linked with social or economic disadvantage. Health disparities negatively affect groups of people who have systematically experienced greater social or economic obstacles to health.

**Health equity** Everyone should have the opportunity to pursue the healthiest life possible, no matter where they live or work, the color of their skin, or the amount of money they have (as defined by the Robert Wood Johnson Foundation).

**Health in all policies** A comprehensive approach where private and public entities, across sectors, work toward common goals to achieve improved health for all and reduce health inequities.

**Health inequalities** Differences, variations, and disparities in the health achievements of individuals and groups of people.

**Health inequity** A difference or disparity in health outcomes that is systematic, avoidable, and unjust.

**Health insurance exchanges** Internet-based marketplaces to obtain health insurance for those who are not eligible for other forms of insurance.

**Health literacy** The degree to which individuals have the capacity to obtain, process, and understand basic health information and services needed to make appropriate health decisions.

**Health navigation** Assistance to individuals to enable them to effectively utilize the public health, health care, and health insurance systems

**Health-related quality of life (HRQOL)** A health status measure that reflects the number of unhealthy days due to physical plus mental impairment. HRQOL provides an overall quality of health measure, but it does not incorporate the impact of death.

**Health system** The healthcare system plus the public health system.

**Healthcare delivery system** A linkage of institutions and healthcare professionals that together take on the responsibility of delivering coordinated care.

**Healthcare disparity** Racial or ethnic differences in the quality of health care that are not due to access-related factors or clinical needs, preferences, and appropriateness of intervention.

**Healthcare safety net** The provision of services for those who cannot afford to purchase the healthcare services.

**Healthcare system** A healthcare delivery system plus the financial system that pays for the delivery of health care.

**Healthy communities** A Robert Wood Johnson Foundation program that aims to create "a culture of health" which addresses a wide range of social issues form housing to employment; to crime, social interactions, and recreational opportunities.

**Herd immunity** Protection of an entire population from a communicable disease by obtaining individual immunity through vaccination or natural infections by a large percentage of the population (synonym: population immunity).

**Heuristics** Rules of thumb for decision making that often allow more rapid decision making based on a limited amount of information.

**High-risk approach** A public health approach that focuses on those with the highest probability of developing disease and aims to bring their risk close to the levels experienced by the rest of the population.

**Home rule** Authority granted to local jurisdictions, such as cities or counties, by state constitutions or state legislative actions.

**Hospitalist** A physician whose primary professional focus is the general medical care of hospitalized patients.

**Human–animal bond** A mutually beneficial and dynamic relationship between people and animals that is influenced by behaviors that are essential to the health and well-being of both.

**Human microbiome** Microbial organisms which normally live in association with human beings, especially in the gastrointestinal track.

**Immunization** The strengthening of the immune system to prevent or control disease through exposure to antigens or administration of antibodies.

**Imposed risk** A potential threat to the health of individuals and populations that is not under their direct control, such as exposure to environmental toxins from a local factory.

**Improving-the-average approach** A public health approach that assumes that everyone is at some degree of risk and health can be improved by reducing the risk for the entire population.

**Inactivated vaccine** Injection of a nonliving organism or antigens from an organism designed to develop antibodies to protect an individual from the disease (synonym: dead vaccine).

**Incidence** Rates that measure the chances of occurrence of a disease or other condition over a period of time, usually one year.

**Incomplete penetrance** In relationship to genetics, indicates that not all those with a genetic mutation for a specific disease will develop the disease.

**Incremental cost-effectiveness** A measurement of the additional cost relative to the additional net-effectiveness (see: net-effectiveness).

**Incubation period** Time between exposure and the development of symptoms of a disease.

**Infant mortality rate** A population health status measure that estimates the rate of death in the first year of life.

**Infection** Invasion of host's bodily tissues by an organism such as bacteria or a virus.

**Infectious disease** A disease caused by an organism such as bacteria or a virus. Here used to include communicable diseases as well as other infections that are not communicable from human to human or animals to humans.

**Infectivity** The ability of a pathogen to enter and multiply in a susceptible host.

**Inference** A statistical term used to imply the drawing of conclusions about a population based upon data from a sample using statistical significance testing.

**Influences** As used in systems thinking, factors or determinants that interact with each other to bring about outcomes, such as disease or the results of disease.

**Inform of decision** A decision-making approach in which a clinician is merely expected to inform the patient of what is planned.

**Informed consent** A decision-making approach in which a clinician is expected to provide information and obtain agreement to proceed from the patient.

**Inpatient facility** A healthcare facility in the United States in which an individual may remain for more than 24 hours. Examples include hospitals and nursing homes.

**Institutional review board (IRB)** An institution-based group that is mandated by federal regulations to review human research conducted at the institution and determine whether it meets federally defined research standards.

**Intentional injuries** Injuries that are brought about on purpose, whether the injury is self-inflicted or meant for others.

**Interaction analysis** An approach to environmental health assessment that looks at the consequences of two or more exposures.

**Interventions** The full range of strategies designed to protect health and prevent disease, disability, and death.

**Judicial law** Law made by courts when applying statutory or administrative law to specific cases (synonyms: case law, common law).

**Justice** An ethical principle based on a sense of fairness in distribution of what is deserved.

**Koch's postulates** Four postulates that together definitely establish a cause and effect for a communicable disease: the organism must be shown to be present in every case of the disease; the organism must not be found in cases of other diseases; once isolated, the organism must be capable of replicating the disease in an experimental animal; and the organism must be recoverable from the animal (see: Modern Koch's postulates).

**Lead-time bias** The situation in screening for disease in which early detection does not alter outcome but only increases the interval between detection of the disease and occurrence of the outcome, such as death.

**Legislative statutes** In the United States, the type of law that includes statutes passed by legislative bodies at the federal, state, and local levels.

**Leverage points** Points or locations in a system at which interventions can have substantial impacts (synonym: control points).

**Licensure** Granted by a governmental authority that provides permission to engage in an activity, such as the practice of a health profession.

**Life expectancy** A population health status measure that summarizes the impact of death in an entire population utilizing the probability of death at each age of life in a particular year in a particular population.

**Live vaccines** Use of a living organism in a vaccine. Living organisms included in vaccines are expected to be attenuated or altered to greatly reduce the chances that they will themselves produce disease (synonym: attenuated vaccines).

**Long-shot effect** A decision-making attitude in which a decision maker perceives the status quo as intolerable and is willing to take an action with only a small chance of success and a large chance of making the situation worse.

**Mainstream factors** Factors affecting behavior that result from the relationship of an individual with a larger group or population, such as peer pressure to smoke or the level of taxation on cigarettes.

**Market justice** The philosophy that market forces should be relied upon to organize the delivery of healthcare services.

**Medicaid** A federal–state program that covers groups defined as categorically needy as well as groups that may be covered at the discretion of the state, including those defined as medically needy, such as those in need of nursing home care.

**Medical home** A concept of primary care that includes a team approach as part of a larger healthcare system.

**Medical loss ratio** The ratio of benefit payments paid to premiums collected, indicating the proportion of the premiums spent on medical services.

**Medical malpractice** A body of state civil law, as well as federal law, designed to hold practitioners accountable to patients for the quality of health care.

**Medicare** A federal health insurance system that covers most individuals 65 and older as well as the disabled and those with end-stage renal disease.

**Medigap** A supplemental health insurance linked to Medicare and designed to cover all or most of the charges that are not covered by Medicare, including the 20% copayment required for many outpatient services.

**Mental health** A state of successful performance of mental function, resulting in productive activities, fulfilling relationships with other people, and the ability to adapt to change and to cope with challenges.

**Micronutrients** Vitamins and minerals that in small quantities are considered essential to good health.

**Model** A combination of ideas and concepts taken from multiple theories and applied to specific problems in particular settings.

**Modern Koch's postulates** A set of criteria for establishing that an organism is a contributory cause of a disease, requiring evidence of an epidemiological association, isolation, and transmissions (see: Koch's postulates).

**Morbidity** A public health term to describe the symptoms produced by a disease or other condition; at times distinguished from disability, which is defined in terms of function.

**Mortality** A public health term to describe the frequency of deaths produced by a disease or other condition.

**Multiple risk factor reduction** Simultaneous efforts to reduce more than one risk factor.

**Multiplicative interaction** A type of interaction between two or more exposures such that the overall risk when two or more exposures are present is best estimated by multiplying the relative risk of each of the exposures.

**Natural experiment** A change that occurs in one particular population but not another similar population without the intervention of an investigator.

**Necessary cause** If the "cause" is not present, the disease or "effect" will not develop.

**Negative constitution** The principle that the U.S. Constitution allows but does not require government to act to protect public health or to provide healthcare services.

**Negligence law** A body of law designed to protect individuals from harm.

**Net effectiveness** A measure of the benefits minus the harms of an intervention (synonym: net-benefit).

**No-duty principle** The standard of U.S. law that healthcare providers, either individuals or institutions, do not have an obligation to provide health services.

**N-of-1 trial** A clinical trial in which a single individual is the entire trial. The individual is often exposed to an intervention and after an outcome is observed, the exposure is then terminated. If safety permits, the individual is re-exposed to determine whether the outcome recurs.

**Nongovernmental organization (NGO)** Any nonprofit, voluntary citizens' group which is organized on a local, national or international level.

**Nutritional transition** Countries frequently move from poorly balanced diets often deficient in nutrients and calories to a diet of highly processed food including fats, sugars, and salt.

**Odds ratio** A measure of the strength of the relationship that is often a good approximation of the relative risk. This ratio is calculated as the odds of having the risk factor if the disease is present divided by the odds of having the risk factor if the disease is absent.

**Off-label prescribing** Prescription written for FDA-approved products for indications, dosages, or durations other than those specifically approved by the FDA.

**One Health** The relationship between human health, animal health, and the health of the ecosystem.

**Outbreak** An increased number of cases of a disease over a defined time period in which affected individuals share a characteristic in common.

**Outcome measures** Measures of quality that imply a focus on the result of health care, ranging from rates of infection to readmissions with complications.

**Out-of-pocket expenses** Payments for health services not covered by insurance that are the responsibility of the individual receiving the services.

**Outpatient facility** A healthcare facility in the United States in which patients can remain for fewer than 24 hours. These facilities include the offices of clinicians, general and specialty clinics, emergency departments, and a range of new types of community-based diagnostic and treatment facilities.

**Pandemic** An epidemic occurring worldwide, or over a very wide area, crossing international boundaries and affecting a large number of people.

**Passive immunity** Short-term protection against a disease provided by administration of antibodies.

**P.E.R.I.E. process** A mnemonic that comes from the first letters in the steps of the evidence-based public health approach.

**Phases 1, 2, 3, and 4** The FDA steps of drug approval. The initial three steps occur prior to approval, while the fourth step, often referred to as postmarket surveillance, occurs after the drug is approved by the FDA.

**Place** In social marketing, the location of the target audience(s) and how to reach them.

**Point of service plans (POS)** A type of health plan that is a modification of staff model HMOs. These plans allow enrollees to obtain care outside the HMO but require that the patient pay for a portion of the cost of the care received.

**Police powers** Authority of governmental public health based on the power of state government to pass legislation and implement actions to protect the common good.

**Policy development** A core public health function that includes developing evidence-based recommendations and other analyses of options, such as health policy analysis, to guide implementation, including efforts to educate and mobilize community partnerships to implement these policies.

**Population comparisons** A type of investigation in which groups are compared without having information on the individuals within the group (synonym: ecological study).

**Population health approach** As used here, an evidence-based approach to problem solving that considers a range of possible interventions, including health care, traditional public health, and social interventions (synonyms: ecological approach, socioecological approach).

**Population health status measures** Quantitative summary measures of the health of a large population, such as life-expectancy and HALEs.

**Population pyramid** Graphic display of the age distribution of a population divided into males and females.

**Portability** The ability to continue employment-based health insurance after leaving employment, usually by paying the full cost of the insurance. A federal law known as COBRA ensures this continued health insurance.

**Posttest probability of disease** The probability of the disease after the results of the test are known.

**PRECEDE-PROCEED** A planning framework that provides a structure to design and evaluate health education and health promotion programs through a diagnostic planning process followed by an implementation and evaluation process.

**Prediction rule** A quantitative formula designed to increase the ability to predict the outcome of a condition and thereby guide the use of interventions.

**Predictive value of a negative** The posttest probability that the disease is absent when the test results are negative.

**Predictive value of a positive** The posttest probability of the disease when the test results are positive.

**Preferred provider organization (PPO)** An insurance system that works with a limited number of clinicians. These providers agree to a set of conditions that usually includes reduced payments and other conditions. Patients may choose to use other clinicians, but they often need to pay more out of pocket.

**Premium** The price paid by the purchaser for the insurance policy on a monthly or yearly basis.

**Preponderance of the evidence** A legal term implying that a trial is decided based upon the conclusion that the evidence is more supportive of the plaintiff than the defendant or vice versa.

**Pretest probability of disease** The probability of the disease before the test results are known. An estimate based on prevalence of the disease, the presence of risk factors for the disease, and, if present, signs or symptoms suggestive of the disease.

**Prevalence** A measurement of the number of individuals who have a disease at a particular point in time divided by the number of individuals who could potentially have the disease.

**Price** As used in social marketing, refers to the benefits, the barriers, and financial costs of a behavior or innovation.

**Primary care** Traditionally refers to the first contact providers of care who are prepared to handle the great majority of common problems for which patients seek care.

**Primary intervention** An intervention that occurs before the onset of the disease.

**Procedural due process** A form of due process that prohibits governments from denying individuals a right in an arbitrary or unfair way.

**Process measures** Measurements of quality that focus on the procedures and formal processes that go into delivering care, from procedures to ensure credentialing of health professionals to procedures to ensure timely response to complaints.

**Product** As used in social marketing, refers to the behavior or innovation being marketed.

**Proof of concept** In the context of FDA drug testing, evidence from a phase 2 investigation which suggests that a drug has efficacy.

**Proportion** A fraction in which the numerator is made up of observations that are also included in the denominator.

**Promotion** As used in social marketing, refers to organizing a campaign or program to reach the target audience(s).

**Protective factor** A factor that is associated with a reduced probability of disease.

**Provider** A term used to include a wide range of health professionals who provide health services.

**Proximal cause** A legal concept of causation that asks whether the injury or other event would have occurred if the negligent act had not occurred.

**Public health assessment** A formal assessment that incorporates risk assessment but also includes data on the actual exposure of a population to a hazard.

**Public health emergency of international concern** A formal statement by the Director of the World Health Organization which may be issued under the International Health Regulations.

**Public health surveillance** Collection of health data as the basis for monitoring and understanding health problems, generating hypotheses about etiology, and evaluating the success of interventions (synonym: surveillance).

**Quality adjusted life-year (QALY)** A measurement that asks about the number of life-years saved by an intervention rather than the number of lives.

**Quarantine** The compulsory physical separation of those with a disease or at high risk of developing a disease from the rest of the population.

**R naught ($R_0$)** The number of new cases one individual with the disease generates on average over the course of the disease's communicable period (synonym: reproduction number, reproduction ratio).

**Randomization** As part of a randomized clinical trial, assignment of participants to study and control groups using a chance process in which the participants are assigned to a particular group with a known probability (synonym: random assignment).

**Randomized controlled trial** An investigation in which individuals are assigned to study or control groups using a process of randomization (synonym: experimental study).

**Rates** Used here as a generic term to describe measurements that have a numerator and a denominator.

**RE-AIM** A mnemonic that comes from the first letters of the steps in a fully developed evaluation process.

**Reciprocal determinism** A component of social cognitive theory describing the dynamic interplay among personal factors, the environment, and behavior.

**Recommendations** Statements based upon evidence indicating that actions, such as cigarette cessation, will improve an outcome, such as reducing lung cancer.

**Reductionist thinking** An approach to problem solving that looks at each of the components of a problem one at a time.

**Relative risk** A ratio of the probability of the outcome if a factor known as a risk factor is present compared to the probability of the outcome if the factor is not present.

**Respect for persons** An ethical principle that incorporates two ethical convictions: first, that individuals should be treated as autonomous agents, and second, that persons with diminished autonomy are entitled to protection.

**Reverse causality** The situation in which the apparent "cause" is actually the "effect."

**Rights** Protections afforded to individuals on the basis of the U.S. Constitution, a state constitution, or legislative actions.

**Ring vaccination** As used in the smallpox eradication program, immediate vaccination of populations in surrounding geographic areas after identification of a case of disease.

**Risk assessment** A process used in environmental health to formally assess the potential for harm due to a hazard, taking into account factors such as the likelihood, timing, and duration of exposure.

**Risk avoider** A decision maker who consistently favors avoiding an action even when a decision analysis utilizing probabilities, utilities, and timing argues for the action.

**Risk characterization** A step in risk assessment that looks at the extra risk of health problems in an exposed population.

**Risk factor** A characteristic of individuals or an exposure that increases the probability of developing a disease. It does not imply that a contributory cause has been established.

**Risk indicator** A characteristic, such as gender or age, that is associated with an outcome but is not considered a contributory cause (synonym: risk marker).

**Risk taker** A decision maker who consistently favors taking an action even when a decision analysis utilizing probabilities, utilities, and timing argues against the decision.

**Risk-taking attitudes** A decision-making attitude in which an individual or group consistently favors taking actions or avoiding actions that differ from the recommendations of a decision analysis utilizing probabilities, utilities, and the timing of events.

**RNA virus** A virus that has ribonucleic acid as its genetic material.

**Route of transmission** The anatomical and physiological methods for transmission from person to person or from animal species to humans.

**Score** In the context of evidence-based recommendations, a measurement of the quality of the evidence and a measurement of the magnitude of the impact.

**Screening** As used here, testing individuals who are asymptomatic for a particular disease as part of a strategy to diagnose a disease or identify a risk factor.

**Secondary care** Refers to specialty care provided by clinicians who focus on one or a small number of organ systems or on a specific type of service, such as obstetrics or anesthesiology.

**Secondary intervention** Early detection of disease or risk factors and intervention during an asymptomatic phase.

**Self-imposed risk** A potential threat an individual knowingly and willingly takes on through his or her own actions, such as choosing not to wear a motorcycle helmet while riding a motorcycle.

**Sensitive** In decision analysis, indicates that changes in a particular factor within a realistic high and realistic low range result in changes in the recommendation of the decision analysis.

**Sensitivity** The probability of a positive test when the disease is present.

**Sequential testing** A screening strategy that uses one test followed by one or more additional tests if the first test is positive (synonym: consecutive testing).

**Shared decision making** A decision-making approach in which a clinician is expected to directly or indirectly provide information and options for intervention to a patient and then rely on the patient to synthesize the information and make his or her own decision.

**Simultaneous testing** A screening strategy that uses two tests initially, with follow-up testing if either test is positive (synonym: parallel testing).

**Single payer** A healthcare system with one source of payment, usually a governmental source.

**Skimming** Enrolling predominating healthy individuals into a health plan to reduce the costs to the plan.

**Social cognitive theory** An interpersonal theory of behavior change that focuses on the interaction between individuals and their social systems.

**Social determinants of health** The complex, integrated, and overlapping social structures and economic systems including the social environment, physical environment, health services, and structural and societal factors.

**Social justice** A philosophy that aims to provide fair treatment and a fair share of the reward of society to individuals and groups.

**Social marketing** The use of marketing theory, skills, and practice to achieve social change, for example, in health promotion.

**Socioeconomic gradient** A phenomenon describing the hierarchical differences in health outcomes among a population based on the value that society places on certain characteristics, whether it be income, job, educational attainment, etc.

**Socioeconomic status** In the United States, a measurement using scales reflecting education, income, and professional status.

**Source traceback** A process used in foodborne outbreak investigations to trace the origin of food suspected of causing an outbreak.

**Specificity** The probability of a negative test when the disease is absent.

**Spontaneous reporting system** An FDA system for reporting adverse events that occur while taking medications.

**Stages of change model** A model of behavioral change that hypothesizes five steps in the process of behavioral change, including precontemplation, contemplation, preparation, action, and maintenance (synonym: transtheoretical model).

**Standard population** The age distribution of a population that is often used as the basis for comparison with other populations. The age distribution of the U.S. population in the year 2000 is generally used.

**State Child Health Insurance Program (SCHIP)** A federally funded health insurance program that provides funds to the states to use to expand or facilitate the operation of Medicaid or for other uses to serve the health needs of lower income children.

**Strength of the relationship** Supportive or ancillary criteria indicating that the measurement of the magnitude of an association, such as a relative risk or odds ratio, is large or substantial.

**Structure measures** Measure of quality of health care focused on the physical and organizational infrastructure in which care is delivered.

**Substantive due process** A type of due process in which state and federal governments must justify the grounds for depriving an individual of life, liberty, and property.

**Sufficient cause** If the "cause" is present, the disease or "effect" will occur.

**Surrogate endpoint** Use of substitute measures of outcomes that do not necessarily reflect the clinically important outcomes that a drug or other therapy intends to improve (synonym: surrogate outcome).

**Syndemic** A systems thinking approach that focuses attention on how health problems interact as part of larger systems.

**Syndrome** A pattern of risk factors or symptoms that tend to occur together.

**System** An interacting group of items forming a unified whole.

**System error** Problems resulting from deficiencies in the system for delivering health care or other services.

**Systems analysis** A variety of methods that operationalize the investigation of systems.

**Systems diagram** A graphic means of displaying the way we understand systems to be structured and/or to function.

**Systems thinking** An approach that examines multiple influences on the development of an outcome or outcomes and attempts to bring them together in a coherent whole.

**Tertiary care** A type of health care often defined in terms of the type of institution in which it is delivered, often an academic or specialized health center. This type of care may also be defined in terms of the type of problem that is addressed, such as trauma centers, burn centers, or neonatal intensive care.

**Tertiary intervention** An intervention that occurs after the initial occurrence of symptoms but before irreversible disability occurs.

**Theory** A set of interrelated concepts that presents a systematic view of relationships among variables in order to explain and predict events and situations.

**Theory of planned behavior** A theory of behavior change that posits that behavioral intention is influenced by individuals' attitudes toward performing a behavior, their beliefs about whether people important to them approve or disapprove of the behavior, and their beliefs about their control over performing the behavior.

**True positive** Individuals who have a positive result on a screening test and turn out to have the disease.

**True rate** A measurement that has a numerator that is a subset of the denominator and a unit of time, such as a day or a year, over which the number of events in the numerator is measured.

**Unaltered environment** The natural environment.

**Uncontrollability effect** Perception of increased probability of occurrence of an event due to the perceived inability of an individual to control or prevent the event from occurring.

**Under-5 mortality** A population health status measure that estimates the probability of dying during the first 5 years of life.

**Undergraduate medical education** Refers to the four years of medical school leading to a MD or DO degree, despite the fact that an undergraduate, or bachelor's, degree is generally required for admission.

**Unfamiliarity effect** Perception of increased probability of an event due to an individual's absence of prior experience with the event.

**Unintentional injuries** Injuries that occur not on purpose, such as most motor vehicle collisions, drowning, falls, fires, and poisonings.

**Upstream factors** Factors affecting behavior that are grounded in social structures and policies, such as government-sponsored programs that encourage tobacco production.

**Utility scale** A scale that goes from zero to one, with zero reflecting immediate death and one reflecting full health. This scale is used to measure the value or importance that an individual or a group places on a particular outcome.

**Victim blaming** Placing the responsibility or blame for a bad outcome on the individual who experiences the bad outcome due to his or her behavior.

**Vulnerable populations** Groups at higher than average risk of developing disease and/or bad outcomes of disease.

**Zoonotic disease** Disease that exists in animals but can be transmitted to humans.

# Index

Note: Page numbers followed by *b*, *f*, *t*, and *n* indicate material in boxes, figures, tables, and footnotes respectively.

## A

AA. *See* Alcoholics Anonymous
absolute risk, 33*n*
ACA. *See* Affordable Care Act
academic health center, 209*n*
accelerated approval, drugs, 275
access to healthcare, 101
    social determinants of health, 85
Accountable Care Organizations (ACOs), 216*b*
accreditation, 253
    of health professionals, 192
acetaminophen (Tylenol), 87, 277*b*
ACOs. *See* Accountable Care Organizations
action stage, of change model, 90*t*
activities of daily living, 210
actual causes, 126, 126*t*
acute life-threatening condition, 275
administrative processes, 216
administrative regulations, 103*b*
adolescents, continuing problem, 50
adverse effects, of drug, 275
Affordable Care Act (ACA), 227
    legislation, 225
aflatoxins, 268
age
    adjustment/distribution of, 29*b*
    elderly driver (case study), 123
    groups, leading causes of death and disability by, 13, 13–14*t*
    impact on healthcare costs, 233
    as public health issue, 22–23*b*
Agency for Healthcare Research and Quality (AHRQ), 255*t*
Agency for Toxic Substances and Disease Registry (ATSDR), 255*t*
aging society, 48–50
agriculture, and infectious diseases, 302
AHRQ. *See* Agency for Healthcare Research and Quality
AIDS. *See* HIV/AIDS
air quality, 4
Air Quality Index (AQI), 165
    for particle pollution, 166*t*
alcohol abuse, 143–144*b*
Alcoholics Anonymous (AA), 144*b*

alienation, social determinants of health, 83
"all-hazards" approach, 176
allergic reactions, 155*n*
allied health practitioner, 192
allopathic physicians, 195
altered environment, impact on disease, 164
Alzheimer's disease, 142
American Cancer Association, 260
American Heart Association, 260
American Lung Association, 260
American Public Health Association (APHA), 7
    role in making health policy, 104–106
amyloid-B, 143
ancillary criteria, 31–32, 34*t*
animal testing, 272
anthrax, 178*b*
antibiotics, 146, 155, 162
    history of public health and, 7
    resistant of, 146, 315–316
antibody, 153
APHA. *See* American Public Health Association
apprentice system, in medical education, 198*b*
AQI. *See* Air Quality Index
artifactual, group associations, 28
asbestos, 168
aspirin, 283
assessment, as core public health function, 248, 249*t*
associations, 27
assurance, as core public health function, 248–249, 250*t*
asthma
    determinants of, 17–18*b*
    environmental factors in, 166*b*
asymptomatic individuals, screening and, 131
at-risk population, 26*b*
"atrial fibrillation," 239
ATSDR. *See* Agency for Toxic Substances and Disease Registry
attributable risk percentage, 37*n*
authoritative decisions, in health policy, 104

## B

baby boomers, 22*b*
Bacillus Calmette-Guérin (BCG) vaccine, 149*b*
Back-to-Sleep campaign, 87
bacteria, resistant strains of, 146
bacterial diseases, 305
balance billing, 224*b*
bar charts, 63*b*
barriers, to communicable diseases, 152–153
Bayes' theorem, 133, 134*b*
BCG vaccine. *See* Bacillus Calmette-Guérin vaccine
behavioral change
    ability to change health behavior, 86–87
    cigarette smoking (case study), 121–122
    easy versus difficult changes, 87
    history of public health and, 8
    individual, 87
    stages in, 88
behavioral economics, 97*b*
behavioral sciences, public health related to, 77–78, 78*t*
behaviors, as determinant of disease, 16
behind-the-counter drugs, 276*b*
Belmont Report, 111
beneficence, in ethical research, 111–112
benzene, risk assessment and, 168, 168–169*b*
BIG GEMS framework, 16
Bill and Melinda Gates Foundation, 260
bioethics, 112*n*
    of healthcare and public health, 101
    principles of, 109–110
biological plausibility, 33, 34*t*
bioterrorism, 178*b*
black box warnings, 278
BMI. *See* body mass index
body mass index (BMI), 268
bottlenecks, 286
    identifying, 287, 288*t*, 294
branding, social marketing and, 95
BRCA1. *See* breast cancer gene variant
breakthrough drugs, 276*b*